Perfect Home Remedies
(Constipation, Piles & Fissures)

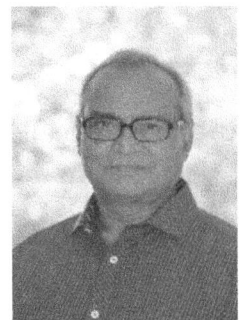

Author: Ram Babu Sao

Born in a poor family in small village, I was sickly and weak throughout my childhood and also struggled with poverty, sickness and malnutrition. At the age of 15, I approached an Ayurveda Practitioner in my village only and joined his clinic to improve my health as well as to provide services to the people to provide Ayurvedic medicines. In villages, everybody is poor and can't afford allopathic medicines much. I am an educationist, a tireless social worker and a very humble but cordial humanist and have endeavoured upon the age old inheritance in an altogether new version. I learned that how effectively and steadily Ayurveda Medicine can improve the common man health. I have been sharing best home remedies practices and techniques with other for their benefits. India is the only country in the world with a full faculty of Biomedicine, Acupressure, Yoga, Pranayama, Ayurvedic medicines and research, a full of ayurvedic hospital and several clinical units where home remedies and ayurvedic medicines are prescribed. Modalities used in this book include herbs, nutrition, exercise, acupressure, counselling of Ayurveda energy work, mind-body medicine; breathe work (Pranayama), yoga, and aromatherapy. My accomplishments are detailed in this book **"Perfect Home Remedies (Constipation, Piles & Fissures)"** for the benefit of the common man. I am a scholar and learnt Ayurveda based on Ayurveda teachings and Articles on Home Remedies for prevention of Constipation, files and Fissures. This technique truly works for real patients to help them improve their quality of life, their health, and their well-being, which is a truly integrative path. I have studied many books and magazines on Ayurvedic and Natural treatment of diseases. I thought of the necessity of a consolidated and concise book covering all the different aspects and topics on the subject matters pertaining to Home Remedies at one place. I am trying to bring home remedies to the light between the common men and women of this society.

Contact: **Mobile: 9819506068 Email: rbsao8844@yahoo.co.in**

@   Copyright: Author-2017

CAUTION

Disclaimer

The book **"Perfect Home Remedies (Constipation, Piles & Fissures)"** is not a writer's whole & sole product. It is a combination of the knowledge and expertise of the author and the Data collected from different Books and Articles on home remedies to prevent constipation & Bowel Movement, specially researched to meet the objective and to enhance the knowledge of natural healing. Wherever necessary, the reference of the other books has been given in this book. The Data in this book provides only information, knowledge, guidance and reference to practice for natural. I don't permit anybody to claim that this book is the only best book on "Perfect Home Remedies for Constipation & Bowel Movement". However, it is important to remember that home remedies are not a substitute for medical care. This book is for information only and should not be used for the diagnosis or treatment of medical conditions. This book makes no warranty as to its accuracy. Consult a doctor or other health care professional for diagnosis and treatment of medical conditions. Be sure to consult with your general practitioner or medical specialist for any issues or problems you may have.

ISBN-13: 978-1542589031

ISBN-10: 1542589037

First Edition: January, 2017

Publisher: Amazon.in

Preface

Constipation and irregular bowel movements appears to be quite a problem for a lot of people from infants to the elderly and interfere with health and vitality. The symptoms of constipation are obvious and include infrequent bowel movements, hard stools, and difficulty in passing stools. The side effects of constipation commonly include Abdominal Discomfort, Headaches, Nausea, Anal cancer, Anal fissures, Bowel perforation, Colon and Colorectal cancer, Colorectal disorder, Crohn's disease, Diverticulitis, Haemorrhoids, Ischemic colitis, Kidney damage and infections, Rectal prolapsed, Ulcerative colitis and Fatigue.

Constipation is a symptom, not a disease and effective treatment of constipation may require first determining the cause. The treatments mainly include sufficient exercises and yoga, sufficient fibre diet, sufficient liquid intake, sufficient probiotic and stomach acid, magnesium balancing, solar plexus balancing, body detoxifying, maintaining eating habit and changes in dietary habits, minimum use of laxatives and enemas, and in particular surgery. Constipation is common and in the general population rates of constipation varies from 30-50 percent. In elderly people, the rate of constipation is 50–75 percent.

Constipation means different things to different people. For many people, it simply means infrequent bowel movement. For others, however, constipation means hard stools, difficulty in passing stools (straining), or a sense of incomplete emptying after a bowel movement. Constipation refers to bowel movements that are infrequent or hard to pass stool. Constipation is a common cause of painful defecation. It means either going to the toilet less often than usual to empty the bowels, or passing hard or painful stools (faeces).

Constipation most commonly occurs when waste or stool moves too slowly through the digestive tract or cannot be eliminated effectively from the rectum, which may cause the stool to become hard and dry. Constipation is one of the most common gastrointestinal (GI) problems, affecting about 75 million people. Constipation is common among all ages. Constipation is a symptom with many causes.

Many people have chronic constipation, which include passing fewer than three stools a week, having lumpy or hard stools, straining to have bowel movements, feeling as though there's a blockage in your rectum that prevents bowel movements, feeling as though you can't completely empty the stool from your rectum, needing help to empty your rectum, such as using your hands to press on your abdomen and using a finger to remove stool from your rectum. Chronic constipation person has at least passing fewer stools three days per month for more than three months associated with abdominal discomfort, which is often diagnosed as irritable bowel syndrome (IBS) when no obvious cause is found. Complications may include necrosis and ulcers of the rectal tissue. Loss of appetite can also occur. The number of bowel movements generally decreases with age. Most adults have bowel movements between three and 14 times per week, and this would be considered normal. The most common pattern is one bowel movement a day, but this pattern is seen in less than half the people. Moreover, most people are irregular and do not have bowel movements every day or the same number of bowel movements each day.

There is a belief that "toxins" accumulate when bowel movements are infrequent or that constipation leads to many diseases. It is important to distinguish acute (recent onset) constipation from chronic (long duration) constipation. Acute constipation requires urgent assessment because a serious medical illness may be the underlying cause like tumours of the colon, Anal cancer, Anal fissures, Bowel perforation, Colon and Colorectal cancer, Colorectal disorder, Crohn's disease, Diverticulitis, Haemorrhoids, Ischemic colitis, Kidney damage and infections, Rectal prolapsed, Ulcerative colitis. Constipation also requires an immediate assessment if it is accompanied by worrisome symptoms such as rectal bleeding, abdominal pain and cramps, nausea and vomiting involuntary loss of weight. Colonic propagating pressure wave sequences (PSs) are responsible for discrete movements of the bowel contents and are vital for normal defecation. Haemorrhoids are swollen and inflamed veins around your anus or in your lower rectum. You can develop haemorrhoids if you strain to have a bowel movement. If you have haemorrhoids, you may have bleeding in your rectum. You have bleeding in the rectum when you see bright red blood in your stool, on toilet paper, or in the toilet after a bowel movement. Anal fissures are small tears in your anus that may cause itching, pain, or bleeding.

Constipation is common among all ages and populations likely to be and include, people taking medicines to relieve broken bone, a pulled tooth, or back pain; medicines to treat depression; people who just had surgery; people with lower incomes; and women especially during pregnancy or after giving birth. The causes of constipation can be divided into congenital, primary, and secondary. The most common cause is primary and not life-threatening. In the elderly, constipation causes include: 1). Lack of Fibrous Food/Diet: A fibre-rich diet supports the growth of beneficial bacteria, which make their home in the intestinal tract. 2). Inadequate Intake of Water/Liquid: Intake of Water/Liquid help in softening the stool. 3). Lack of Magnesium Intake: Magnesium is a mineral that supports your body's overall health. It plays a key role in muscle function, which may explain why it can be so helpful for individuals who suffer from constipation. After all, your GI tract is one long muscle that must be healthy in order to produce consistent bowel movements. 4). Missing Lifestyle: In addition to dietary considerations, lifestyle may play a significant role in constipation, especially in stubborn cases of chronic irregularity. 5). Lack of Regular exercise: Regular exercise is one of the best ways to get your bowels moving. Walking and other rhythmic exercise massages the intestinal tract and stimulates peristalsis. Regular exercise also helps alleviate the stress that can contribute to constipation. 6). Lack of Yoga/Meditation, Asana, Mudra, and Pranayama Practice: They improve your overall health. 7). Imbalance of Solar Plexus (Mani Chakra): 8). Laziness or missing in regular toilet routine: Establishing a regular toilet routine helps constipation. Ignoring your body's signals is an often-overlooked cause of constipation. Instead of postponing the urge to "go," always heed these signals as quickly as possible. 9). Thyroid or Hypothyroidism function: Constipation is also one of the symptoms of hypothyroidism, and thyroid function should be evaluated. 10). Food allergies: Food allergies can be at the root of chronic constipation as well; the most common problematic food is pasteurized dairy products, but soy, beef, peas, legumes, beans, tomatoes, oranges, and black tea can also be problematic. 11). Emotions: Even emotions have been found to play a role along with Ischemic colitis; Low fibre diets; medications; Multiple sclerosis; Narrowing of the colon (bowel stricture); neurological problems affecting the nerves; abdominal cancer that presses on the colon; Parkinson's disease; poor bowel habits; possibly abuse of laxatives; problems with the pelvic muscles involved in having a bowel movement; spinal cord injury; stroke; disorders to the colon; ulcerative colitis; barium enema; antacid medicines containing calcium and aluminium; certain calcium channel blockers such as nifedipine and verapamil; changes in physical activities; changes in your usual diet; childhood chronic constipation; decreased physical activity; dieting; slimming diets; eating a lot of dairy products; eating habit disorders; hypothyroidism; inadequate fluid intake; insufficient dietary fibre intake; excessive use of laxatives; metabolic and muscular problem; not being active; not drinking enough water; psychological-voluntary withholding of the stool; rarely heavy metal toxicity; side effects of medications; specific diseases - like amyloidosis, celiac disease, lupus, and scleroderma, hypothyroidism; and structural and functional abnormalities. Constipation is usually easier to prevent than to treat by maintenance of the body with adequate exercise, fluid intake, and high-fibre diet, electrolytes which include calcium, chloride, potassium, magnesium and sodium regulating a number of body functions. This book **"Perfect Home Remedies (Constipation, Piles & Fissures)"** is my accomplishment for the benefit of the common man. I have learnt about home remedies based on Ayurveda teachings and many other articles on "Home Remedies for prevention of Constipation" and have given the concise matters in this book. This technique truly works for real patients, to help them improve their quality of life, their health, and their well-being, which is a truly integrative path. He has studied many books and magazines on Vedic treatment by acupressure. He thought of the necessity of a consolidated and concise book covering all the different aspects and topics on subject matters pertaining to "Home Remedies for Constipation" at one place. I am trying to bring this information in light between the common men and women of this society.

Contents

Introduction

1.1   General

Constipation means different things to different people. For many people, it simply means infrequent bowel movement. For others, however, constipation means hard stools, difficulty in passing stools (straining), or a sense of incomplete emptying after a bowel movement. Constipation refers to bowel movements that are infrequent or hard to pass. Constipation is a common cause of painful defecation. It means either going to the toilet less often than usual to empty the bowels, or passing hard or painful stools (faeces). Constipation most commonly occurs when waste or stool moves too slowly through the digestive tract or cannot be eliminated effectively from the rectum, which may cause the stool to become hard and dry. Constipation is one of the most common gastrointestinal (GI) problems, affecting about 75 million people. Constipation is common among all ages. Constipation is a symptom with many causes. Severity of constipation, flatulence and bloating was summarized into four categories (severe, moderately severe, mild and no symptoms).

Many people have chronic constipation, which include passing fewer than three stools a week, having lumpy or hard stools, straining to have bowel movements, feeling as though there's a blockage in your rectum that prevents bowel movements, feeling as though you can't completely empty the stool from your rectum, needing help to empty your rectum, such as using your hands to press on your abdomen and using a finger to remove stool from your rectum. Chronic constipation person has at least passing fewer stools three days per month for more than three months associated with abdominal discomfort, which is often diagnosed as irritable bowel syndrome (IBS) when no obvious cause is found. There can be faecal incontinence and paradoxical or overflow diarrhoea as liquid stool passes around the obstruction. Complications may include necrosis and ulcers of the rectal tissue. Abdominal pain and bloating could also be present depending on the severity of the condition. Loss of appetite can also occur. The number of bowel movements generally decreases with age. Most adults have bowel movements between three and 14 times per week, and this would be considered normal. The most common pattern is one bowel movement a day, but this pattern is seen in less than half the people. Moreover, most people are irregular and do not have bowel movements every day or the same number of bowel movements each day.

Medically speaking, constipation usually is defined as fewer than three bowel movements per week. Severe constipation is defined as less than one bowel movement per week. There is no medical reason to have a bowel movement every day. Going without a bowel movement for two or three days does not cause physical discomfort, only mental distress for some people. Contrary to popular belief, there is a belief that "toxins" accumulate when bowel movements are infrequent or that constipation leads to cancer. It is important to distinguish acute (recent onset) constipation from chronic (long duration) constipation. Acute constipation requires urgent assessment because a serious medical illness may be the underlying cause like tumours of the colon. Constipation also requires an immediate assessment if it is accompanied by worrisome symptoms such as rectal bleeding, abdominal pain and cramps, nausea and vomiting involuntary loss of weight. The evaluation of chronic constipation may not be urgent, particularly if simple measures bring relief. Colonic propagating pressure wave sequences (PSs) are responsible for discrete movements of the bowel contents and are vital for normal defecation. Deficiencies in PS frequency, amplitude, and extent of propagation are all implicated in severe defecator dysfunction (SDD). Chronic, or long-lasting, constipation can lead to health problems such as haemorrhoids, anal fissures, and rectal prolapsed or faecal impaction. Haemorrhoids are swollen and inflamed veins around your anus or in your lower rectum. You can develop haemorrhoids if you strain to have a bowel movement. If you have haemorrhoids, you may have bleeding in your rectum. You have bleeding in the rectum when you see bright red blood in your stool, on toilet paper, or in the toilet after a bowel movement. Anal fissures are small tears in your anus that may cause itching, pain, or bleeding.

Constipation is common among all ages and populations likely to be and include: Non-Caucasians; Older adults; People taking medicines to relieve broken bone, a pulled tooth, or back pain; People taking medicines to treat depression; People who just had surgery; People with lower incomes; and Women especially during pregnancy or after giving birth. Constipation is a symptom, not a disease, effective treatment of constipation may require first determining the cause. The causes of constipation can be divided into congenital, primary, and secondary.

1.1　Constipation in children:

Constipation in children usually occurs at three distinct points in time: After starting formula or processed foods (while an infant), during toilet training in toddlerhood, soon after starting school (as in at kindergarten).After birth, most infants pass 4-5 soft liquid bowel movements a day. Breast-fed infants usually tend to have more bowel movements compared to formula-fed infants. Some breastfed infants have a bowel movement after each feed, whereas others have only one every 2–3 days. Infants who are breastfed rarely develop constipation. By the age of two years, a child will usually have 1–2 bowel movements per day and by four years of age; a child will have one bowel movement per day. The six-week period after pregnancy is called the postpartum stage. During this time, women are at increased risk of being constipated. Constipation can cause discomfort for women, as they are still recovering from the delivery process especially if they have had a perinea tear or underwent an episiotomy. Haemorrhoids are common in pregnancy and also may get exacerbated when constipated. Women sometimes get enemas during labour that can also alter bowel movements in the days after having given birth. However, there is insufficient evidence to make conclusions about the effectiveness and safety of laxatives in this group of people. No special diet or medications are necessary for children with constipation (colonic hypo motility, a type of constipation). Their tendency towards constipation helps them to remain clean between enemas. The real challenge is to find an enema capable of cleaning the colon completely. Soiling episodes or "accidents" occur when there is an incomplete cleaning of the bowel. The group of children with loose stools and diarrhoea (colonic hyper motility) has an overactive colon. There is rapid transit of stool results in frequent episodes of diarrhoea. This means that even when an enema cleans the colon rather easily, stool keeps on passing fairly quickly from the cecum to the descending colon and the anus. To prevent this, a constipating diet and/or medications to slow down the colon are necessary. Eliminating foods that further loosen bowel movements will help the colon to slow down. Those who experience hyper motility may have to follow a constipating diet and avoid laxative foods. The diet is rigid and includes food such as banana, apple, baked bread, white pasta with no sauce, boiled meat, and others, while fried foods and dairy products are avoided.

1.2 Glossary:

The following are health and medical definitions of terms that appear in the Constipation:

Abdomen: The belly, that part of the body that contains all of the structures between the chest and the pelvis. The abdomen is separated anatomically from the chest by the diaphragm, the powerful muscle spanning the body cavity below the lungs. The abdomen includes a host of organs including the stomach, small intestine, colon, rectum, liver, spleen, pancreas, kidneys, appendix, gallbladder, and bladder. The abdomen includes a host of organs including the stomach, small intestine, colon, rectum, liver, spleen, pancreas, kidneys, appendix, gallbladder, and bladder.

Abdominal pain: Pain in the belly. Abdominal pain can be acute or chronic. It may reflect a major problem with one of the organs in the abdomen, such as appendicitis or a perforated intestine, or it may result from a fairly minor problem, such as excess build-up of intestinal gas. Absorption: Uptake. For example, intestinal absorption is the uptake of food (or other substances) from the digestive tract.

Abdominal: Relating to the abdomen, the belly, that part of the body that contains all of the structures between the chest and the pelvis. The abdomen is separated anatomically from the chest by the diaphragm, the powerful muscle spanning the body cavity below the lungs.

Acid reflux: When acid from the stomach leaks up into the oesophagus (the throat) and may cause symptoms such as heartburn or leave an unpleasant taste. Acne: Acne is a skin condition predominantly affecting the face, chest and back. It causes pustules and papules (and spots) which can be painful and irritating. Acne is most common in teenagers and young adults, but is also commonly seen in adults in their thirties and forties. It is understood that there are a number of different triggers for acne including hormone imbalances, constipation and food intolerances.

Acupressure: A traditional Chinese medicine bodywork technique based on the principles of acupuncture. Acupressure is the application of pressure rather than needles on specific points on the body to control symptoms such as pain or nausea.

Anaemia: Abnormally low levels of blood or red blood cells in the bloodstream. Most cases are caused by iron deficiency, or lack of iron.

Anal Fissure: Short-term constipation or intermittent bouts of constipation are unlikely to cause any long-term problems. Sometimes a split or tear in the anal skin (Anal fissure) can occur with the passage of particularly big or hard stools (faeces). This is very painful and there may be a small amount of fresh red blood on the toilet paper. Treatment of an anal fissure involves lifestyle measures (exercises and enough liquid intake and fibrous diet) to keep the stools soft, and perhaps laxatives too, to keep the stools really easy to pass. Local anaesthetic ointment or glycerol trinitrate (GTN) ointment can be prescribed by your GP to ease the pain and help relax the muscles around the back passage (anus), to help the fissure to heal.

Anaphylaxis: Anaphylaxis is a serious allergic reaction that is quick to develop and may, in severe cases, cause death. Common causes include shellfish, nuts, insect bites or stings and some medications.

Androgen is a hormone that is sometimes known as the 'male hormone', but both men and women carry it. In men it plays an important role in male traits and reproductive activity, and in women one of its main roles it to be converted into the female hormone, oestrogen.

Antibacterial: An antibacterial is an agent that inhibits the growth of bacteria, or indeed kills it.

Antibiotics: Medicines can kill bacteria in the colon, used to cure some cases of colitis. Antibiotics may also be used for attacks of inflammatory bowel disease.

Antibody: An antibody, also known as an immunoglobulin, is a Y-shaped protein that is used by the immune system to identify and neutralize foreign objects such as bacteria and viruses.

Anti-inflammatory medicines: Various drugs can slow down immune system function, easing symptoms of inflammatory bowel disease.

Antioxidant: An antioxidant is a substance found in food that is used by the body to protect against free radicals - highly unstable molecules that can affect our health.

Antiviral: An antiviral is an agent that helps prevent or stops viral replication within cells, for example a common cold virus.

Anus: The anus is the opening at the end of the digestive tract, found at the bottom. Its main function is to control the elimination of stools. This is the opening of the rectum to the outside of the body.

Anxiety: Anxiety is a state of inner turmoil whereby one has feelings of fear, worry and uneasiness, often accompanied by nervous behaviour such as pacing or insomnia.

Barium enema: An enema using a white, chalky solution containing barium, in preparation for series of X-ray images of the lower intestine (colon). The barium outlines the colon on the X-ray film.

Bifid bacteria: Bifid bacteria are a group of bacteria that make up the majority of bacteria found in the intestines. It is possible to take certain strains of bifid bacteria in probiotic supplement form to boost levels of good bacteria in the gut which may help relieve digestive symptoms such as constipation.

Bile: Bile is a bitter fluid, yellow to green in colour. It is produced by the liver and helps us to digest fat in the small intestine for excretion as faeces.

Bowel management: Bowel management is a medical approach to manage faecal incontinence or constipation. Bowel control is often a challenge for children who are born with anomalies in their anus or rectum, Hirschsprung's disease, and/or spina bifida. Some patients have a poor prognosis and will never be able to control their bowel, and so benefit from bowel management techniques. Bowel management is mainly achieved through a daily fibrous diet, exercise, yoga and enema which empty the colon to prevent unwanted and uncontrolled bowel movements that day. Some people also use laxatives and a controlled diet as part of their bowel management regimen. Another alternative is transanal irrigation. Children who suffer from faecal incontinence after the repair of an imperforate anus are usually those born with a bad prognosis type of defect and severe associated defects (defect of the sacrum, poor muscle complex). However, such children can still achieve a good quality of life when treated with the bowel management program. Children operated on for imperforate anus and who suffer from faecal incontinence can be divided into two groups that require individualized treatment plan.

Bowel: The bowel is another name for the intestines or gut.

Bypass diarrhoea: Bypass diarrhoea (also known as Overflow Diarrhoea) is diarrhoea typically caused by constipation. It occurs when a hard plug of stool in the lower bowel, caused by faecal impaction, prevents proper evacuation and liquid faeces escapes from the rectum.

Cancer: An abnormal growth of cells which tend to proliferate in an uncontrolled way and, in some cases, to metastasize (spread). Cancer is not one disease. It is a group of more than 100 different and distinctive diseases. Cancer can involve any tissue of the body and have many different forms in each body area. Most cancers are named for the type of cell or organ in which they start. If a cancer spreads (metastasizes), the new tumour bears the same name as the original (primary) tumour.

Chronic: In medicine, lasting a long time. A chronic condition is one that lasts 3 months or more. Chronic diseases are in contrast to those that are acute (abrupt, sharp, and brief) or sub acute (within the interval between acute and chronic).

Colon biopsy: During a colonoscopy, a small piece of colon tissue may be removed for testing. A colon biopsy can help diagnose cancer, infection, or inflammation.

Colon bleeding (haemorrhage): Multiple potential colon problems can cause bleeding. Rapid bleeding is visible in the stool, but very slow bleeding might not be.

Colon cancer: A malignant tumour arising from the inner wall of the large intestine (the colon). In the US, colon cancer is the third leading type of cancer in males and the fourth in females. Risk factors for cancer of the colon and rectum (colorectal cancer) include colon polyps, long-standing ulcerative colitis, and genetic family history. Most colorectal cancers develop from polyps. Removal of colon polyps can prevent colorectal cancer. Colon polyps and early colon cancer can have no symptoms. Therefore, regular screening is important, starting at age 50 (or earlier, if added risk factors are present). Diagnosis can be made by barium enema or by colonoscopy, with biopsy confirmation of cancer tissue. Surgery is the most common treatment for colorectal cancer.

Colon Conditions: Inflammation of the colon is Colitis. Inflammatory bowel disease or infections are the most common causes.

Colon polyps: Polyps are small growths. Some of these develop into cancer, but it takes a long time. Removing them can prevent many colon cancers.

Colon surgery: Using open or laparoscopic surgery, part or the entire colon may be removed (colostomy). This may be done for severe bleeding, cancer, or ulcerative colitis.

Colon: The colon is also called the large intestine. The ileum (last part of the small intestine) connects to the cecum (first part of the colon) in the lower right abdomen. The colon is the long, coiled, tube like organ that removes water from digested food. The remaining material, solid waste called stool, moves through the colon to the rectum and leaves the body through the anus. It is also known as large bowel and large intestine. The colon is divided into four parts:

The ascending colon travels up the right side of the abdomen.
• The transverse colon runs across the abdomen.

• The descending colon travels down the left abdomen.

• The sigmoid colon is a short curving of the colon, just before the rectum. The colon removes water, salt, and some nutrients forming stool. Muscles line the colon's walls, squeezing its contents along. Billions of bacteria coat the colon and its contents, living in a healthy balance with the body.

Colon: The long, coiled, tube like organ that removes water from digested food. The remaining material, solid waste called stool, moves through the colon to the rectum and leaves the body through the anus. It is also known as large bowel and large intestine.

Colonoscopy: A procedure whereby a physician inserts a viewing tube (colonoscopy) into the rectum for the purpose of inspecting the colon. During colonoscopy, polyps can be removed, bleeding can be cauterized, and a biopsy can be performed if abnormal areas of the colon are seen.

Colonoscopy: An exam of the entire colon using a small, lighted instrument.

Complete Prolapsed: The entire wall of the rectum slides out of place and usually sticks out of the anus. At first, this may occur only during bowel movements. Eventually, it may occur when you stand or walk. And in some cases, the prolapsed tissue may remain outside your body all the time.

Constipation: Infrequent and frequently incomplete bowel movements. Constipation is the opposite of diarrhoea and is commonly caused by irritable bowel syndrome (IBS), diverticulitis, and medications. Paradoxically, constipation can also be caused by overuse of laxatives. Colon cancer can also narrow the colon and thereby cause constipation. A high-fibre diet can frequently relieve constipation. If the diet is not helpful, medical evaluation is warranted. Constipation is a digestive condition which is medically defined by the following symptoms; Stool is hard or lumpy in more than 25% of bowel movements. Stool is produced less than three times a week. The sufferer has to strain on more than 25% of bowel movements. The bowel does not feel fully emptied

Criteria: The Rome II Criteria for constipation require at least two of the following symptoms for 12 weeks or more over the period of a year: 1) Straining with more than one-fourth of defecations; 2) Hard stool with more than one-fourth of defecations; 3) Feeling of incomplete evacuation with more than one-fourth of defecations; 4) Sensation of anorectic obstruction with more than one-fourth of defecations; 5) Manual manoeuvres to facilitate more than one-fourth of defecations; and 6) Fewer than three bowel movements per week.

Crohn's disease: An inflammatory condition that usually affects the colon and intestines. Abdominal pain and diarrhoea (which may be bloody) are symptoms. Crohn's disease favours the ileum (the lower part of the small intestine) but can occur anywhere along the intestinal tract while, by contrast, ulcerative colitis affects the colon (the large intestine) alone. The inflammation in Crohn's disease involves the entire thickness of the bowel wall, whereas in ulcerative colitis the inflammation is confined to the mucosa (the inner lining) of the intestine.

Dehydration: Dehydration is the excessive loss of bodily water and generally becomes noticeable when 2% of the body's normal water content has been lost. Symptoms include constipation, dizziness, fatigue and headaches. Diseases of the gastrointestinal tract that cause vomiting or diarrhoea may lead to dehydration. There are a number of other causes of dehydration including heat exposure, prolonged vigorous exercise, kidney disease, and medications that cause voiding (diuretics). One clue to dehydration is a rapid drop in weight. A loss of over 10% (15 pounds in a person weighing 150 pounds) is considered severe.

Depression: Depression is a state of low mood with feelings of sadness, anxiety, emotionless, hopelessness, worry, worthless, guilt, etc. Depressed people often lose interest in activities and themselves, and may have difficulty in remembering details or have feelings of self harm or suicide.

Diagnosis: The diagnosis is essentially made from the patient's description of the symptoms. Bowel movements that are difficult to pass, very firm, or made up of small hard pellets (like those excreted by rabbits) qualify as constipation, even if they occur every day. Other symptoms related to constipation can include bloating, distension, abdominal pain, headaches, a feeling of fatigue and nervous exhaustion, or a sense of incomplete emptying. Inquiring about dietary habits will often reveal a low intake of dietary fibre, inadequate amounts of fluids, poor ambulation or immobility, or medications that are associated with constipation. During physical examination, scybala (manually palpable lumps of stool) may be detected on palpation of the abdomen. Rectal examination gives an impression of the anal sphincter tone and whether the lower rectum contains any faeces or not. Rectal examination also gives information on the consistency of the stool, the presence of haemorrhoids, admixture of blood and whether any tumours, polyps or abnormalities are present. Physical examination may be done manually by the physician, or by using a colonoscopy. X-rays of the abdomen, generally only performed if bowel obstruction is suspected, may reveal extensive impacted faecal matter in the colon, and confirm or rule out other causes of similar symptoms.

Diarrhoea: A common condition that involves unusually frequent and liquid bowel movements, which is opposite of constipation. There are many infectious and non-infectious causes of diarrhoea. Persistent diarrhoea is both uncomfortable and dangerous to the health because it can indicate an underlying infection and may mean that the body is not able to absorb some nutrients due to a problem in the bowels. Treatment includes drinking plenty of fluids to prevent dehydration and taking over-the-counter remedies. People with diarrhoea that persists for more than a couple days, particularly small children or elderly people, should seek medical attention. Diarrhoea is a loosening of bowel movements and is accompanied by increased frequency and urgency. Stools that are frequent, loose, or watery are commonly called diarrhoea. Most diarrhoea is due to self-limited, mild infections of the colon or small intestine.

Dietary Fibre: Also known as "roughage", dietary fibre is the indigestible portion of food which aids in moving faeces through the gastrointestinal tract. Lack of dietary fibre often contributes to constipation.

Digestive Disorders: Digestive disorders are a source of irritation and discomfort that may cause them to drastically limit their lifestyles and frequently miss work, such as, Gastrointestinal Tract. The gastrointestinal (GI) tract is a long muscular tube that functions as the food processor for the human body. The digestive system includes the following organs: mouth and salivary glands, stomach, small and large intestines, colon, liver, pancreas, and gallbladder. Irritations or inflammation of the various sections of the GI tract are identified as gastritis (stomach), colitis (colon), ileitis (ileum or small intestines), hepatitis (liver), and cholecystitis (gallbladder). The GI tract is not a passive system. Rather, it has the capability to sense and react to materials passed through it. For a healthy digestive system, every person requires different food selections that match their GI tract capacity.

Digestive enzymes: Digestive enzymes are found within the digestive system and are enzymes that help to break down food molecules into smaller components so that they can be absorbed and used by the body.

Digestive juices: Digestive juices are secretions of the digestive system (such as saliva, gastric juice and bile) that break down food.

They are secreted by different organs and play different roles in the digestive process as they vary in their chemical composition.

Digestive system: The system of organs responsible for getting food into and out of the body and for making use of food to keep the body healthy. The digestive system includes the salivary glands, mouth, esophagus, stomach, liver, gallbladder, pancreas, small intestine, colon, and rectum. The digestive system's organs are joined in a long, twisting tube from the mouth to the anus. Inside this tube is a lining called the mucosa? In the mouth, stomach, and small intestine, the mucosa contains tiny glands that produce juices to help digest food. Two solid organs, the liver and the pancreas (both of which are embryo logically derived from the digestive tract), produce digestive juices that reach the intestine through small tubes known as ducts. In addition, parts of other organ systems (for instance, nerves and blood) play a major role in the digestive system. Our digestive system is a complex series of organs and glands that work together to process and breakdown our food from the minute it enters our mouth all the way through to excretion via the anus.

Diverticulitis: Small weak areas in the colon's muscular wall allow the colon's lining to protrude through, forming tiny pouches called diverticulitis. Diverticulitis usually causes no problems, but can bleed or become inflamed or infected. When diverticulitis become inflamed or infected, diverticulitis results. Abdominal pain, fever, and constipation are common symptoms.

Electrolyte: A substance that dissociates into ions in solution and acquires the capacity to conduct electricity. Sodium, potassium, chloride, calcium, and phosphate are examples of electrolytes, informally known as lutes. Electrolyte replacement is needed when a patient has prolonged vomiting or diarrhoea, and as a response to strenuous athletic activity. Commercial electrolyte solutions are available, particularly for sick children (solutions such as Pedialyte) and athletes (sports drinks, such as Gatorade). Electrolyte monitoring is important in treatment of anorexia and bulimia. Electrolytes is a medical terms for salts, specifically ions. They are important to our body as they are needed by our cells (especially nerves, the heart and muscles) to function and carry out electrical impulses such as nerve impulses and muscle contractions.

Enema: A term for pushing liquid into the colon through the anus. Enemas can deliver medicines to treat constipation or other colon conditions. Enemas can be used to provide a form of mechanical stimulation. However, enemas are generally useful only for stool in the rectum, not in the intestinal tract. An enema is a procedure which involves introducing liquid into the intestines via the anus. It is used by the medical profession as a remedy for severe constipation, or as a complementary therapy by Colonic Hydro therapists to 'flush' out material and toxins from the colon. It is the liquid injected into the rectum. An enema may be used for therapeutic (such as to stimulate evacuation of the bowels or heal inflammation of colon called colitis) or diagnostic (such as imaging studies of the gastrointestinal tract - barium enema) purposes.

Epidemiology: Constipation is the most common digestive complaint as per survey data. Depending on the definition employed, it occurs in 2% to 20% of the population. It is more common in women, the elderly and children. The reason it occurs more frequently in the elderly is felt to be due to an increasing number of health problems as human's age and decreased physical activity. 12% of the population worldwide reports having constipation. Chronic constipation accounts for 3% of all visits annually to paediatric outpatient clinics.

Esophagus: A tube that connects the mouth with the stomach.

Faecal impaction: A faecal impaction is a solid, immobile bulk of human faeces that can develop in the rectum as a result of chronic constipation. A related term is faecal loading which refers to a large volume of stool in the rectum of any consistency. Individuals who have had one faecal impaction are at high risk of future impactions. Therefore, preventative treatment should be instituted in patients following the removal of the mass. Patients shall increase dietary fibre, fluid intake, exercising daily, and attempting regularly to defecate every morning after eating should be promoted in all patients. Often underlying medical conditions cause faecal impactions; these conditions should be treated to reduce the risk of future impactions. Many types of medications (most notably opioid pain medications, such as codeine) reduce motility of the colon, increasing the likelihood of faecal impactions. If possible, alternate medications should be prescribed that avoid the side effect of constipation. Given that all opioids can cause constipation, it is recommended that any patient placed on opioid pain medications should be given medications to prevent constipation before it occurs. Daily medications can also be used to promote normal motility of the colon and soften stools. Daily use of laxatives should be avoided by most individuals as it can cause the loss of normal colon motility. However, for patients with chronic complications, daily medication under the direction of a physician may be needed. Polyethylene glycol 3350 can be taken daily to soften the stools without the significant risk of adverse effects that are common with other laxatives. In particular, stimulant laxatives should not be used frequently because they can cause dependence in which an individual loses normal colon function and is unable to defecate without taking a laxative. Frequent use of osmotic laxatives should be avoided as they can cause electrolyte imbalances. Faecal impaction happens when hard stool packs your intestine and rectum so tightly that the normal pushing action of your colon is not enough to push the stool out. Faecal impaction occurs most often in children and older adults.

Faecal impaction: Faecal impaction is a condition often caused by long-term constipation. It occurs when a large lump of hard stool is difficult to pass and remains stuck in the rectum. It may take place after laxative use when the muscles of the intestines forget how to naturally move the stool.

Faecal Incontinence: Faecal incontinence is when someone is unable to control their bowel movements. Unlike diarrhoea, the consistency and frequency of stool does not necessarily have to change when suffering from incontinence. This condition can sometimes be caused by long-term (chronic) constipation.

Faecal incontinence: The medical definition of faecal incontinence is the incapacity to voluntarily hold faeces in the rectum. There are two subgroups to those with faecal incontinence: real faecal incontinence and pseudo incontinence.

Faecal: Relating to the faeces, the stool. The excrement discharged from the intestines.

Faeces: Faeces are another term used to describe stools, and is the waste product expelled from the digestive tract via the anus.

Fats: Plural of the word "fat". See the definition of fat.

FDA: Food and Drug Administration.

Fibre: The parts of fruits and vegetables that cannot be digested. Fibre is of vital importance to digestion; it helps the body move food through the digestive tract, reduces serum cholesterol, and contributes to disease protection and is also known as bulk and roughage.

Fissure: A cleft or groove. A fissure can be normal or abnormal.

Flatulence: Flatulence is the term used to explain passing intestinal wind or 'breaking wind', which is completely normal but can cause embarrassment or discomfort in some people.

Flatulence: Excess gas in the intestinal tract. But excess flatulence is difficult to define without a yardstick to measure the "normal" frequency of gas passages. Symptom-free individuals have recorded approximately 14 passages of gas per 24 hours.

Gastrointestinal Tract: The gastrointestinal tract is the entire route that food takes from the mouth to the rectum, including the stomach and the intestines. The term is not synonymous with "digestive system" because it only describes the route that food takes, rather than all the organs involved in digesting food. The causes of blood in the stool range from harmless, annoying conditions of the gastrointestinal tract such as haemorrhoids to very serious conditions such as cancer. Blood in the stool should be evaluated by a healthcare professional.

Gastrointestinal: Adjective referring collectively to the stomach and small and large intestines.

Haemorrhoids: Dilated (enlarged) veins in the walls of the anus and sometimes around the rectum, usually caused by untreated constipation but occasionally associated with chronic diarrhoea. Symptoms start with bleeding after defecation. If untreated, haemorrhoids can worsen, protruding from the anus. Treatment involves changing the diet to prevent constipation and avoid further irritation, the use of topical medication, and sometimes surgery. It is also known as piles.

Hormones: Substances made in the body by cells or organs that control the function of cells or organs. An example is estrogens, which controls the function of female reproductive organs.

Hypothyroid: Deficiency of thyroid hormone which is normally made by the thyroid gland which is located in the front of the neck.

If you have further questions, contact your obstetrician–gynaecologist.

Immune System: The body's natural defence system against foreign substances and invading organisms, such as bacteria that cause disease.

Inflammatory bowel disease: A group of chronic intestinal diseases characterized by inflammation of the bowel -- the large or small intestine. The most common types of inflammatory bowel disease (IBD) are ulcerative colitis and Crohn's disease.

Internal Prolapsed (intussusceptions): One part of the wall of the large intestine (colon) or rectum may slide into or over another part, like the folding parts of a toy telescope. The rectum does not stick out of the anus. Intussusceptions are most common in children and rarely affect adults. In children, the cause is usually not known. In adults, it is usually related to another intestinal problem, such as a growth of tissue in the wall of the intestines (such as a polyp or tumour).

Intestinal obstruction: Blockage of the intestine by infolding (intussusceptions), malformation, tumour, digestive problems, a foreign body, or inflammation. Symptoms can include cramp abdominal pain, lack of ability to eliminate normal faeces, and eventually shock. On examining the abdomen, the doctor may feel a mass. Abdominal X-rays may suggest intestinal obstruction, but a barium enema may be needed to show the actual cause. Treatment depends on the cause of the obstruction. See also: Intussusceptions.

Intestine: The long, tube like organ in the abdomen that completes the process of digestion. It consists of the small and large intestines.

Kefir: Kefir is a type of fermented milk drink (it can also be made with water). It is made using kefir "grains" which are not related to grains, but are a combination of lactic acid bacteria and yeasts, which act as a fermentation starter. It is easy to digest and contains high levels of vitamins and minerals as well as live cultures which are thought to help reduce digestive problems.

Lactose Intolerant: Being unable to digest lactose, a sugar found in many dairy products.

Laxative: A product that is used to empty the bowels.

Laxative: Something that promotes emptying of the bowels. Laxatives are used to combat constipation. They are sometimes overused, producing diarrhoea. Laxatives include milk of magnesia and many others. Medicines and herbs and some salts can stimulate the bowel muscles or bring more water into the bowel to relieve constipation. Some laxatives are not safe with long term use.

Magnesium: A mineral involved in many processes in the body including nerve signalling, the building of healthy bones, and normal muscle contraction. About 350 enzymes are known to depend on magnesium. Magnesium is contained in all unprocessed foods. High concentrations of magnesium are contained in nuts, whole grains, and dark-green leafy vegetables, legumes such as peas and beans, and fruit. Magnesium is thus readily available in foods that form the basis of a healthful diet.

Nerve: A bundle of fibres that uses electrical and chemical signals to transmit sensory and motor information from one body part to another. The fibrous portions of a nerve are covered by a sheath called myelin and/or a membrane called neurilemma. (Note that entries for specific nerves can be found under the names of the particular nerves. For example, the optic nerve is not under 'nerve, optic' but rather under 'optic nerve.')

Nutrients: Nourishing substances supplied through food, such as vitamins and minerals.

Osteoporosis: A condition in which the bones become so fragile that they break more easily.

Partial Prolapsed (also called Mucosal prolapsed): The lining (Mucous membrane) of the rectum slides out of place and usually sticks out of the anus. This can happen when you strain to have a bowel movement. Partial prolapsed is most common in children younger than 2 years.

Pelvic muscles: Pelvic muscles inability to relax the pelvic muscles to allow for a bowel movement (animus). Pelvic muscles don't coordinate relaxation and contraction correctly (dyssynergia). Weakened pelvic muscles are conditions that affect hormones in the body. Hormones help balance fluids in your body. Diseases and conditions that upset the balance of hormones may lead to constipation, including, Diabetes, Overactive parathyroid gland (hyperparathyroidism), Pregnancy and Underactive thyroid (hypothyroidism).

Polypectomy: During colonoscopy, removal of a colon polyp is called polypectomy.

Probiotics: Microbes are important for the health of the colon. Probiotics are supplements of healthy microbes which may have benefit for some conditions like Crohn's colitis.

Prognosis: Complications that can arise from constipation include haemorrhoids, anal fissures, and rectal prolapsed and faecal impaction. Straining to pass stool may lead to haemorrhoids. In later stages of constipation, the abdomen may become distended, hard and diffusely tender. Severe cases ("faecal impaction" or malignant constipation) may exhibit symptoms of bowel obstruction (vomiting, very tender abdomen) and encopresis, where soft stool from the small intestine bypasses the mass of impacted faecal matter in the colon.

Pseudo incontinence: In cases of pseudo incontinence, a child is believed to suffer from faecal incontinence. However, investigation shows that he or she suffers from severe constipation and faecal impaction. When the impaction is treated and the patient receives enough laxatives to pass stool, he or she becomes continent.

Psyllium (Ispaghula): Psyllium or Ispaghula is mainly used as a dietary fibre to relieve symptoms of both constipation and mild diarrhoea and occasionally as a food thickener and in reducing cholesterol levels. Psyllium is mainly used as a dietary fibre, which is not absorbed by the small intestine. The purely mechanical action of psyllium is to absorb excess water while stimulating normal bowel elimination. Although its main use has been as a laxative, it is more appropriately termed a true dietary fibre and as such can help reduce the symptoms of both constipation and mild diarrhoea and as a gastro retentive. The laxative properties of psyllium are attributed to the fibre absorbing water and subsequently softening the stool. It is also one of the few laxatives that do not promote flatulence. Psyllium is arabinoxylan and hemicelluloses and is often referred to as husk, or psyllium husk. The milled seed mucilage is a white fibrous material that is hydrophilic, meaning that its molecular structure causes it to attract and bind to water. Upon absorbing water, the clear, colourless, mucilaginous gel that forms increases in volume by tenfold or more. This drug may also be used to help relieve the symptoms of irritable bowel syndrome. Psyllium is taken with adequate water as it thickens in the throat, so take it with a full glass of water or other liquid (10 ounces/300 millilitres), stir completely, and drink right away, so that it will not swell in the throat, not causing choking. You may add more liquid to the mixture if it becomes too thick. Dosage is based on your age, medical condition, and response to treatment. Do not increase your dose or take this drug more often than directed. Take Psyllium at least 2 hours from your other medications. It may take 1 to 3 days before this medication starts working. Use this medication regularly to get the most benefit from it. To help you remember, take it at the same time(s) each day. Do not take this medication for more than 7 days unless directed by your doctor. Tell your doctor if your condition persists or worsens, or if bleeding from the rectum occurs. Side Effects of psyllium: Gas or stomach cramping may occur. If any of these effects persist or worsen, tell your doctor or pharmacist promptly. Many people using this medication do not have serious side effects. A very serious allergic reaction to this drug is rare. Precaution for psyllium: Stop using psyllium and call your doctor at once if you have: Choking or trouble swallowing; Severe stomach pain, cramping, nausea or vomiting; Constipation that lasts longer than 7 days; Rectal bleeding; or Itchy skin rash.

Real faecal incontinence: For a child with real faecal incontinence, the normal mechanism of bowel control is not working. Alterations of the muscles that surround the anorectic canal along with poor sphincters (those muscles which control the anus) are responsible for faecal incontinence in children operated on for anorectic with a bad prognosis. Some patients operated on for Hirschsprung's disease have this anatomic problem as do those with spinal problems. The supply of nerve connections of these muscles is important for their correct function. A deficit of nerve connections occurs in anorectic anomalies as well as in other conditions. In cases of spina bifida, or following spinal cord injury, the contraction and relaxation of the muscles, as well as sensation, are deficient. The presence and the passage of faeces and the perception of the difference between solid and liquid faeces and gas are limited.

Rectal Bleeding (Blood in Stool, Hematochezia): Rectal bleeding (known medically as hematochezia) refers to passage of bright red blood from the anus, often mixed with stool and/or blood clots. Most rectal bleeding comes from the colon, rectum, or anus. Blood in the stool can be bright red, maroon in colour, black and tarry, or occult (not visible to the naked eye). The gastrointestinal tract such as haemorrhoids and anal tears from straining against hard stools with constipation, such as cancer, are the main causes of blood in the stool, which range, from harmless to annoying conditions. Blood in the stool should be evaluated by a health-care professional. The colour of the blood during rectal bleeding often depends on the location of the bleeding in the gastrointestinal tract. Generally, the closer the bleeding site is to the anus, the blood will be a brighter red. Thus, bleeding from the anus, rectum, and the sigmoid colon tend to be bright red, whereas bleeding from the transverse colon and the right colon (transverse and right colon are several feet away from the anus) tend to be dark red or maroon colour. In some patients, bleeding can be black and "tarry" (sticky) and foul smelling. The black, smelly, and tarry stool is called Melina. Melina occurs when the blood is in the colon long enough for the bacteria in the colon to break it down into chemicals (haematin) that are black. Therefore, Melina usually signifies bleeding is from the upper gastrointestinal tract (for example, bleeding from ulcers in the stomach or the duodenum or from the small intestine) because the blood usually is in the gastrointestinal tract for a longer period of time before it exits the body. Sometimes Melina may occur with bleeding from the right colon. On the other hand, blood from the sigmoid colon and the rectum usually does not stay in the colon long enough for the bacteria to turn it back. Rarely, massive bleeding from the right colon, from the small intestine, or from ulcers of the stomach or duodenum can cause rapid transit of the blood through the gastrointestinal tract and result in bright red rectal bleeding. In these situations, the blood is moving through the colon so rapidly that there is not enough time for the bacteria to turn the blood black. Sometimes, bleeding from the gastrointestinal tract can be too slow to cause either rectal bleeding or Melina. In these patients, bleeding is occulting (not visible to the naked eye). The blood is found only by testing the stool for blood (faecal occult blood testing) in the laboratory. Occult bleeding has many of the same causes as rectal bleeding and may result in the same symptoms as rectal bleeding. It is often associated with anaemia that is due to loss of iron along with the blood (iron deficiency anaemia).

Rectal prolapsed: Rectal prolapsed happens when your rectum slips so that it sticks out of your anus. Rectal prolapsed can happen if you strain during bowel movements, among other reasons. Rectal prolapsed may cause mucus to leak from your anus. Rectal prolapsed is most common in older adults with a history of constipation, and is also more common in women than men, especially postmenopausal women. In severe cases of rectal prolapsed, a section of the large intestine drops from its normal position as the tissues that hold it in place stretch. Typically there is a sharp bend where the rectum begins. With rectal prolapsed, this bends and other curves in the rectum may straighten, making it difficult to keep stool from leaking out (faecal incontinence). Rectal prolapsed is most common in children and older adults, especially women. Many things increase the chance of developing rectal prolapsed. Risk factors for children include:

Rectum: The final part of the digestive tract.

Rectum: The last 6 to 8 inches of the large intestine. The rectum stores solid waste until it leaves the body through the anus.

Remedy: Something that consistently helps treat or cure a disease.

Renal: Having to do with the kidney. For example, renal cancer is cancer of the kidneys.

Risk factors for adults include: Risk factors for adults include as, straining during bowel movements because of constipation; tissue damage due to surgery or childbirth; and weakness of pelvic floor muscles that occurs naturally with age.

Salmonellosis: The bacteria Salmonella can contaminate food and infect the intestine. Salmonella causes diarrhoea and stomach cramps, which usually resolve without treatment.

Shigellosis: The bacteria Shigella can contaminate food and invade the colon. Symptoms include fever, stomach cramps, and diarrhoea, which may be bloody.

Sigmoidoscopy: An endoscope is inserted into the rectum and advanced through the left side of the colon. Sigmoidoscopy cannot be used to view the middle and right sides of the colon.

Stomach cramp: When a muscle in our digestive suddenly contracts and cannot relax, causing pain.

Stool occult blood testing: A test for blood in the stool. If blood is found in the stool, a colonoscopy may be needed to look for the source.

Stool softeners: Over-the-counter and prescription medicines can soften the stool; stool softeners can affect constipation, but not always.

Stool: Stool is synonymous with faeces or excrement. Stool is essentially the indigestible waste matter from the food you eat after it passes through the digestive system. It is the solid matter that is discharged in a bowel movement.

Strain: A strain is a subset of a bacteria species, which often offers different functions. As a result when considering probiotics, it is important to note that all strains of beneficial bacteria are not the same and some may possess a specific health benefit. It is an injury to a tendon or muscle resulting from overuse or trauma.

Symptom: Any subjective evidence of disease. In contrast, a sign is objective. Blood coming out a nostril is a sign; it is apparent to the patient, physician, and others. Anxiety, low back pain, and fatigue are all symptoms; only the patient can perceive them.

Syndrome: A combination of symptoms and signs that together represent a disease process.

1.3   Does and Don'ts:

Does:

1. Make a habit of bowel evacuation early morning everyday
2. Drink 8 to 10 glasses of water regularly
3. Exercise regularly, preferably yoga.
4. Develop a regular eating habit and chew the food before swallowing
5. Intake plenty of leafy vegetables and salads
6. Eat fibre-rich fruits and vegetables like papaya, orange, beans, asparagus etc
7. Drinking lemon juice mixed with warm water in the morning useful in cleaning the bowel.

Don'ts:

1. Exert pressure to empty your stomach
2. Intake of fried foods and beans and vegetables like cabbage, cauliflower, potatoes. Nuts and dried foods should be avoided along with non-vegetarian foods
3. Avoid smoking and alcoholism and also avoid drinking strong coffee/tea
4. Don't take excess stress or tension
5. Say no to processed foods

Curing constipation through exercises is the best option to get relief from this unpleasant disease.

Exercises given here are for otherwise healthy patients. If you have multiple medical conditions please are cautioned that some exercises may not be suitable at all.

1.4   References:

A Natural Approach to Healthy Bowel Movements & Constipation Prevention: by Be Whole

Best Natural Haemorrhoids Treatments At Home: by Shelly Rayner

How to Cure Constipation: The Complete Constipation Diet And Exercise: by Barney Fraser

High Potency Supplement for Healthy Immune System Colon Bowel Digestive Constipation Nature: by Doctor Health

Perfect Digestion: The Complete Mind-Body Programme for Overcoming Digestive Disorders: by Dr Deepak Chopra

Constipation: How To Treat Constipation: by Ace McCloud

Constipation Remedies, Symptoms, Causes and Cures by Ashley Rose bloom

Constipation: Remedies to get rid of chronic constipation by K.M. Kassi

Constipation: How To Cure Constipation: by Barney Fraser

Healing Digestive Illness: by Russell Mariani MD FAAFP

Constipation: by Amanda Hollingsworth

Perfect Digestion: by Dr Deepak Chopra

Constipation: by Barney Fraser

Constipation: by Ace McCloud

Constipation: by K.M. Kassi

3 Steps to Prevent Chronic Constipation: by Nicky Sandra

CONSTIPATION: by DR ARPITA SINGH and ALABHYA SINGH

Constipation: Constipation Remedies, Symptoms: by Ashley Rose bloom

Allens' Keynotes: Rearranged and Classified with Leading Remedies of the Materia Medica and Bowel Nosodes by Henry Clay Allen

Gut: the inside story: by Giulia Enders

Gut Reactions: by Justin Sonnenburg and Erica Sonnenburg

Shackelford's Surgery of the Alimentary Tract (Shackelfords Surgery of the Alimentary Tract): by Charles J. Yeo, David W McFadden, John H. Pemberton and Jeffrey H. Peters

Emergency Medicine Secrets: by Vincent J. Markovchick, Peter T. Pons and Katherine A. Bakes

Paediatric Gastrointestinal and Liver Disease: by Robert Wyllie and Jeffrey S. Hyams

How to Poop Like A Pro: by David Koski

Bowel Movement Journal: by Health & Wellness Books Import

Bowel Movements: A Humorous Look at Taking a Dump: by Kelly Patrick Gray

Constipation: Constipation Diet Guide To Constipation Relief with Constipation Diet Strategies for Improved Bowel: by Amanda Hollingsworth

Books" abnormal bowel" Showing all results:

2

Constipation

2.0   General:

Constipation refers to bowel movements that are infrequent or hard to pass. Constipation is a common cause of painful defecation. It means either going to the toilet less often than usual to empty the bowels, or passing hard or painful stools (faeces). Constipation most commonly define that the stool moves too slowly through the digestive tract or cannot be eliminated effectively from the rectum because of the stool becomes hard and dry. Constipation is one of the most common gastrointestinal (GI) problems, affecting about 75 million people. Constipation is common among all ages. Severity of constipation, flatulence and bloating is summarized into four categories, such as, severe, moderately severe, mild and chronic.

Many people have chronic constipation, which include passing fewer than three stools a week, having lumpy or hard stools, straining to have bowel movements, feeling as though there's a blockage in your rectum that prevents bowel movements, feeling as though you can't completely empty the stool from your rectum, needing help to empty your rectum, such as using your hands to press on your abdomen and using a finger to remove stool from your rectum. Chronic constipation person has at least passing fewer stools three days per month for more than three months associated with abdominal discomfort, which is often diagnosed as irritable bowel syndrome (IBS) when no obvious cause is found. Abdominal pain and bloating could also be present depending on the severity of the condition. Loss of appetite can also occur. The number of bowel movements generally decreases with age. Most adults have bowel movements between three and 14 times per week, and this would be considered normal constipation. The most common pattern is one bowel movement a day, but this pattern is seen in less than half the people. Severe constipation is defined as less than one bowel movement per week. Going without a bowel movement for two or three days does not cause physical discomfort, only mental distress for some people. It is important to distinguish acute (recent onset) constipation from chronic (long duration) constipation. Acute constipation requires urgent assessment because a serious medical illness may be the underlying cause like tumours of the colon. Constipation also requires an immediate assessment if it is accompanied by worrisome symptoms such as rectal bleeding, abdominal pain and cramps, nausea and vomiting involuntary loss of weight. The evaluation of chronic constipation may not be urgent, particularly if simple measures bring relief. Colonic propagating pressure wave sequences (PSs) are responsible for discrete movements of the bowel contents and are vital for normal defecation. Deficiencies in PS frequency, amplitude, and extent of propagation are all implicated in severe defecator dysfunction (SDD). Chronic or long-lasting, constipation can lead to health problems such as haemorrhoids, anal fissures, and rectal prolapsed or faecal impaction. Haemorrhoids are swollen and inflamed veins around your anus or in your lower rectum. You can develop haemorrhoids if you strain to have a bowel movement. If you have haemorrhoids, you may have bleeding in your rectum. You have bleeding in the rectum when you see bright red blood in your stool, on toilet paper, or in the toilet after a bowel movement. Anal fissures are small tears in your anus that may cause itching, pain, or bleeding.

Constipation is common among all ages and populations likely to be and include: Non-Caucasians; Older adults; People taking medicines to relieve broken bone, a pulled tooth, or back pain; People taking medicines to treat depression; People who just had surgery; People with lower incomes; and Women especially during pregnancy or after giving birth. Constipation is a symptom, not a disease, effective treatment of constipation may require first determining the cause. The causes of constipation can be divided into congenital, primary, and secondary.

2.1 Symptoms of mild Constipation:

Constipation means hard stools, difficulty in passing stools (straining), or a sense of incomplete emptying after a bowel movement. It means either going to the toilet less often than usual to empty the bowels, or passing hard or painful stools (faeces). Symptoms of Constipation are often associated with irritable bowel syndrome (IBS). The key symptom of IBS is abdominal pain. The pain is associated with a change in the frequency or consistency of bowel habit. The altered bowel habit may be chronic or recurrent constipation, or diarrhoea. In addition, symptom occurrence can fluctuate over time. There can be periods when symptoms flare-up as well as periods when they diminish or disappear. Doctors usually define constipation as hard pellet-like stools. The pain from a blockage comes from the bowels stretching, says Chukka, and left alone, this can lead to a bowel perforation. (That's when a hole forms through the stomach, large bowel, or small intestine. Doctor would put a tube down the nose to suck everything out and decompress the bowel. Being constipated means your bowel movements are tough or happen less often than normal. Almost everyone goes through it sooner or later. Although it's not usually serious, you'll feel much better when your body is back on track. The normal length of time between bowel movements varies widely from person to person. Some people have them three times a day. Others have them only once or twice a week. Going longer than 3 or more days without one, though, is usually too long. After 3 days, the stool or faeces become harder and more difficult to pass. Constipation is a common problem. It means either going to the toilet less often than usual to empty the bowels, or passing hard or painful stools (faeces).

This is because they may cause abdominal bloating and discomfort without doing much to clear a lot of faeces which are stuck further down the gut. The most common symptoms of constipation are infrequency, irregularity or difficulty in elimination of the hard facial matter. The other symptoms include

- Acidity
- Bleeding as a result of straining
- Bloating of the abdomen, and possibly a "rumbling" noise
- Bowel movements with stools that are hard, dry, and small, making them painful or difficult to pass.
- Coated tongue
- Constant fullness in the abdomen
- Dark circles under the eyes
- Depression
- Difficulty during defecation (straining during more than 25% of bowel movements.
- Dizziness
- Don't have a bowel movement every day.
- Fewer than three bowel movements a week.
- Foul breath
- Gas
- Hard or small stools.

- Hard, dry stools that are difficult to pass
- Having three bowel movements a week.
- Headache
- Heart burn
- Passing blood from bowel or stool
- Weight gain;
- Indigestion
- Infrequent bowel movements
- Insomnia.
- Straining on more than 75% of passing stool.
- Loss of appetite
- Nausea
- non-Caucasians;
- getting older as an adults;
- Pain in the lumbar region
- Pain or pressure in the belly
- Sensation of hard stools;
- Sensation that the bowels haven't completely emptied
- Sense that everything didn't come out.
- Straining in this context is a strong effort to push out stool often by holding one's breath and by pushing the respective muscles in the abdominal area hard
- Swollen belly or belly pain.
- The sensation of incomplete bowel evacuation.
- Throwing up belly.
- Ulcer in the mouth

2.2.1   Symptoms   of   Severe Constipation:

- Severe Constipation is defined as less than one stool per week. Some of the symptoms of constipation include:
- Lower abdominal discomfort.
- Infrequent bowel movements.
- Straining to have a bowel movement,
- Hard or small stools,
- rectal bleeding
- anal fissures caused by hard stools,
- physiological distress,
- Obsession with having bowel movements.

- Constipation (failure to pass stools or gas)
- Life threatening faecal impaction.

2.2.2 Symptoms of Chronic Constipation:

Chronic constipation can result in faecal impaction. This is something that is more likely in the elderly and infirm. Basically, a large mass of hard faeces blocks the rectum. The mass is too big to pass and the rectum is stretched and enlarged, so the muscles within it don't work so well to push faeces out. Chronic constipation can interfere with their ability to go about their daily tasks. Chronic constipation may also cause excessive straining to have a bowel movement and other signs and symptoms. Sometimes people with this problem think that they have diarrhoea. This is because liquid faeces, from above the blockage, leak around the big lump of faeces and out of the anus. This is known as overflow diarrhoea. In this situation, you may also have faecal incontinence - that is, you have no control over this liquid faeces leaking out. Faecal impaction with overflow diarrhoea is likely if you have been getting progressively more constipated, and then have liquid faeces, possibly explosive, and without much control. Chronic, or long-lasting, constipation can lead to health problems such as haemorrhoids, anal fissures, and rectal prolapsed or faecal impaction.

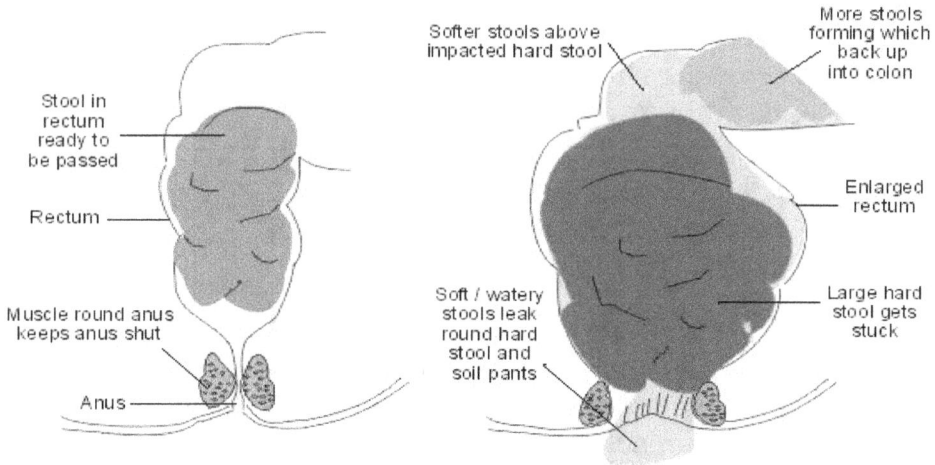

Normal   Faecal impaction with overflow diarrhoea

Constipation may be considered chronic if you've experienced two or more of these symptoms for the last three months. Consult your doctor if you experience unexplained and persistent changes in your bowel habits. Medical evaluation of constipation should be done when constipation is of sudden onset, severe, worsening, associated with other worrisome symptoms such as loss of weight, or is not responding to simple, safe and effective treatments. Haemorrhoidsare swollen and inflamed veins around your anus or in your lower rectum. You can develop haemorrhoids if you strain to have a bowel movement. If you have haemorrhoids, you may have bleeding in your rectum. You have bleeding in the rectum when you see bright red blood in your stool, on toilet paper, or in the toilet after a bowel movement. Anal fissures are small tears in your anus that may cause itching, pain, or bleeding. Chronic constipation has many possible causes. Symptoms of chronic constipation include:

- A large or hard stool can cause tiny tears in the anus.
- Abdominal pain and bloating could also be present depending on the severity of the condition.
- Accumulation of hardened stool that gets stuck in your intestines.
- Feeling as though there's a blockage in your rectum that prevents bowel movements,
- Feeling as though you can't completely empty the stool from your rectum,
- Having lumpy or hard stools,
- Intestine that protrudes from the anus (rectal prolapsed).
- Loss of appetite can also occur.
- Needing help to empty your rectum using your hands to press on your abdomen and using a finger to remove stool from your rectum.
- Passing fewer than three stools a week,
- Stool that can't be expelled (faecal impaction).
- Straining to have a bowel movement, which can cause a small amount of the rectum to stretch and protrude from the anus.
- Swollen veins in your anus (haemorrhoids).
- Torn skin in your anus (anal fissure).

2.3   Cause of Constipation

In general, constipation may be caused by not eating enough fibre, or not drinking enough fluids. Constipation appears to be quite a problem for a lot of people. From infants to the elderly, irregular bowel movements interfere with health and vitality. The symptoms of constipation are obvious and include infrequent bowel movements, hard stools, and difficulty passing stools. The side effects of constipation commonly include abdominal discomfort, bloating, gas, bad breath, headaches, nausea, and fatigue. It's no wonder laxative sales are big business. Conventional stimulant laxatives force your digestive tract into overdrive, which deprives your body of nutrients as food is rushed along. Massive quantities of gelatinous fibre drinks, swallowed in an attempt to prevent constipation, can cause problems of their own with spasms, bloating and irritation of the gut lining. Consider the gentler, easier methods to help your digestive tract perform both naturally and optimally. It makes perfect sense that the primary causes for constipation are related to diet. It can also be a side-effect of certain medicines, or related to an underlying medical condition. In many cases, the cause is not clear. Laxatives are a group of medicines that can treat constipation. Ideally, laxatives should only be used for short periods of time until symptoms ease. Note: there is a separate leaflet on constipation in children. Not eating enough fibre (roughage) is a common cause. 18 gram per day is recommended by the British Nutrition Foundation. Fibre is the part of plant food that is not digested. It remains in your gut. It adds bulk to the stools (faeces) and helps your bowels to work well. Foods high in fibre include fruit, vegetables, cereals and wholemeal bread. Not drinking much may make constipation worse. Stools are usually soft and easily passed if you eat enough fibre and drink enough fluid. However, some people need more fibre and/or fluid than others in order to avoid constipation. Some special slimming diets are low in fibre and may cause constipation.

In order to experience such promising side effects (in essence, results) of confidence, feeling great, looking great, happiness, overall health and success on a daily basis, we must be clean from the inside out, exercise regularly, drink water, stress less, bulk up on high fibrous foods, and implement healthier eating habits. This could mean you have to eliminate, or at least reduce the following items you consume on a daily basis.

When you eliminate all of these foods, which cause constipation from your diet, you are proactively reducing the chance of constipation and hence the number of constipation side affects you experience is less. They impact your overall digestive health badly.

It is important to remember that constipation is not a disease; it is a symptom of a much larger issue. We will all experience constipation symptoms at some point in our life. When we have a majority of people consuming tempting, delicious and perhaps taste addictive foods on a daily basis, these statistics become a disappointing reflection of how far we are in making our health a priority. Unless you're looking to prevent being a statistic, then that is exactly what will happen. Due to the environment in which we all live, every day we come in contact with many industrial chemicals, heavy metals and other substances that can be detrimental to our health. Our body absorbs an abundance of toxins from genetically modified foods, pesticides, soy, white flour, MSG, refined sugar and artificial sweeteners. These impurities contaminate nearly everything we eat, drink, touch, or breathe and they are the root cause of many dangerous health conditions. If you have added weight of an impacted colon, you will be suffering more through irregular, uncomfortable, and painful bowel movements because of constipation. A healthy digestive system alone has a challenging time ridding the body of all these toxins, much less a digestive system plagued by constipation.

Some people have a good diet, drink a lot of fluid, do not have a disease or take any medication that can cause constipation; however, they still become constipated. Their bowels are said to be underactive. This is quite common and is sometimes called functional constipation or primary constipation. Most cases occur in women. This condition tends to start in childhood or in early adulthood and persists throughout life. Do not ignore the feeling of needing the toilet. Some people suppress this feeling if they are busy. It may result in a backlog of stools which is difficult to pass later. When you go to the toilet, it should be unhurried, with enough time to ensure that you can empty your bowel. Chronic constipation can be more difficult to treat.

Chronic constipation is sometimes complicated by a backlog of hard faeces building up in the bowel (faecal loading) or even partially blocking it (impaction).

This is normal and tends to settle down after a few weeks as the gut becomes used to the increase in fibre or bulk-forming laxative. Occasionally, bulk-forming laxatives can make symptoms worse if you have very severe constipation. Constipation is a symptom, not a disease, effective treatment of constipation may require first determining the cause. The causes of constipation can be divided into congenital, primary, and secondary. Constipation with no known organic cause, i.e. no medical explanation, exhibits gender differences in prevalence: females are more often affected than males. The most common cause is primary and not life-threatening. In the elderly, constipation causes include: Primary or functional constipation is ongoing symptoms for greater than six months not due to any underlying cause such as medication side effects or an underlying medical condition. It is not associated with abdominal pain, thus distinguishing it from irritable bowel syndrome. Constipation is common; in the general population rates of constipation varies from 2–30 percent. In elderly people living in care homes the rate of constipation is 50–75 percent. There is no one cause of constipation, but many cases can be tied to it. Causes of Constipation include:

- Alcoholic beverages
- Antacid medicines containing calcium and aluminium.
- Anticonvulsants used for epilepsy
- Antidepressants tablets
- Anxiety, depression and grief
- Bowel obstructions, such as a tumour or benign growth
- Bowel problems like haemorrhoids, irritable bowel syndrome, or diverticulitis
- Caffeinated Drinks, such as, sodas, coffee, energy drinks
- Calcium channel blockers such as nifedipine and verapamil, which can cause severe constipation due to dysfunction of motility in the recto sigmoid colon.
- Calcium Supplements
- Carbonated Drinks High in Sugar, such as, sodas, energy drinks
- Celiac disease.
- Changes in Physical activities
- Changes in your usual diet
- Childhood chronic constipation can be manifested as intolerance to cow's milk.
- Chronic kidney failure
- Colon and rectum problem
- Colonic inertia
- Consumption of meat in large quantities, excessive use of strong tea and coffee, inadequate chewing, overeating and wrong combination of foods, irregular habits of eating and drinking May all give to poor bowel function.
- Cough and cold medications containing dextromethorphan
- Crohn's disease,
- cystic fibrosis,
- Dairy Products, such as, milk, butter, ice-cream
- Decreased physical activity,
- Dehydration
- Delaying the urge to go to the toilet
- Depression
- diabetes mellitus,
- Diet deficient in leafy, green vegetables and salads

- Diet low in fibre (lacking whole grains, bran, fresh fruit and vegetables)
- Diet, particularly if you're eating one high in processed foods low in fibre.
- Dieting: Constipation can be caused or exacerbated by a dieting. Slimming diets are low in fibre and may cause constipation.
- Difficulty with the muscles involved in elimination.
- Diseases primarily of other parts of the body that also affect the colon.
- Diuretics, antidepressants and antihistamines
- Diverticulitis,
- Eating habit disorders.
- Enriched White Flour, such as, white bread, doughnuts, some varieties of tortillas
- Excessive intake of animal protein
- Excessive intake of tea and coffee
- Excessive use of Prescription and over-the-counter (OTC) medications
- Excessive use of strong tea and coffee.
- Faecal impaction, a condition in which stool hardens in the rectum and prevents the passage of any stool (although occasionally diarrhoea may occur even with the obstruction due to colonic fluid leaking around the impacted stool).
- Fast & Fried Foods, such as, pizza, burgers, tacos, fried chicken
- faulty and irregular habit of defecation, frequent use of purgatives, weakness of abdominal muscles due to sedentary habits, lack of physical activity, and emotional anxiety and strain.
- Habitual use of laxatives and enemas (leading to a rebound the effect)
- Heart medications such as calcium-channel blockers
- Heavy intake of dairy products, meats, refined sugar and eggs
- High levels of estrogens and progesterone during pregnancy,
- Hormonal changes
- Hormonal disorders,
- hypocalcaemia,
- hypothyroidism,
- Ignoring the urge to go. If you consistently ignore the urge to have a bowel movement, for instance, to avoid using a public toilet, eventually you may stop feeling the urge.

- Illness
- Imbalance of Solar plexus or third Chakra or Manipura Chakra
- Improper lifestyle
- Inactive lifestyle
- Insufficient dietary fibre intake/Lack of fibrous diet,
- Insufficient intake of liquids such as water or pure juice
- Intake of alcohol
- Intestinal obstruction
- Iron supplements or increased blood calcium levels are also potential causes. Spinal cord injury is a common cause.
- Iron tablets
- Irritable bowel syndrome (IBS),
- Irritable colon and rectum
- Ischemic colitis,
- Lack of exercise or any other physical activity, or negligence of the recommended constipation exercise.
- Laxatives use for a long time: Laxatives are a group of medicines that can treat constipation. Ideally, laxatives should only be used for short periods of time until symptoms ease. Stools (faeces) become hard and difficult or painful to pass due to lack of liquid intake.
- Lead poisoning
- Lifestyle habits
- Long bed rest
- Low intake of water
- Low fibre diets,
- Magnesium deficiencies
- Mature age - older adults often suffer from constipation due to a combination of poor diet, insufficient fluids, poor bowel habits or the side effects of prescription medication
- Meals without enough leafy and green vegetables, salads etc in the diet
- Medical conditions such as irritable bowel syndrome (IBS), underactive thyroid gland (hypothyroidism), spinal injury, multiple sclerosis, kidney failure, colon or rectal cancer, too much calcium in the blood, tumours and lesions of the bowel
- Medications such as painkillers (especially codeine), antacids, antispasmodic drugs, antidepressants or iron tablets
- Medicines (even some common ones like pain killers)
- Multiple sclerosis.

- Narcotic medications like Codeine and oxycodone
- Narrowing of the colon (bowel stricture).
- Nerve diseases
- Neurologic disorders such as Parkinson's disease, multiple sclerosis, or spinal cord injury
- Not being able to go to the toilet because of poor mobility
- Not being active.
- not doing enough exercise
- Not drinking enough - always drink more when you increase fibre in your diet
- Not eating enough fibre (whole grain food, fruits and vegetables, wholemeal, high fibre cereals)
- Not having enough roughage diet
- Not having enough roughage or high fibre food in diet
- Nutritional deficiencies
- Other abdominal cancer that presses on the colon.
- Over eating and insufficient chewing.
- Overuse of laxative and suppositories (use to soften stool)
- Overweight
- Pain killer medications such as codeine and morphine
- Parkinson's, fissures and pelvic dysfunction
- Poor bowel habits such as ignoring the urge to have bowel movements
- Poor diet or sudden changes in diet
- Pregnancy - hormonal changes and pressure on the bowel by the heavy womb can cause prolonged constipation which can in turn result in the development of anal fissures or haemorrhoid.
- Problems like hypocalcaemia, hypothyroidism and diabetes
- Problems with the nerves around the colon and rectum.
- Problems with the pelvic muscles involved in having a bowel movement may cause chronic constipation.
- Rectal cancer.
- Rectal or colon cancer
- Rectal trauma,
- Rectum bulge through the back wall of the vagina (rectocele).
- Red, Fatty Meats, such as, steak, veal, brisket, pork
- Refined Sugars, such as, chocolate, cake, pie, candy-bars, alcohol, beer, wine, mixed drinks
- Rtia and pelvic floor dysfunction.
- Slow movement of stool through the colon.

- Slow transit bowel which means it takes longer for the faeces to travel all the way to the rectum, so more water is removed over time and constipation is much more likely. This occurs where there is nerve damage such as with stroke, Parkinson's, multiple sclerosis or trauma.
- Spinal cord injury.
- Stress and anxiety
- Stroke.

2.3.1 Insufficient dietary fibres intake:

Fibre is the part of plant food that is not digested. It remains in your gut. It adds bulk to the stools (faeces) and helps your bowels to work well. Foods high in fibre include fruit, vegetables, cereals and wholemeal bread. Not eating enough fibre or eating less than 18 gram fibre per day in your diet may cause Constipation. A fibre-rich diet supports the growth of beneficial bacteria, which make their home in the intestinal tract. These bacteria encourage regular bowel movements. A diet that relies heavily on processed foods lacks fibre, and a certain amount of fibre is essential for regular, effortless elimination. A diet based on whole, unprocessed foods provides the necessary bulk to keep waste material moving smoothly through the intestinal tract which helps to decrease the body's load of toxins. The more sluggish the bowels, the longer the body are exposed to toxins to be shed. Fibre is the indigestible part of plants, and vegetables and fruits are the best fibre sources, rather than grains. Although grains are often recommended, they can actually cause problems because of their anti-nutrient coatings and greater potential for allergies. Fruits and vegetables are also rich in carotenoids and other phytonutrients, which help keep the mucosal lining of the large intestine healthy. A fibre-rich diet supports the growth of beneficial bacteria, which make their home in the intestinal tract. These bacteria encourage regular bowel movements. Some studies show that improving the population of friendly intestinal flora is enough to cure stubborn cases of constipation. Supplementing your diet with naturally lacto-fermented foods such as pickles, sauerkraut, kefir, and yogurt helps replenish the supply of these beneficial microorganisms. It may also be necessary to supplement your diet with concentrated sources of probiotics, particularly if constipation is chronic or internal flora has been disrupted by the use of antibiotics.

Dietary fibre refers to the edible parts of plants or carbohydrates that cannot be digested. Fibre is in all plant foods, including fruits, vegetables, grains, nuts, seeds, and legumes. You can also find a form of fibre called chitin in the shells of crustaceans such as crab, lobster, and shrimp.

No, some fibres are soluble in water and others are insoluble. Soluble fibre slows digestion and helps you absorb nutrients from food. Insoluble fibre adds bulk to your stool, helping the stool pass more quickly through the intestines. Most plant foods contain some of each kind of fibre. Foods containing high levels of soluble fibre include dried beans, oats, oat bran, rice bran, barley, citrus fruits, apples, strawberries, peas, and potatoes. Foods high in insoluble fibre include wheat bran, whole grains, cereals, seeds, and the skins of many fruits and vegetables. Go for whole-grain breads, cereals, and pastas. Cereal fibres generally have cell walls that resist digestion and retain water within the cellular structures. Wheat bran can be highly effective as a natural laxative. Eat plenty of fresh fruits, vegetables, and legumes such as beans and lentils. The fibre found in citrus fruits and legumes stimulate the growth of colonic flora, which increases the stool weight and the amount of bacteria in the stool. Encouraging the growth of certain bacteria in the colon may help promote a healthy intestine.

2.3.2 Inadequate Intake of Liquid:

Not drinking enough water may cause Constipation. Not drinking much liquid make constipation worse. Stools are usually soft and easily passed if you eat enough fibre and drink enough fluid. However, some people need more fibre and/or fluid than others in order to avoid constipation. Adequate water intake or liquid is a way to manage constipation. Water is important for our digestion. It keeps the food we eat moving along through our intestines and it keeps our intestines smooth and flexible, too. Dehydration is one of the most common causes of chronic constipation. The food we eat makes its way from our stomach to the large intestine, or colon. If we don't have enough water in our body already or if we are dehydrated, the large intestine soaks up water from our food waste. This makes hard stools that are difficult to pass. Watch the amount of fluid we drink, listen to our body, and drink more liquids during exercise and hot weather. Dehydration happens when our body gets rid of more fluids, usually through sweating or going to the bathroom more than normal, than it absorbs. Drinking too little water during exercise, hot weather, or daily activities can also cause the body to use up its stored water. Extra fluids help keep the stool soft and easy to pass, but drinking more liquids does not cure constipation.

When it comes to thirst, most experts say "let our body be your guide." The Institute of Medicine's Food and Nutrition Board suggests that women need 91 ounces of water each day and men need 125 ounces. Remember, this recommendation includes the fluids in your food. In general, for healthy, average people, 3 litres a day is a good goal. Fruit and vegetable juices, clear soups, and herbal teas are also good sources of fluids. But, stay away from alcohol. It is a diuretic, which gets rid of water from our body and leads to dehydration. Caffeinated drinks like coffee, tea, and colas are also diuretics and leads to dehydration, but as long as you drink moderate amounts, they probably won't cause dehydration.

Fluid losses induced by diarrhoea and febrile illness alter water balance and promote constipation. The improvement of constipation by increasing water intake is effective when fluid consumption is lower than normal for all age and activity level. In the elderly, low fluid intake, which may be indicative of hypo hydration, was a cause of constipation and a significant relationship between liquid deprivation from 2500 to 500 ml per day and constipation was reported. Dehydration is also observed when saline laxatives are used for the treatment of constipation if fluid replacement is not maintained and may affect the efficacy of the treatment. While sulphate in drinking water does not appear to have a significant laxative effect, but fluid intake and magnesium sulphate-rich mineral waters were shown to improve constipation. In conclusion, fluid loss and fluid restriction and thus dehydration or hypo hydration increase constipation. It is thus important to maintain rehydration as a prevention of constipation.

Fluid intake is vital for good general health and particularly to maintain bladder and bowel health, since bladder health is linked to an adequate daily urine output which, in turn, is influenced by fluid intake. Low fluid intake can contribute to constipation. Maintaining an appropriate intake is therefore important for patients with bladder or bowel dysfunction. Some authors have identified that long-term care settings can influence the amount of fluid consumed. Since older people are particularly vulnerable to inadequate intake a campaign has been initiated to improve the fluid intake among residents of care homes in England. Ensuring patients have an appropriate fluid intake has many implications for nursing practice. The patients with bladder and bowel problems are given general advice about healthy living, which should include information about drinking appropriate fluids in sufficient quantities. The giving of advice on fluids is therefore a crucial nursing role that has the potential to contribute greatly to reducing continence problems, bladder infections and constipation and to promoting general wellbeing.

Some older people, or those who have frequency problems, may restrict fluid intake in the belief that this will reduce their problem. In fact, fluid restriction can exacerbate symptoms of urgency, frequency and incontinence, as concentrated urine can irritate the bladder and, over time, poor urine volumes may result in the bladder needing to empty when it is only partially full. The reduced volumes, more concentrated urine and less frequent bladder emptying associated with inadequate intake may also increase the risk of urine infection and bladder cancer.

Appropriate Liquid intake

Water: Constipation is related to dehydration in the colon, you need to make sure you are drinking lots of water. When your body is properly hydrated, less water will be withdrawn from the colon. This will keep your stool soft and easy to pass. The general consensus is that the average healthy adult needs a daily fluid intake of 1.5 L to replace natural loss over and above 3 L of body requirement, but the ideal amount varies between individuals. This may depend on several factors, which include illness and disease, age, weight, activity level and external factors such as hot weather. The type and timing of the fluid taken can also have an effect on bladder and bowel function. One of the easiest causes of constipation to address is dehydration. Our body has a very sophisticated system for regulating how much water it absorbs and how much it excretes; if we aren't drinking enough water, our body clings on to every last drop because it needs all that fluid to maintain blood volume and perform other important functions. Since we don't have any fluid left over for less essential needs like pooping, the poop in our colon becomes very dehydrated and hard, which makes it difficult to pass and often painful on the way out. If we increase our water intake, our body will have more to excrete, so our faeces will become softer and easier to pass.

There is no magic amount of water necessary for proper bowel function (it varies from person to person depending on age, activity level, and other factors), but since drinking more is such an easy and non-invasive remedy, it's worth a try if you think it might be even a remotely plausible explanation.

Herbal teas: These are an increasingly popular alternative to tea and coffee, but they are not suitable for everyone, as they have a range of different properties, such as,

- Nettle can have a diuretic effect;
- Chamomile may relax bladder spasm;
- Ginger and peppermint may relieve wind;
- Liquorice may relieve constipation;
- Rosehip, orange and rhubarb should be avoided by people with loose stools.

As with all herbal medicines, patients should seek further information before taking herbal teas and excessive intake should be avoided.

Fruit juices: Fruit Juices are generally good for health but some specific properties should be noted. Grapefruit juice should be avoided with some medications; for example, antihistamines, statins and calcium channel blockers, so it is important to consult the leaflets supplied with all medications; Orange juice is rich in vitamin C, but excessive consumption can cause diarrhoea; High intake of acidic juices may exacerbate the symptoms of rheumatoid arthritis, gastric irritation and interstitial cystitis.

2.3.3   Magnesium Deficiencies:

Magnesium is a mineral that supports your body's overall health. It plays a key role in muscle function, which may explain why it can be so helpful for individuals who suffer from constipation. After all, your GI tract is one long muscle that must be healthy in order to produce consistent bowel movements. We get enough Magnesium from Magnesium rich Foods. Magnesium deficiency is dramatically under-diagnosed because it doesn't show up on a normal blood test. Only 1 percent of the magnesium in our body is stored in our blood, and the majority of its stored in our bones. Magnesium-rich foods are essential for cellular health and over 300 biochemical functions in the body. Our body has 3,751 magnesium binding sites. This indicates that magnesium benefits are far greater. Our body requires and uses magnesium for so many different functions; we can quickly become low in magnesium especially if we are not consuming enough high magnesium foods. Some of the major functions in our body require magnesium. Some of the main health challenges that have been linked to a magnesium deficiency include:

- Protein synthesis
- Nerve function
- Blood sugar control
- Neurotransmitter release
- Blood pressure regulation
- Energy metabolism

- Production of the antioxidant glutathione
- Hormone imbalance and PMS
- Fibromyalgia
- Heart attack
- Type 2 diabetes
- Osteoporosis
- Constipation
- Tension or migraine headaches
- Anxiety and depression
- Chronic fatigue

Best Food Sources of Magnesium:

Increasing intake of high magnesium foods is essential to our health. Magnesium is more crucial than Calcium. The foods that are highest in magnesium are green leafy vegetables, which are packed with chlorophyll. Chlorophyll is known as the "life blood" of a plant and has the ability to absorb the sun's light and turn it into energy. One major difference between human blood and chlorophyll is that human blood has iron at the centre of the cell, but plants have magnesium at the centre of the cell. Green leafy vegetables aren't the only foods rich in magnesium and chlorophyll. Here are the top 10 foods high in magnesium that we should want to add into our diet. Men RDA are 400 milligrams and Women RDA are 310 milligrams a day.

Magnesium is found in such foods as green leafy vegetables, avocados, bananas, melon, legumes, nuts, seeds and certain whole grains. A good rule of thumb is that if a food contains dietary fibre, it also probably provides magnesium. Magnesium is also added to some cereal grains (although this isn't the preferred source, since refining the grains removes important, naturally occurring nutrients from the grain's germ and bran). Percentages based on the RDA for adult women of 320 mg/day:

Almonds ¼ cup: 97 mg (30%)
Avocado 1 raw: 39 mg (12%)
Bananas 1 banana: 37 mg. (11%)
Black Beans 1 cup cooked: 120 mg. (37%)
Broccoli 1 cup cooked: 32 mg. (10%)
Brussels Sprouts 1 cup cooked: 32 mg. (10%)
Cashews ¼ cup: 91 mg (28%)
Chard — 1 cup: 154 milligrams (38%)
Dark Chocolate — 1 square: 95 milligrams (24%)
Figs — ½ cup: 50 milligrams (13%)
Mung Beans 1 cup cooked: 97 mg. (30%)

Potatoes 1 large: 85 mg. (26%)
Pumpkin Seeds 1/4 cup: 42 mg 13%
Spinach 1 cup cooked: 157 mg. (49%)
Swiss chard 1 cup cooked: 150 mg. (47%)
Yogurt or curd — 1 cup: 50 milligrams (13%)
Other foods that are also high in magnesium include: salmon, coriander, goat cheese, Beans, Nuts, Whole grains such as brown rice and whole wheat flour, Green leafy vegetables, fish and artichokes. Here are five key areas where magnesium has been proven effective:
1)   Cardiovascular;
2)   Fibromyalgia;
3)   Type 2 Diabetes;
4)   Osteoporosis;
5)   Migraine Headaches.   Magnesium content in Magnesium-reach food: The following a list of the magnesium content in common food sources of magnesium is sorted by milligrams magnesium per gram of food content.

Table: Magnesium content in common food sources

Foods	Serving Size, Common Units	Serving Size, Grams	Milligrams Magnesium	Milligrams Magnesium per Gram	% Daily Value (DV)
Cocoa, unsweetened	2 tbsp.	10	52	5.24	14%
Bran Breakfast Cereal, ready to eat	1 oz.	28	78	2.78	19%
Almonds	1 oz.	28	75	2.68	19%
Cashews, dry roasted	1 oz.	28	73	2.61	18%
Pumpkin Seeds, roasted	1 oz.	28	73	2.61	18%
Molasses	1 tbsp.	20	48	2.42	12%
Peanuts, dry roasted	1 oz.	28	49	1.75	12%
Peanut Butter	2 tbsp.	32	49	1.53	12%

Whole Wheat Bread (Roti), homemade	1 slice	28	37	1.32	9%
Halibut	3 oz.	85	91	1.07	23%
Navy Bean Sprouts, raw	1 oz.	28	28	1.01	7%
Mackerel	3 oz.	85	83	0.97	21%
Spinach, boiled	1/2 cup	90	79	0.87	20%
Whole Wheat Bread, store bought	1 slice	28	23	0.82	6%
Coffee, espresso	2 oz.	60	48	0.80	12%
Spinach, raw	1 cup	30	24	0.79	6%
Quinoa, cooked	1/2 cup	92.5	59	0.64	15%
Milk Chocolate	1 oz.	28	18	0.63	4%
Soybeans, boiled	1/2 cup	90	54	0.60	14%
Black-Eyed Peas (Cowpeas), boiled	1/2 cup	87.5	46	0.52	12%
Buckwheat Grouts (Kasha), cooked	1/2 cup	84	43	0.51	11%
Parsley, raw	1 oz.	28	14	0.50	3%
Lima Beans, boiled	1/2 cup	94	40	0.43	10%
Acorn squash, baked	1/2 cup	102.5	44	0.43	11%
Swiss Chard	1/2 cup	175	75	0.43	19%
Egg	1	46	18	0.39	3%
Tofu	1/2 cup	126	47	0.37	12%
Bacon, pan-fried	3 oz.	85	31	0.36	8%
Pork	3 oz.	85	31	0.36	8%

43

Tenderloin, broiled					
Okra, boiled	1 cup	160	58	0.36	14%
Bulgur Wheat, cooked	1/2 cup	91	29	0.32	8%
Salmon	3 oz.	85	26	0.31	7%
Whole Wheat Spaghetti	1/2 cup	70	21	0.30	6%
Parsnips, boiled	1/2 cup	78	23	0.29	6%
Chicken Breast, roasted	3 oz.	85	24	0.29	6%
Ground Beef, pan browned	3 oz.	85	24	0.28	6%
Oatmeal	1/2 cup	117	32	0.27	8%
Broccoli, boiled	1/2 cup	78	16	0.21	4%
Pasta Sauce	1/2 cup	128	27	0.21	7%
Potatoes, boiled without skin	1 cup	156	31	0.20	8%
Lettuce	2 leaves	34	4	0.12	1%
Milk, 2%	1 cup	244	27	0.11	7%
Apple	1 medium	182	9	0.05	3%
Coffee, from grounds	6 oz.	178	5	0.03	1%

[Source: http://www.ars.usda.gov/, www.nutritiondata.com]

Magnesium supplements can take one to four hours to produce a bowel movement, but if constipation is severe it may take longer or possibly not work at all. It is important to note that a magnesium and constipation can be related by way of taking excess calcium as a supplement. If this is the case, then magnesium is needed to balance the calcium on the digestive tract. For this reason some people, such as menopausal women, might be better to take a calcium supplement that also contains magnesium. Always consult your physician about these types of changes to your diet or supplement regimen.

Adequate Magnesium consumption can come from foods, generally, whole grain food, fruit and vegetable is more than adequate to supply the body's magnesium needs.

- Green vegetables---Leafy types are the highest
- Legumes (All types of beans and Peanuts)
- Fruits and berries in general
- grains
- nuts
- wheat germ
- cornmeal
- Soy products
- honey
- fish
- cabbage
- avocados
- peas
- prunes
- soy milk
- Hard tap water
- dairy products

Types of Magnesium Supplements:

Magnesium is naturally present in some foods, synthetically added to other food products and available as a dietary supplement. Additionally, it's found in some over-the-counter medicines, such as antacids and laxatives. Magnesium supplements are available in a variety of forms. The absorption rate of magnesium supplements differs depending on the kind – usually types that dissolve in liquid are better absorbed in the gut than less soluble forms.

Considering all of the important roles that magnesium plays in the body – and the fact that a magnesium deficiency is one of the leading nutrient deficiencies in adults, with an estimated 80 percent being deficient in this vital mineral – it's a good idea to consider taking magnesium supplements regularly and eating magnesium-rich foods. For many people, a magnesium deficiency causes noticeable negative symptoms – including muscle aches or spasms, poor digestion, anxiety, and trouble sleeping. Yet, magnesium deficiency is often overlooked and rarely tested. Therefore, magnesium may be one of the most underutilized but most necessary supplements. It's believed that magnesium in the form of Mag Phos, citrate, chelate and chloride forms are absorbed well than magnesium supplements in oxide and magnesium sulphate form. Here's a bit about the different types of magnesium supplements that you'll likely come across:

(1) Mag Phos: Mag Phos - 6x is a homeopathic medicine supplement for Magnesium. Mag Phos 6x 4-10 tabs dissolved in hot water before breakfast reduces sugar level fantastically. Mag Phos is especially effective, when taken early morning empty stomach dissolved in hot water. Mag Phos helps body in increasing blood flow and relaxing muscles. Diabetics have low blood flow and body cells unable to absorb insulin. Mag Phos - 6x is doing wonders in control of Diabetes and constipation.

Magnesium Phos -6X is a Cell Salt, and is a wonderful remedy for constipation, muscle spasms, whether affecting back, leg, abdomen or calf muscles. Using Magnesium Phos 6X in the evening for a peaceful night sleep without charley horses relaxes tight back muscles. Supports intestinal health, and is beneficial for abdominal spasms and intestinal problems such as colitis or constipation. Magnesium Phos calms agitated nerves for pain relief of headache, writer's cramp, sciatica, neuralgia. Use before and after dental work to calm tooth pain. Spasmodic is a key symptom and Magnesium Phos calms spasmodic coughs, hiccups and menstrual cramps. Magnesium helps with abdominal pains improved by eating. Magnesium Phos is from magnesium, an important mineral that is involved in over 300 enzyme reactions in the body. Homeopathic Magnesium Phos goes quickly into the system for prompt relief. Studies have shown that most adults are deficient in the mineral magnesium. Refined foods, pollution, non-absorption and insufficient ability of the body to utilize magnesium in the body are some of the causes. It is especially recommended that diabetics, individuals with heart disease and those with high blood pressure have their magnesium levels checked.

Magnesium Phos, especially in low potency 6X, can help your body utilize magnesium in the body and from food and is completely safe (unlike 500 mg supplements that can cause bowel overload with resulting diarrhoea). This is homeopathic potency of minerals used within the cells. Cell Salts can improve the body's ability to absorb Magnesium. If lacking in Magnesium Phos, nerves are on edge with the inability to relax emotionally (showing as anxiety, nervous disorders, depression) and physically (showing as muscle problems, fibromyalgia-worse with even a light touch, nerve sensitivity-even the skin may feel overly sensitive).

Deficiency symptoms include stress, pain, anxiety, depression, muscle spasms, migraine headaches, PMS headaches, agitation, irritability, constipation, fatigue. Magnesium Phos is found inside the cells of muscles, nerves, bones, the brain and spine. Deficiency affects muscle fibres and nerve endings. Magnesium is one of the trios including Potassium and Calcium involved in muscle function. Magnesium deficiency has been linked with CFS (Chronic Fatigue Syndrome). Consider Magnesium Phos when there has been nerve injury or damage. Speed injury recovery with Magnesium Phos. Magnesium Phos is indicated when nerve pain is shooting, darting, or spasmodic. Couple this with magnesium's presence in the brain and you'll see Magnesium Phos importance in neuralgias and headaches. Magnesium Phos is the Cell Salt to use for nerve pain. Magnesium Phos is indicated for migraines, fatigue, hearing disorders, neuralgia, panic attacks.

This works successfully with other therapies and absorbs instantly, great for people with digestion difficulties. People using the Cell Salts and remedies feel 90% better. This is helpful in Abdominal problem, such as, intestinal problems, calms spasmodic abdominal cramping, useful for colic with much gas and belching, without relief, helpful for menstrual cramps that are relieved by onset of flow, shooting, darting pains and useful for leg cramps and writer's cramp This is useful for irritable bowel syndrome, intestinal symptoms, anxiety, PMS headaches. Magnesium Phos is also known under the following names, spellings and abbreviations: Magnesia Phosphorus, Magnesia Phosphorica, Magnesia Phos, Magnesium Phosphate, Magnesium Phosphorus, Mag Phos, Mg Ph. Magnesium Phos is one of the 12 Homeopathic Cell Salts also termed Tissue Salts or Biochemic Salts.

This is a biochemical Cell Salts, instant melt tablets. Cell Salts means minerals for cell health. Biochemistry developed by Dr. Schussler is use of minerals in homeopathic potency. Cell Salts are used successfully because minerals are the foundational nutrition for the body's enzyme activities and energy cycles and Cell Salts are instantly bio available. Mag Phos - 6x is Magnesium and Phosphates. Magnesium ions are good in manipulating important biological polyphosphate compounds like ATP, DNA, and RNA. Innumerable enzymes thus require magnesium ions to function. The lack of functioning, ill functioning, malfunctioning of the subtle airs, liquids, and subatomic particles are fundamental to all morbid conditions. If they are from the RNA and DNA or genetically mutated, they do convert to chronic ailments like Diabetes, heart ailments, constipation and syndromes of various kinds, and various levels of developmental problems like autism, spastic children and the like. In homeopathy the ionisation through dilution and potencies, do act at much more subtle energy levels.

When we talk about cramps we are talking about muscles, we are talking about water, and hydration or dehydration; we are talking about solubility of Magnesium in water and therefore its capacity to attract water into the intercellular space averting a situation of cramps from dehydration. Magnesium Phosphate has a wider role to play. Magnesium phosphate is found in the brain, spinal cord, heart, liver, lungs, spleen, pancreas, kidneys, intestines, thyroid gland, as well as the nerve and muscle cells. That itself shows that Mag Phos is capable of correcting the problems and ailments and morbid conditions in those areas. That includes the pancreases, and therefore some cases of diabetic would respond to the therapy of Magnesium phosphate in a large way.

The fundamental symptom of Mag Phos in homeopathy is pain and that too drawing pain or radiating pain or neuralgia. Meaning mostly the nerve is involved and pain is of course caused by the blockage of subtle air. Thyroid, spleen or pancreases damages or imbalances all other glands, when it is imbalanced or damaged. Inversely, when there is a genetic mutation as visible in the absence of Mag phos in the DNA and RNA which are major regions of its function, it should be understood that those defects would blossom into unbalancing or damaging the whole endocrine system. And the same Mag phos which is cause would become the cure when used in ionised subatomic particles as we do in homeopathic potency or the succession method in homeopathy.

(2) Magnesium Chelate: Magnesium Chelate is highly absorbable by the body and the kind found in foods naturally. This type is bound to multiple amino acids (proteins) and used to restore magnesium levels.

(3) Magnesium Citrate: This is Magnesium combined with citric acid. This may have a laxative effect in some cases when taken in high doses, but is otherwise safe to use for improving digestion and preventing constipation.

(4) Magnesium Chloride Oil: Magnesium Chloride Oil is an oil form of magnesium that can be applied to skin. It's also given to people who have digestive disorders that prevent normal absorption of magnesium from their food. Athletes sometimes use magnesium oil to increase energy and endurance, to dull muscle pain, and to heal wounds or skin irritation.

(5) Magnesium Glycinate: Magnesium Glycinate is highly absorbable; this is recommended for anyone with a known magnesium deficiency and less likely to cause laxative effects than some other magnesium supplements.

(6) Magnesium Threonate: Magnesium Threonate has a high level of absorbability since it can penetrate the mitochondrial membrane. This type is not as readily available, but as more research is conducted, it may become more widely used.

These are the current RDAs for magnesium depending on your age and gender according to the NIH:

Infants–6 months: 30 mg

7–12 months: 75 mg

1–3 years: 80 mg

4–8 years: 130 mg

9–13 years: 240 mg

14–18 years: 410 mg for men; 360 mg for women

19–30 years: 400 mg for men; 310 mg for women

Adults 31 years and older: 420 mg for men; 320 mg for women

Pregnant women: 350-360 mg

Women who are breastfeeding: 310-320 mg

Magnesium is connected to other nutrients within the body, including calcium, vitamin K and vitamin D. Experts believe that one of the reasons magnesium supplements are so beneficial is because they help counterbalance high levels of calcium that can accumulate in the body when people take calcium supplements regularly. Similarly, taking vitamin D in high levels, or being deficient in vitamin K2, can lower magnesium stores in the body and contribute to a deficiency.

This is why it's important to be careful when using any supplement, including magnesium supplements. Consuming any supplement in doses that are too high can create an imbalance in other nutrients and toxicity. Hence, I usually recommend getting magnesium or other nutrients from food sources, as foods naturally contain other important balancing nutrients. In the case of deficiency, a person may need to take a supplement for a certain period of time. However, if possible, try to use food-based supplements in these cases, or be aware of how nutrients, such as calcium and magnesium work together.

Health Benefits of Magnesium:

Magnesium has many benefits throughout all the body's critical functions. From nerves to cells to muscles, magnesium is hard at work regulating and promoting proper function.

1. Increase Energy: Magnesium is used to create "energy" in your body by activating adenosine tri-phosphate, also known as ATP. This means that without enough magnesium, you don't have the energy you need and can suffer from fatigue more easily. Inadequate magnesium intake also means you tire more quickly and need a higher level of oxygen during exercise. One study conducted by the ARS Community Nutrition Research Group found that when magnesium-deficient women exercised, they needed more oxygen to complete low-level activities and had a higher heart rate compared to when their magnesium levels were higher.

2. Calms Nerves & Anxiety: Magnesium is vital for GABA function, an inhibitory neurotransmitter that produces "happy hormones" like serotonin. Certain hormones regulated by magnesium are crucial for calming the brain and promoting relaxation, which is one reason why a magnesium deficiency can lead to sleeplessness or insomnia.

3. Treats Insomnia & Helps You Fall Asleep: Magnesium supplements can help quiet a racing mind and make it easier to get a good night's sleep. Our circadian rhythms shift, especially as we age, because of our decreased nutrient consumption and a lower nutrient absorption, which puts many of us at risk for insomnia. Example: When 46 patients were either given magnesium supplements or a placebo over an eight-week period, the group taking magnesium supplements experienced a significant increase in sleep time, an easier time falling asleep, higher concentrations of melatonin (the hormone responsible for inducing sleepiness) and lower levels of cortical which are associated with stress.

4. Helps with Digestion by Relieving Constipation: Magnesium helps to relax muscles within the digestive tract, including the intestinal wall, which controls your ability to go to the bathroom. Because magnesium helps neutralize stomach acid and moves stool through the intestines, taking magnesium supplements is a natural way to help you poop. When researchers from the National Institute of Health and Nutrition in Tokyo studied the effects of magnesium in the diet of 3,800 women, low magnesium intake was associated with significant increases in the prevalence of constipation. Another study found that when elderly patients experiencing constipation took magnesium supplements, they were more efficient at reducing constipation than

the use of bulk-laxatives. Keep in mind, however, that if you experience a laxative effect when taking magnesium supplements, you may be taking too high of a dose. Taking the proper dose of magnesium should help you go to the bathroom easily on a normal schedule, but shouldn't cause discomfort or diarrhoea.

5. Relieves Muscle Aches and Spasms: Magnesium has an important role in neuromuscular signals and muscle contractions. When you don't acquire enough magnesium, your muscles can actually go into spasms. Magnesium helps muscles to relax and contract, and also enables you to move around. Additionally, magnesium balances calcium within the body, which is important because overly high doses of calcium, usually from supplements, can cause problems associated with muscle control – including controlling the heart. While calcium is often taken in high quantities, magnesium supplements usually are not taken by most adults. This can result in the potential for intense muscle pains, cramps, contractions and weakness.

6. Regulates Levels of Calcium, Potassium and Sodium: Together with other electrolytes, magnesium regulates diverse biochemical reactions in the body. Magnesium plays a role in the active transport of calcium and potassium ions across cell membranes. This makes magnesium vital to nerve impulse conductions, muscle contractions and normal heart rhythms. Magnesium, working with calcium, also contributes to the structural development of bone and is required for the synthesis of DNA, RNA and the antioxidant glutathione.

7. Support proper blood pressure levels Heart: Magnesium is very important for heart health. The highest amount of magnesium within the whole body is in the heart, specifically within the heart's left ventricle. Magnesium works with calcium to support proper blood pressure levels and prevent hypertension. Without a proper balance of magnesium to other minerals like calcium, a heart attack can even occur due to severe muscle spasms.

8. Prevents Migraine Headaches: Because magnesium is involved in neurotransmitter function and blood circulation, it can help control migraine headache pain by releasing pain-reducing hormones and reducing vasoconstriction, or constriction of the blood vessels that raises blood pressure. Several studies show that when sufferers of migraines supplement with magnesium, their symptoms improve.

9. Prevent Osteoporosis: Magnesium is needed for proper bone formation and influences the activities of osteoblasts and osteoclasts that build healthy bone density.

Magnesium also plays a role in balancing blood concentrations of vitamin D, which is a major regulator of bone homeostasis. A higher

magnesium intake correlates with increased bone mineral density in both men and women according to several studies. Research also shows that women can help prevent or reverse osteoporosis by increasing their magnesium consumption and preventing magnesium deficiency.

2.3.4   Missing Lifestyle:

In addition to dietary considerations, lifestyle may play a significant role in constipation, especially in stubborn cases of chronic irregularity. Lack of exercise not only causes weight gain and other health problems, it can also affect digestion. "Sedentary lifestyle is the thing that I would worry most about," as being inactive can cause constipation. The best thing you can do to move your bowels is wake up, eat a real meal, and do some low-level activity.   Maintain life style to prevent constipation.

Lack of physical activity (Exercise):

No physical inactivity may cause Constipation. Pregnancy (About 1 in 5 pregnant women will become constipated). It is due to the hormonal changes of pregnancy that slow down the gut movements. In later pregnancy, it can simply be due to the baby taking up a lot of room in the tummy and the bowels being pushed to one side. Problems with the nerves and muscles in the digestive system may cause Constipation. Regular exercise is one of the best ways to get your bowels moving. Walking and other rhythmic exercise massages the intestinal tract and stimulates peristalsis. Regular exercise also helps alleviate the stress that can contribute to constipation. The National Institutes of Health, NIH, says that exercising regularly helps keep your digestion system, including your intestines, healthy and active. The NIH recommends getting about 20 to 30 minutes of exercise every day to help prevent constipation. Stress is also a risk factor for constipation, so try activities like yoga or tai chi that combine exercise and stress reduction. If your bowel habits are sluggish and you suffer constipation, maybe some exercise can help speed things up. According to experts, exercise does more than tone your heart and other muscles. Exercise is essential for regular bowel movements. In fact, one of the key risk factors for constipation is inactivity. Exercise helps constipation by decreasing the time it takes food to move through the large intestine, thus limiting the amount of water absorbed from the stool into the body. Hard, dry stools are harder to pass. In addition, aerobic exercise accelerates your breathing and heart rate. This helps to stimulate the natural contraction of intestinal muscles.

Intestinal muscles that contract efficiently help move stools out quickly.

Best Time to Exercise: Morning is the best time for exercise when your stomach is empty or two hour after a big meal before engaging in any rigorous physical activity. After eating, blood flow increases to the stomach and intestines to help the body digest the food. However, if you exercise right after eating, the blood flows toward the heart and muscles instead. Since the strength of the gut's muscle contractions directly relate to the quantity of blood flowing in the area, less blood in the GI tract means weaker intestinal contractions, fewer digestive enzymes, and the food waste moving sluggishly through the intestine. One of the best choices of exercise for constipation relief is a brisk 10- to 20-minute walk. Make walking a habit by taking a stroll after dinner and before bedtime. This can lead to bloating, excess gas, and constipation. So after a big meal, give your body a chance to digest it before you start on that nature hike. The Best Exercises for Constipation is simply getting up and moving in ground. A regular walking regimen, even 10 to 15 minutes several times a day, can help the body and digestive system function optimally. If you are already fit, you might opt for aerobic exercise: running, jogging, swimming, or swing dancing. All these exercises can help keep the digestive tract healthy. Stretching may also help alleviate constipation, as might certain yoga positions. The slowing down of you bowel movements causes your intestines to swell up having an adverse effect on your health. The result is your stomach sticking out leaving only bloated feelings behind as you worry about how you are going to deal with the problem. This bulge in your stomach is different than the fat you shed while dieting. However, that doesn't mean you can exercise and eat healthy to make it go away. In fact, there are ways you can send constipation away fast and easy with very little effort.

People who need to go on a diet and people who are often constipated are in the same boat. One reason why many people suffer from constipation is that they lack exercise. When your stomach muscles are weak your body can't send food through your bowels as swiftly, or not at all, hence the symptoms of constipation. The first step to fixing constipation is exercise. For pregnant women not able to push their bodies as much as they used to, and people lacking exercise because of sitting at the desk all day are said to be develop constipation easier than most. Exercises and healthy foods that can help rid constipation from your body.

In order to treat constipation by exercising, you need to train the muscles around your stomach, i.e. your abs that work to make your intestines function better, producing smoother bowel movements. Although strength training would work the same way; but we all know how hard that would be.

Lack of Yoga and Pranayama:

Constipation is most common digestive problems which is a by product of modern dietary habits and sedentary lifestyle. When the waste matter stays for more time in the colon, toxins and fluids are absorbed in the colon and the faecal matter becomes hard. In this condition, bowel movement is irregular, painful or bowels are not emptied completely when it moves. When we sleep our body keeps working to eliminate waste products from our body. Early dinner coupled with stress free sleep of 7 to 8 hours will help our body in proper elimination of these waste products.

Most of the persons suffering from constipation have mild symptoms which are not attributed to any digestive system abnormality or systemic disease. Simple constipation can get cured by healthy eating, taking proper sleep and yoga. Yoga practice can provide an effective remedy for constipation. Yoga will be more effective if it is supplemented with healthy eating and lifestyle changes. You can also start yoga for constipation in addition to other methods of treatment you are following. The benefit of yoga is you get the cure naturally and gradually you can get rid of any medication or laxatives.

If walking doesn't appeal to you, try yoga. Yoga masters believe that certain yoga positions and breathing exercises aid digestion and strengthen stomach muscles, thus helping to relieve constipation.

Pranayama for Constipation: Yoga breathing exercises help stimulates bowel action. If you suffer from high blood pressure do not attempt Bhastrika and Kapalabhati Pranayama. Agnisaar Pranayama (Abdominal Lifts) is an excellent exercise for getting relief from chronic constipation and indigestion. It also strengthens flabby abdominal muscles. Effective Pranayama for constipation cure are Alom Vilom, Agnisaar, Bhastrika and Kapalabhati.

Asanas Pranayama: It must be remembered that effect of a given asana is not limited to treating a particular disease. Therefore choose a yoga sequence of asanas which you are comfortable and can practice regularly. The Yoga for constipation poses listed here exercises the abdominal organs and restores their normal function. The muscles of large intestine also become stronger and help in easy waste elimination. Simple Poses for Constipation Cure include: Surya

Namaskara (Sun Salutation Pose), Tada Asana, Trikonasana, Pawanamuktasana, Bhujangasana (Cobra Pose), Shalabhasana (Locust Pose), Dhanurasana (Bow Pose), Yoga Mudra, Paschimottansana (Head to Knee Pose), and Vajrasana (Diamond Pose)

Bandha for Pranayama: For constipation relief, Uddiyana Bandha and Mulabandha, done early in the morning are most effective.

Natural Tips/ Remedies for Constipation: If you are doing yoga for constipation, diet control and lifestyle change are a must which will add up to the benefits of yoga for curing constipation. You can benefit by using some or all of the tips/ natural remedies listed below:

Immediately after waking up early in the morning, drink two/ three glasses of water at room temperature. Another better option is to drink fresh lime juice prepared with Luke warm water and by adding one teaspoon of honey. Walk around for 10-15 minutes at a leisurely pace to stimulate bowel action.

If above method does not help, still try to establish a daily routine for bowel movements. Sit on the toilet for 10 minutes at the same time. This may take some time say a month to produce results.

Drink an adequate amount of water each day (six to eight glasses).

Regular physical exercise is also important for maintaining proper bowel movements. Regular yoga practice is the best exercise to avoid constipation.

The diet taken during constipation must be easily digestible so that it does not overload the digestive system. Take light meals including fresh foods, vegetables, sprouts and salads. These will provide natural source of daily requirement of fibre. Psyllium seed husk and wheat bran are good source of natural fibre.

Eat two to three hours before going to sleep, so that the food is digested before you sleep.

Drinking a glass of warm milk before going to bed helps in easy evacuation in the morning. In case of severe constipation, mix two teaspoons of castor oil in the milk.

You should eat food in a relaxed manner. Digestive process depends on how we eat food. If food is eaten in hurry or in a state of stress, anger or fear, it produces a toxic effect in the body and promotes indigestion. Also, chew your food properly and slowly.

A common Ayurvedic medicine for constipation is Triphala Churn. It is a powder made by grinding three kinds of herbs. A teaspoon of this powder taken with warm water or milk at the time going to bed is beneficial. Do only the followings:

- Try to avoid laxatives.

- Sleeping hours should be regulated and efforts should be made to have a sound sleep.
- A warm-water or mineral oil enema can relieve constipation.
- Do not delay going to the toilet when you sense natural urge for defecation, this can result in constipation.
- Foods for Constipation Cure
- Yoga for constipation will be more effective if you can eat a simple diet.
- Eat unrefined food such as whole grain cereals bran, honey and lentils.
- Green leafy vegetables (spinach, French beans, tomatoes, lettuce, onion, cabbage, cauliflower, celery, turnip, pumpkin, peas, beetroot, carrots)
- Fresh fruits (apples, pears, grapes, papayas, mangoes, grapefruit, gooseberries, guava and oranges)
- Milk products (butter, ghee and cream)
- Dry fruits (figs, raisins, apricots, dates)
- An exclusive fruit diet for 7 days would be the best bet for treatment. After the fruit diet, have a balanced diet consisting mostly of raw foods, fresh fruits and whole grain cereals.
- Preferred food for Constipation: To avoid constipation, I will like to get most of my nutrition from fruits, salads and vegetables. Some of these are Apple, Cucumber, Grapes, Lemon, tomatoes, Guava, Papaya and green leafy vegetables.
- Avoid These Foods
- Avoid starch consumption, spices, fats, excessive salt, white flour, rice, bread, pulses, cakes, pastries, biscuits, cheese, and white sugar.
- Thereafter, start yoga for constipation in consultation with a yoga expert. Reduce constipation symptoms by yoga poses

2.3.5 Imbalance of Solar Plexus (Mani Chakra):

Solar plexus imbalances may cause Constipation. Solar plexus imbalances are a common cause of constipation. Solar plexus is a complex of ganglia and radiating nerves of the system at the pit of the stomach. The Solar plexus is also known as "Nabhi Chakra or Mani Chakra" because of its radiating nerve fibres and is a complex network of nerves (a Nerve plexus) located in the abdomen, near the abdominal aorta. It is behind the stomach. Solar plexus is a nerve plexus in the abdomen that is situated behind the stomach and in front of the aorta and contains several ganglia distributing nerve fibres to the viscera or the pit of the stomach and is the controlling centre for all the organs below the diaphragm. It is where we can have a mental understanding of our emotional self.

The Manipura not only governs the emotional and mental aspect of your psyche but also your psychic experiences. Often a feeling of intuition or "gut feeling" in a certain situation will benefit you greatly if you listen to it. All aspects of the digestive tract, including the assimilation of nutrients are controlled by the 3rd Chakra.

When this Chakra is balanced you will be in complete control over your emotions and thoughts. Your ego mind or small mind will have no unwanted influence over your actions. You will know without a doubt, and accept your place in the Universe, have self-love and, in turn, have a great appreciation for all the people in your life and the uniqueness that they bring to world. When in tune, your Solar-plexus will radiate warmth and joy through-out your entire being, and to others who come into contact with you.

Over-active Solar-plexus Chakra: If your chakra is over-active you may be judgemental or critical – and you will easily find fault in others. You may be demanding and have extreme emotional problems, being very rigid or stubborn (it's either your way or no way). Often anger or aggressiveness results from an over-active chakra. You may always be planning to do things, but never doing, and your work or interests become a priority over things you have to do (a workaholic). You may also be a perfectionist and can't settle on something that is already good enough; it always has to be better.

Under-active Solar-plexus Chakra: If this chakra is under active it can cause severe emotional problems. You may have a lot of doubt and mistrust towards the people in your life, and worry too much about what other people might think about you. You may also run on "auto pilot" avoiding your feelings of depression or anxiety; you may feel afraid or alone when you start to look at what you have been avoiding. You also may feel that you are not good enough and be seeking a constant approval of others, this can lead to a need, or dependency on the people in your life.

Symptoms of a Solar-plexus imbalance:

Poor digestion, weight problems, ulcers, diabetes, hypoglycaemia, hyperglycemias, arthritis, pancreas, liver or kidney problems, anorexia, bulimia, hepatitis, intestinal tumours, colon disease.

Healing the Manipura:

There are many ways one can begin to balance their Chakras. Below you will find several useful methods; including colour, nature and sound therapy.

Affirmation for the Solar-plexus:

I am confident in all that I do. I am successful and release my creative energy into this Reality, effortlessly.

Colour of the Solar-plexus: The Manipura is associated with the colour yellow. Picturing a beautiful yellow sunflower where the chakra is located can have an instant affect. Yellow Candles or surrounding yourself with pictures of yellow things can begin to bring this chakra into balance. You will feel a warm glowing from the Manipura when this begins to happen!

Organs/Glands governed by the Solar-plexus: Large Intestine, Stomach, Digestive System, Adrenal Glands,

2.3.6   Thyroid   or Hypothyroidism:

Underactive thyroid (called hypothyroidism) may cause constipation. Hypothyroidism (underactive thyroid) is a condition in which the thyroid gland doesn't produce enough of certain important hormones may cause Constipation. Women, especially those older than age 60, are more likely to have hypothyroidism. Hypothyroidism upsets the normal balance of chemical reactions in your body. It seldom causes symptoms in the early stages, but over time, untreated hypothyroidism can cause a number of health problems, such as obesity, joint pain, infertility and heart disease. Constipation is also one of the symptoms of hypothyroidism, and thyroid function should be evaluated.

2.3.7   Food allergies:

Food allergies can be at the root of chronic constipation as well; the most common problematic food is pasteurized dairy products, but soy, beef, peas, legumes, beans, tomatoes, oranges, and black tea can also be problematic.

Emotions: Even emotions have been found to play a role in constipation.

2.3.8   Medications:

Some medications (especially strong pain drugs such as narcotics, antidepressants, or iron pills) may cause Constipation. Some medicines can cause constipation as a side-effect, such as, painkillers (particularly those with codeine, such as co-codamol, or

58

very strong painkillers, such as morphine), some antacids, some antidepressants (including amitriptyline) and iron tablets. Many medications have constipation as a side effect. Sedatives that reduce intestinal movement may cause faecal matter to become too large, hard and/or dry to expel.

2.3.9 Structural and functional:

Constipation has a number of structural (mechanical, morphological, anatomical) causes, including: spinal cord lesions, Parkinson's, colon cancer, anal fissures, prostates, and pelvic floor dysfunction may cause Constipation.

2.3.10 Specific diseases:

Specific diseases or medical conditions, such as irritable bowel syndrome, neurological disorders, underactive thyroid gland, some gut disorders and conditions that cause poor mobility, particularly in the elderly, diabetes, and autoimmune diseases such as amyloidosis, celiac disease, lupus, and scleroderma, Hypothyroidism, Having a mental health condition such as depression or an eating disorder may cause Constipation.

Unknown (idiopathic): Some people have a good diet, drink a lot of fluid, do not have a disease or don't take any medication, even though they are constipated and are still become constipated. Their bowels are said to be underactive. This is quite common and is sometimes called functional constipation or primary constipation. Most cases occur in women. This condition tends to start in childhood or in early adulthood and persists throughout life.

Risk factors: Factors that may increase your risk of chronic constipation include:

- Being an older.
- Being a woman.

2.4   Side Effect of Constipation

Indeed, constipation is extremely dangerous for your health and life. Constipation affects your quality of life, causes stress, and diminishes your overall sense of well-being. These things tend to self-perpetuate, and profoundly affect the cardiovascular, endocrine, and immune systems. Closer to the end of one's life, chronic constipation strips the large intestine from its thinning, mucosal membrane, and causes flat lesions and polyps that eventually transform into colon cancer. So, as you can see, the connections are plentiful, and I have just scratched the surface. Indeed, constipation is extremely dangerous for your health and life, and you should do everything possible to reverse it while it is still possible, or, at the very least, to manage its after-effects when it has become irreversible. The reasons are that your colon is designed by nature to hold a few pounds of faeces in transit. When a person gets constipated, the colon may be holding 10, 20 or more lbs. The weight by itself isn't the problem, but the volume is – large, heavy stools enlarge and stretch out the colon, irritate the colon mucosa, harm the anal canal, and may produce toxins related to fermentation and rotting.

The gastrointestinal (GI) tract is part of the digestive system, which processes nutrients (vitamins, minerals, carbohydrates, fats, proteins, and water) in foods that are eaten and helps pass waste material out of the body. The GI tract includes the stomach and intestines (bowels). The stomach is a J-shaped organ in the upper abdomen. Food moves from the throat to the stomach through a hollow, muscular tube called the esophagus. After leaving the stomach, partly-digested food passes into the small intestine and then into the large intestine. The colon (large bowel) is the first part of the large intestine and is about 5 feet long. Together, the rectum and anal canal make up the last part of the large intestine and are 6-8 inches long. The anal canal ends at the anus (the opening of the large intestine to the outside of the body).

Indeed, constipation is extremely dangerous for health and life, and one should do everything possible to reverse it while it is still possible, or, at the very least, or to manage its after-effects when it has become irreversible. Chronic acquired constipation is a complex physiological, psychological, and social disorder specific to people in developed societies. Chronic constipation simply doesn't exist in indigenous societies and does not affect so many individuals so early in life. Chronic constipation as a lifestyle disorder doesn't lend itself to simple solutions along the lines of headache, pain reliever, or heartburn or antacid. If, in fact, any simple or even moderately complex solution existed to prevent and eliminate constipation, one wouldn't be suffering this much. There are two approaches like,

(1) The first one immediate, to alleviate the most unpleasant aspects of constipation near instantly, such as hard stools, pain while moving the bowels, anal bleeding, and further damage and suffering.

(a) To cleanse (flush out) the bowels from hard and stale stools. This step replaces bulking fibre, addictive laxatives, expensive colonics, and, in case of faecal impaction, surgical or manual intervention with a safe, non-addictive, inexpensive, reliable, and beneficial supplement.

(b) To initiate a painless bowel movement when it is no longer achievable naturally because of any rectal nerve damage, peristalsis disorders related to an enlarged colon, medication that suppresses bowel movements, pregnancy, or disability, such as spinal cord trauma, stroke, and others.

(c) To maintain proper morphology of stools for unassisted bowel movements (i.e. proper shape, weight, size, density, and moisture content.);

(d) To manage exceptions that disrupts regular bowel movements and contributes to 'psychological' constipation, such as elevated stress, long-distance travel, night shift work and similar others.

(2) The second strategy is long-term. It is intended to eliminate the underlying causes of chronic constipation and attain natural, unassisted bowel movements without fibre, laxatives, laxogenic food, and even supplements, such as Hydro-C.

This goal is achievable only for individuals who suffer from functional or early stage latent constipation. Once the constipation turns organic, unassisted bowel movements aren't likely to be attainable because of the conditions described in the paragraph (b) above.

The recommendations may be too late to restore the bathroom bliss typical in most people's youth, but, at the very least, following them will stop further damage, pain, suffering, and the pernicious fear of approaching the bathroom!

There are serious side of constipation. As you already know, constipation is the slow movement of faeces (stool or body wastes) through the large intestine resulting in infrequent bowel movements and the passage of dry, hard stools. The longer it takes for the stool to move through the large intestine, the more fluid is absorbed and the drier and harder the stool becomes. As a result, when your body is unable to eliminate waste properly to cleanse your digestive system, then you may potentially experience some of the following side effects of constipation.

Constipation predisposes you to all major colorectal disorders and is really dangerous for health for the following reasons:

- Anal cancer,
- Anal fissures.
- Bowel obstruction.
- Bowel perforation.
- Colon cancer,
- Colorectal cancer
- Colorectal disorder.

- Crohn's disease,
- Diverticulitis,
- Dysbacteriosis
- Faecal impaction.
- Faecal incontinence
- Genitourinary health,
- Haemorrhoids.
- Irritable bowel syndrome (IBS),
- Ischemic colitis,
- Kidney damage and infections.
- Multiple sclerosis.
- proctitis,
- Rectal prolapsed.
- Ulcerative colitis,

2.4.1 Colon cancer and treatment:

The colon is another term for the large intestine; it is the lowest part of the digestive system. Inside the colon, water and salt from solid wastes are extracted before the waste moves through the rectum and exits the body through the anus. Colon cancer, also known as colorectal cancer, is the second-leading cause of cancer deaths in both men and women. According to the Centres for Disease Control (CDC), 51,783 Americans died from colon cancer in 2011 (the most recent year for available data). The disease affects slightly more men than women, and risk increases with age. "Colon cancer is a growth in the colon that usually arises from a polyp. Sometimes the polyps look like stalks of cauliflower, sometimes they're flat".

Colon cancer and rectal cancer often occur together and are called colorectal cancer. Colon cancer is the third most common cause of cancer death. Cancer is a class of diseases characterized by out-of-control cell growth. Colon cancer forms when this uncontrolled cell growth happens in the cells of the large intestine. Most colon cancers originate from small, noncancerous (benign) tumours called adenomatous polyps that form on the inner walls of the large intestine. Some of these polyps may grow into malignant colon cancers over time if they are not removed during colonoscopy - a procedure looking at the inner lining of the intestine.

Colon cancer cells will invade and damage healthy tissue that is near the tumour, causing many complications. After malignant tumours form, the cancerous cells may travel through the blood and lymph systems, spreading to other parts of the body. These cancer cells can grow in several places, invading and destroying other healthy tissues throughout the body. Colon cancer is not necessarily the same as rectal cancer, but they often occur together in what is called colorectal cancer. Rectal cancer originates in the rectum, which is the last several inches of the large intestine, closest to the anus.

Symptoms of Colon cancer:

Cancer symptoms are quite varied and depend on where the cancer is located, where it has spread, and how big the timorous.

It is common for people with colon cancer to experience no symptoms in the earliest stages of the disease. However, when the cancer grows, symptoms include:

Change in your bowel habits, including diarrhoea or constipation or a change in the consistency of your stool that lasts longer than four weeks

Feeling that your bowel doesn't empty completely

Changes in stool consistency

Continual urges to defecate

Diarrhoea or constipation

If the cancer spreads, or metastasizes, additional symptoms can present themselves in the newly affected area. Symptoms of metastasis ultimately depend on the location to which the cancer has spread, and the liver is the most common place of metastasis.

If you notice any symptoms of colon cancer, such as blood in your stool or a persistent change in bowel habits, make an appointment with your doctor.

Iron deficiency (anaemia)

Irritable bowel syndrome (IBS)

Many people with colon cancer experience no symptoms in the early stages of the disease. When symptoms appear, they'll likely vary, depending on the cancer's size and location in your large intestine.

Narrow stools

Pain during bowel movements

Pain, cramps, or gas in the abdomen

Persistent abdominal discomfort, such as cramps, gas or pain

Rectal bleeding or blood in the stool

Talk to your doctor about when you should begin screening for colon cancer. Guidelines generally recommend that colon cancer screenings begin at age 50. Your doctor may recommend more frequent or earlier screening if you have other risk factors, such as a family history of the disease.

Unexplained weight loss

Weakness or fatigue

Causes of Colon cancer:

Normal cells in the body follow an orderly path of growth, division, and death. Cancer is ultimately the result of cells that uncontrollably grow and do not die. Programmed cell death is called apoptosis, and when this process breaks down cancer results. Colon cancer cells do not die in the normal way, but instead, continue to grow and divide. In most cases, it's not clear what causes colon cancer. Doctors know that colon cancer occurs when healthy cells in the colon develop errors in their DNA. Healthy cells grow and divide in an orderly way to keep your body functioning normally. But when a cell's DNA is damaged and becomes cancerous, cells continue to divide — even when new cells aren't needed. As the cells accumulate, they form a tumour. With time, the cancer cells can grow to invade and destroy normal tissue nearby. And cancerous cells can travel to other parts of the body. Although scientists do not know exactly what causes these cells to behave this way, they have identified several potential risk factors, which may increase the risk of colon cancer, which include:

Adenomas: can become cancerous but are usually removed during colonoscopy. Hyperplasic polyps: rarely become colon cancer. Inflammatory polyps: usually occur after inflammation of the colon (colitis) and may become cancerous.

African-American race: African-Americans have a greater risk of colon cancer than do people of other races.

Alcohol: Heavy use of alcohol may increase your risk of colon cancer.

Diabetes: People with diabetes and insulin resistance may have an increased risk of colon cancer.

Family history of colon cancer: You're more likely to develop colon cancer if you have a parent, sibling or child with the disease. If more than one family member has colon cancer or rectal cancer, your risk is even greater.

Genes - the DNA type: Cells can experience uncontrolled growth if there is damage or mutations to DNA, and therefore, damage to the genes involved in cell division. Cancer occurs when a cell's gene mutations make the cell unable to correct DNA damage and unable to commit suicide. Similarly, cancer is a result of mutations that inhibit certain gene functions, leading to uncontrollable cell growth.

Genes - the family type: Cancer can be the result of a genetic predisposition that is inherited from family members. It is possible to be born with certain genetic mutations or a fault in a gene that makes one statistically more likely to develop cancer later in life.

Inflammatory intestinal conditions: Chronic inflammatory diseases of the colon, such as ulcerative colitis and Crohn's disease can increase your risk of colon cancer.

Inherited gene mutations: Inherited gene mutations increase the risk of colon cancer can be passed through families, but these inherited genes are linked to only a small percentage of colon cancers. Inherited gene mutations don't make cancer inevitable, but they can increase an individual's risk of cancer significantly.

Inherited syndromes that increase colon cancer risk: Genetic syndromes passed through generations of your family can increase your risk of colon cancer. These syndromes include familial adenomatous polyposis and hereditary nonpolyposis colorectal cancer, which is also known as Lynch syndrome.

Low-fibre, high-fat diet: Colon cancer and rectal cancer may be associated with a diet low in fibre and high in fat and calories. Research in this area has had mixed results. Some studies have found an increased risk of colon cancer in people who eat diets high in red meat and processed meat.

Medical factors: There are several diseases and conditions that have been associated with an increased risk of colon cancer. Diabetes, acromegaly (a growth hormone disorder), radiation treatment for other cancers, ulcerative colitis, and Crohn's disease all increase the risk of colon cancer.

Obesity: People who are obese have an increased risk of colon cancer and an increased risk of dying of colon cancer when compared with people considered normal weight.

Older age: The great majority of people diagnosed with colon cancer are older than 50. Colon cancer can occur in younger people, but it occurs much less frequently.

Personal history of colorectal cancer or polyps: If you've already had colon cancer or adenomatous polyps, you have a greater risk of colon cancer in the future.

Polyps: Colon cancer usually derives from precancerous polyps that exist in the large intestine. The most common types of polyps are:

Radiation therapy for cancer: Radiation therapy directed at the abdomen to treat previous cancers may increase the risk of colon cancer.

Sedentary lifestyle: If you're inactive, you're more likely to develop colon cancer. Getting regular physical activity may reduce your risk of colon cancer.

Smoking: People who smoke may have an increased risk of colon cancer.

Traits, habits, and diet: Age is an important risk factor for colon cancer; around 90 percent of those diagnosed are over 50. Colon cancers are more likely to occur in people with sedentary lifestyles, obese people, and those who smoke tobacco. Diet is an important factor associated with colon cancer. Diets that are low in fibre and high in fat, calories, and red meat and processed meats increase the risk of developing colon cancer. In fact, Western diets increase the risk of colon cancer compared with diets found in developing countries. Heavy alcohol consumption may also increase the risk of colon cancer. Being overweight and physically inactive are also risk factors for developing colon cancer.

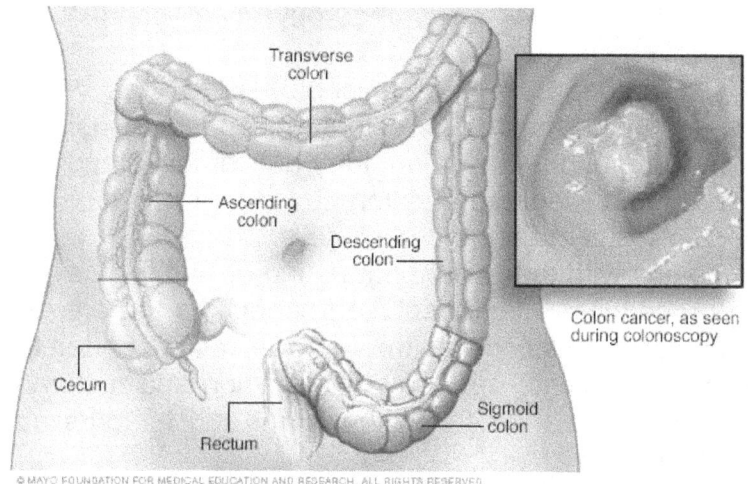

Colon cancer, as seen during colonoscopy

The most common forms of inherited colon cancer syndromes are:
Hereditary non-polyposis colorectal cancer (HNPCC): HNPCC, also called Lynch syndrome, increases the risk of colon cancer and other cancers. People with HNPCC tend to develop colon cancer before age 50.
Familial adenomatous polyposis (FAP): FAP is a rare disorder that causes you to develop thousands of polyps in the lining of your colon and rectum. People with untreated FAP have a greatly increased risk of developing colon cancer before age 40.
FAP, HNPCC and other, rarer inherited colon cancer syndromes can be detected through genetic testing. If you're concerned about your family's history of colon cancer, talk to your doctor about whether your family history suggests you have a risk of these conditions.
Association between diet and increased colon cancer risk: Studies of large groups of people have shown an association between a typical Western diet and an increased risk of colon cancer. A typical Western

diet is high in fat and low in fibre. When people move from areas where the typical diet is low in fat and high in fibre to areas where the typical Western diet is most common, the risk of colon cancer in these people increases significantly. It's not clear why this occurs, but researchers are studying whether a high-fat, low-fibre diet affects the microbes that live in the colon or causes underlying inflammation that may contribute to cancer risk. This is an area of active investigation and research is ongoing.

Diagnosis of colon cancer

In order to diagnose colon cancer, physicians will request a complete physical exam as well as personal and family medical histories. Diagnoses are usually made after the physician conducts a colonoscopy or a barium enema x-ray.

A colonoscopy is a procedure where a long, flexible tube with a camera on one end is inserted into the rectum to inspect the inside of the colon. If polyps are found in the colon, they are removed and sent to a pathologist for biopsy - an examination under a microscope that is used to detect cancerous or precancerous cells.

A barium enema begins with the patient not eating or drinking several hours before the procedure. A liquid solution containing the element barium is then injected into the colon through the rectum. After the barium lines the large intestine, an X-ray of the colon and rectum is taken. The barium will appear white on the X-ray and tumours and polyps will appear as dark outlines.

If a colon cancer diagnosis is made after a biopsy, doctors will often order chest x-rays, ultrasounds, or CT scans of the lungs, liver, and abdomen to see how far the cancer has spread. It is also not uncommon for a doctor to test blood for CEA (carcinoembryonic antigen) - a substance produced by some cancer cells.

Colon cancer prognosis

After a diagnosis is made, doctors determine the stage of the cancer. The stage determines which choices will be available for treatment and informs prognoses.

The standard cancer staging method is called the TNM system:

T - Indicates the size and direct extent of the primary tumour, or degree of invasion into the intestinal wall

N - Indicates the degree to which the cancer has spread to nearby lymph nodes

M - Indicates whether the cancer has metastasized to other organs in the body

A small tumour that has not spread to lymph nodes or distant organs may be staged as (T1, N0, M0), for example.

Colon cancer is also staged from 0 to IV, derived from the TNM classification.

Stage 0 is written as (Tis, N0, M0) where "Tis" stands for carcinoma in situ. This is when the tumour has not grown beyond the inner layer of the colon or rectum and has not invaded deeper tissues nor spread outside of the colon.

Stage IV is written as (Any T, Any N, M1) and describes cancer that has spread to distant sites and other organs throughout the body.

Treatments for colon cancer

Cancer treatment depends on the type of cancer, the stage of the cancer (how much it has spread), age, health status, and additional personal characteristics. There is no single treatment for cancer, but the most common options for colon cancer are surgery, chemotherapy, and radiation therapy. Treatments seek to remove the cancer and/or relieve painful symptoms that the cancer is causing.

Surgery: Surgery to remove part of or the entire colon is called colostomy. During colostomy, a surgeon will remove the part of the colon containing the cancer as well as the marginal area close to the cancer. Also, nearby lymph nodes are also usually removed. Depending on the extent of the colostomy, the healthy portion of the colon will either be reattached to the rectum or attached to an opening in the wall of the abdomen called a stoma. This latter option is called a colostomy, and waste will exit the body through the stoma into a colostomy bag, instead of exiting through the rectum. In addition to invasive surgeries like colostomy, doctors can remove some small, localized cancers using endoscopy.

Laparoscopic surgery (using several small incisions in the abdomen) may also be an option to remove larger polyps.

Palliative surgery might also be employed to relieve symptoms for cancers that are advanced or untreatable. This type of surgery will try to relieve blockage of the colon or to inhibit other conditions to relieve pain, bleeding, and other symptoms.

Chemotherapy

Chemotherapy utilizes chemicals that interfere with the cell division process - damaging proteins or DNA - so that cancer cells will become damaged and die. These treatments target any rapidly dividing cells (not necessarily just cancer cells), but normal cells can usually recover from any chemical-induced damage, while cancer cells cannot.

Chemotherapy is generally used to treat cancer that has spread or metastasized because the medicines travel throughout the entire body. Treatment occurs in cycles so the body has time to heal between doses. However, there are still common side effects such as hair loss, nausea, fatigue, and vomiting. Combination therapies often include multiple types of chemotherapy or chemotherapy combined with other treatment options.

One large-scale study has shown that daily low-dose aspirin improves the survival of patients with certain gastrointestinal cancers, such as colon cancer. While the mechanism is not well understood and aspirin's role in prevention has not been well studied, this information provides another possible adjunctive treatment option.

Radiation

Radiation treatment, also known as radiotherapy, destroys cancer by focusing high-energy rays on the cancer cells. This causes damage to the molecules that make up the cancer cells and leads them to die.

Radiotherapy uses high-energy gamma-rays that are emitted from metals such as radium or high-energy x-rays. Radiotherapy can be used as a standalone treatment to shrink a tumour or destroy cancer cells; it is also used in combination with other cancer treatments.

Radiation treatments are not often used for early stage colon cancers, but may be employed if early stage rectal cancer has penetrated the wall of the rectum or travelled to nearby lymph nodes.

Side effects of radiation therapy may include mild skin changes resembling sunburn or suntan, nausea, vomiting, diarrhoea, and fatigue. Patients also tend to lose their appetites and have trouble maintaining weight, but most side effects subside a few weeks after completing treatment.

Prevention of colon cancer

Colon cancer is the third most common cause of cancer death.

The American Cancer Society suggests screening tests, particularly colonoscopy, for early detection of colon cancer. Colonoscopy is the best method, because it will visualize the entire colon and can remove polyps during the procedure. Other screening tests include faecal occult blood tests (annually), stool DNA testing, flexible sigmoidoscopy (every 5 years), and CT colonography (every 5 years). These frequency recommendations depend, however, on a person's particular risk of colon cancer due to other risk factors.

In general, physicians recommend standard preventive measures such as keeping a healthy weight, exercising, and increasing consumption of fruits, vegetables, and whole grains while decreasing saturated fat and red meat intake. In addition, people are recommended to limit alcohol consumption and quit smoking.

2.4.2   Colon   polyps   and treatment:

A colon polyp is a small clump of cells that forms on the lining of the colon. Most colon polyps are harmless. But over time, some colon polyps can develop into colon cancer, which is often fatal when found in its later stages.

Anyone can develop colon polyps. You're at higher risk if you're 50 or older, are overweight or a smoker, or have a personal or family history of colon polyps or colon cancer.

Colon polyps often don't cause symptoms. It's important to have regular screening tests, such as colonoscopy, because colon polyps found in the early stages can usually be removed safely and completely. The best prevention for colon cancer is regular screening for polyps.

Types of Colon polyps:

There are several types of colon polyps, including:

Adenomatous: About two-thirds of all polyps are adenomatous. Only a small percentage of them actually become cancerous. But nearly all malignant polyps are adenomatous.

Serrated: Depending on their size and location in the colon, serrated polyps may become cancerous. Small serrated polyps in the lower colon, also known as hyperplasic polyps, are rarely malignant. Larger serrated polyps — which are typically flat (sessile), difficult to detect and located in the upper colon — are precancerous.

Inflammatory: These polyps may follow a bout of ulcerative colitis or Crohn's disease of the colon. Although the polyps themselves are not a significant threat, having ulcerative colitis or Crohn's disease of the colon increases your overall risk of colon cancer.

Causes

Healthy cells grow and divide in an orderly way. Mutations in certain genes can cause cells to continue dividing even when new cells aren't needed. In the colon and rectum, this unregulated growth can cause polyps to form.

Polyps can develop anywhere in your large intestine. In general, the larger is a polyp, the greater the likelihood of cancer.

Symptoms

Colon polyps often cause no symptoms. You might not know you have a polyp until your doctor finds it during an examination of your bowel. But some people with colon polyps experience:

Rectal bleeding: This can be a sign of colon polyps or cancer or other conditions, such as haemorrhoids or minor tears in your anus.

Change in stool colour: Blood can show up as red streaks in your stool or make stool appear black. A change in colour may also be caused by foods, medications and supplements.

Change in bowel habits: Constipation or diarrhoea that lasts longer than a week may indicate the presence of a large colon polyp. But a number of other conditions can also cause changes in bowel habits.

Pain, nausea or vomiting: A large colon polyp can partially obstruct your bowel, leading to cramp abdominal pain, nausea and vomiting.

Iron deficiency anaemia: Bleeding from polyps can occur slowly over time, without visible blood in your stool. Chronic bleeding robs your body of the iron needed to produce the substance that allows red blood cells to carry oxygen to your body (haemoglobin). The result is iron deficiency anaemia, which can make you feel tired and short of breath.

Age 50 or older: You have risk factors, such as a family history of colon cancer. Some high-risk individuals should begin regular screening much earlier than age 50.

Colonic polyp's diagnosis

Polyps can be found on a number of tests. These tests may include:

Colonoscopy: During this procedure, a camera attached to a thin, flexible tube is threaded through the anus. This allows your doctor to view the rectum and colon. If a polyp is found, your doctor can remove it immediately or take tissue samples for analysis.

Sigmoidoscopy: This screening method is similar to a colonoscopy, but it can only be used to see the rectum and lower colon. It can't be used to take a biopsy, or a sample of tissue. If your doctor detects a polyp, you'll need to schedule a colonoscopy to have it removed.

Barium enema: For this test, your doctor injects liquid barium into your rectum and then uses a special X-ray to take images of your colon. Barium makes your colon appear white in the pictures. Since polyps are dark, they're easy to identify against the white colour.

CT colonography: This procedure uses a CT scan to construct images of the colon and rectum. After the scan, a computer combines the images of the colon and rectum to produce both 2- and 3-D views of the area. A CT colonography is sometimes called a virtual

colonoscopy. It can show swollen tissues, masses, ulcers, and polyps.

Stool test: Your doctor will give you a test kit and instructions for providing a stool sample. You'll return the sample to your doctor's office for analysis, especially to test for microscopic bleeding. This test will show if you have blood in your stool, which can be a sign of a polyp.

Colonic polyp's treatment

The best way to treat colonic polyps is to remove them. Your doctor will likely remove your polyps during a colonoscopy. The polyps are then examined under the microscope to see what type of polyp it is and if there is any cancer cells present. Doctors can usually get rid of polyps without performing surgery.

However, you may need surgery to remove the polyps if they're large and can't be removed during a colonoscopy. In most cases, this can be done by laparoscopic surgery. This type of surgery is minimally invasive and uses an instrument called a laparoscope. A laparoscope is a long, thin tube with a high-intensity light and a high-resolution camera at the front. The instrument is inserted through an incision in the abdomen. Once your surgeon has a visual of your colon, they'll remove the polyps using a special tool.

Colonic polyps are usually noncancerous and considered harmless. They usually don't cause any symptoms unless they're very large. Removing polyps can reduce or eliminate any related symptoms. It can also help prevent colon cancer from developing in the future.

If you have polyps, you have a higher risk of developing more polyps in the future. Your doctor will recommend repeat screening in three to five years.

Colonic polyp's prevention

Maintaining a healthy diet can help prevent the development of colonic polyps. This includes eating more fruits, vegetables, whole grains, and lean meat. You may also be able to prevent polyps by increasing your intake of vitamin D and calcium. Foods that are rich in vitamin D and calcium include:

- broccoli
- yogurt
- milk
- cheese
- eggs
- liver

- fish

You can further lower your risk for colonic polyps by reducing your intake of high-fat foods, red meat, and processed foods. Quitting smoking and exercising regularly are also important steps to prevent the development of colonic polyps.

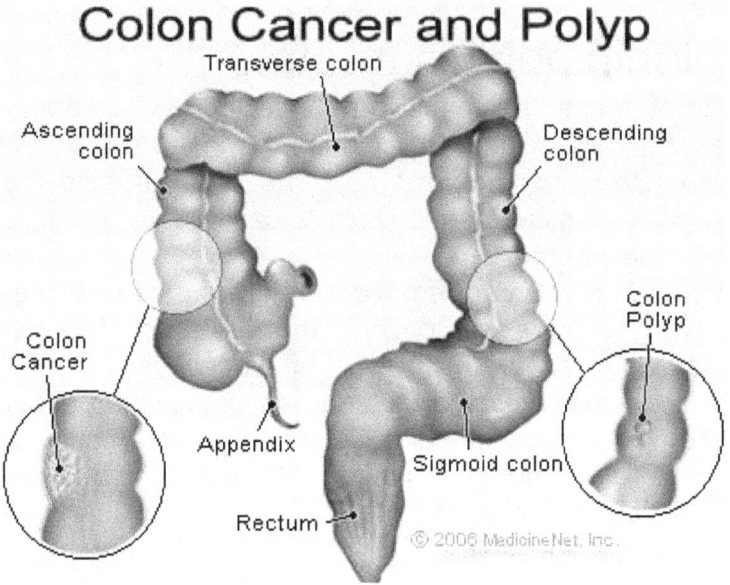

2.4.3   Cholecystitis (gallbladder inflammation) and treatment:

Chronic cholecystitis is a serious condition that is considered a medical emergency. Surgery is often the course of action. A typical bout can last two or three days. Symptoms vary from person to person.

Cholecystitis is the sudden inflammation of your gallbladder. If this condition persists over time, such as for months, with repeated attacks, or if there are recurrent problems with gallbladder function, it's known as chronic cholecystitis.

The gallbladder is a small, pear-shaped organ located on the underside of your liver. It stores bile made by the liver and sends it to the small intestine via the common bile duct (CBD) to aid in the digestion of fats. The CBD connects the liver, the gallbladder, and the pancreas to the small intestine. Gallstones blocking the CBD are the leading cause of cholecystitis. This blockage causes bile to build up in the gallbladder, and that build up causes the gallbladder to become inflamed.

If this happens acutely in the face of chronic inflammation, it is a serious condition. The gallbladder could rupture if it's not treated properly, and this is considered a medical emergency. Treatment usually involves antibiotics, pain medications, and removal of the gallbladder.

Causes of chronic cholecystitis

This condition usually begins with the formation of gallstones in the gallbladder. Gallstones may depend on several factors, including:

* genetic predisposition
* weight
* gallbladder activity
* dietary habits

Gallstones form when substances in the bile form crystal-like particles. They can range from the size of a grain of sand to the size of a golf ball. The presence of gallstones causes pressure, irritation, and may cause infection. The walls of the gallbladder begin to thicken over time. Eventually, the gallbladder starts to shrink. These changes make it harder for the gallbladder to function properly.

In addition to gallstones, cholecystitis can be due to:

* infection of the CBD drainage system
* a CBD blockage
* excess cholesterol in the gallbladder, which can happen during pregnancy or after rapid weight loss
* decreased blood supply to the gallbladder because of diabetes
* tumours in the liver or pancreas
* tumours in the gallbladder, which is rare
* When you experience repeated or prolonged attacks of cholecystitis, it becomes a chronic condition.
* Factors affecting cholecystitis
* A number of factors increase your chances of getting cholecystitis:
* Gallstones are more common in women than in men. This makes women more likely than men to develop cholecystitis.
* The changing of hormones can often cause it. Pregnant women or people on hormone therapy are at greater risk.
* Age: The risk of developing this condition increases after age 40.
* Hispanics and Native Americans have a higher risk of developing gallstones than other people.
* People who are obese are also more likely to get this condition.

- Rapid weight loss or weight gain can bring upon the disorder.
- If you have diabetes, you are at risk of getting cholecystitis.

Symptoms of cholecystitis

Symptoms of cholecystitis can appear suddenly or develop slowly over a period of years. These symptoms appear after a meal that is high in fat. Symptoms include:

- abdominal cramping and bloating
- chills
- fever
- itching
- jaundice, which is when your skin and the whites of your eyes turn yellow
- loose, light-colour stools
- nausea
- Pain that radiates from to your right shoulder or back
- pain that spreads to your back or below your right shoulder blade
- severe abdominal pains that may feel sharp or dull
- Severe pain in your upper right abdomen
- Tenderness over your abdomen when it's touched
- vomiting

A typical attack can last two or three days, but symptoms of cholecystitis vary widely from person to person. The symptoms appear on the right or middle upper part of your stomach. The pain will usually last for 30 minutes. Complications can include:

- pancreatitis, an inflammation of the pancreas
- perforation of the gallbladder as a result of infection
- enlarged gallbladder due to inflammation
- infection may cause the bile to build up
- cancer of the gallbladder (this is a rare, long-term complication)
- death of gallbladder tissue (this can lead to a tear and ultimately a burst of the organ)

The symptoms of cholecystitis can be treated at home with pain medication and rest, if you have been properly diagnosed. It's important that you talk to your doctor first before making the decision to treat at home. You may also take antibiotics and avoid fatty foods.

You should always seek medical attention if you are getting severe pains in your abdomen or if your fever does not break.

Cholecystitis diagnosis

Your doctor will take your medical history and conduct a physical exam. The symptoms of cholecystitis are similar to those of other conditions, so they must rule out those conditions.

There are tests that can help diagnose cholecystitis:

The CT scan uses X-rays to produce very detailed pictures of your abdomen. This is the most sensitive test, and is likely the best bet in locating the problem.

Your doctor may use an abdominal ultrasound to view your gallbladder and liver. This will help them visualize stones and duct obstructions.

Blood tests can identify infections in the bloodstream.

In cholescintigraphy, or a HIDA scan, an injection of a small amount of radioactive material can help identify abnormal contractions or obstructions of your gallbladder and bile ducts. This is also an accurate method of locating the problem. It can take anywhere from an hour to four hours to get your results back.

Endoscopic retrograde cholangio-pancreatography involves using an endoscope (a long, flexible tube inserted down your throat), dye, and an X-ray to thoroughly examine your organs and find defects or problems.

In a percutaneous transhepatic cholangiography, your doctor will insert contrast dye into your liver with a needle. This allows your doctor to see your bile ducts on X-ray.

Treatment options for cholecystitis

The specific cause of your attack will determine the course of treatment. Your doctor will also consider your overall health when choosing your treatment. The options include:

Broad-spectrum antibiotics for fighting infection

Oral dissolution therapy using medications to help dissolve gallstones (this is typically a last resort, reserved for individuals who cannot undergo surgery)

Pain relievers for controlling pain during treatment

Surgery is often the course of action in cases of chronic cholecystitis. Today, gallbladder surgery is generally done laparoscopically. Your surgeon will make small incisions in your abdomen and insert small surgical tools to perform the surgery. In most cases, the surgery is an outpatient procedure, which means a shorter recovery time.

Your healthcare team will advise you about lifestyle and dietary guidelines that can also improve your condition.

Lifestyle and diet changes

Having cholecystitis means you should make important changes to your diet. Upon recovery, eating five to six smaller meals a day is recommended. This allows the bile in your digestive tract to normalize. One big meal can throw off the system and produce a spasm in the gallbladder and bile ducts.

Stick to a low-fat diet with lean proteins, such as poultry or fish. Avoid fatty meats, fried food, and any high-fat foods, including whole milk products.

When treated properly, the long-term outlook is quite good. You don't need a gallbladder to live or to digest food. Without your gallbladder, bile will flow directly from your liver into your small intestine.

Chronic cholecystitis prevention

If you've had one or more bouts of cholecystitis, speak to your doctor to learn about changes you can make to avoid chronic cholecystitis. Ask about dietary guidelines that may include reducing how much fat you eat. Regular exercise is often helpful.

Gallstones are the main cause of cholecystitis. You can lower your risk of developing more gallstones by maintaining a healthy weight. If you need to lose weight, try to do it slowly because rapid weight loss can increase your risk of developing gallstones.

Recovery time

Recovery from gallbladder surgery depends upon the type of surgery you have. Individuals who undergo the laparoscopic procedure will recover faster than those who have traditional surgery, where an abdominal incision is made. Regardless of the type of surgery you have, recovery guidelines can be similar, and expect at least six weeks for full healing. Always follow your surgeon's specific recommendations. Common care instructions include:

• avoid lifting greater than 10 pounds
• eat a low-fat diet with small frequent meals
• expect fatigue, so get plenty of rest
• stay hydrated
• monitor all surgical wounds for redness, drainage, or increased pain

Having gallstones is the main risk factor for developing cholecystitis.

2.4.4 Diverticulitis (a bulging pouch on the wall of the intestine) and treatment:

Diverticulitis is a bulging pouch on the wall of the intestine. Diverticulitis happens when pouches (diverticulitis) form in the wall of the colon. If these pouches get inflamed or infected, it is called diverticulitis. Diverticulitis can be very painful.

Causes of diverticulitis

Doctors aren't sure what causes diverticulitis in the colon (diverticulitis). But they think that a low-fibre diet may play a role. Without fibre to add bulk to the stool, the colon has to work harder than normal to push the stool forward. The pressure from this may cause pouches to form in weak spots along the colon. Doctors aren't sure what causes diverticulitis. Bacteria grow in the pouches, and this can lead to inflammation or infection.

Symptoms of diverticulitis

Symptoms of diverticulitis may last from a few hours to a week or more. Symptoms include:

Belly pain, usually in the lower left side, is sometimes worse when you move. This is the most common symptom.

- Fever and chills.
- Bloating and gas.
- Diarrhoea or constipation.
- Nausea and sometimes vomiting.
- Not feeling like eating.

Treatment of diverticulitis

The treatment you need depends on how bad your symptoms are. You may need to have only liquids at first, and then return to solid food when you start feeling better. Your doctor will give you medicines for pain and antibiotics. Take the antibiotics as directed. Do not stop taking them just because you feel better.

For mild cramps and belly pain: Use a heating pad, set on low, on your belly. Relax. For example, try meditation or slow, deep breathing in a quiet room. Take medicine, such as acetaminophen (Tylenol, for example). Be safe with medicines. Read and follow all instructions on the label. You may need surgery only if diverticulitis doesn't get better with other treatment, or if you have problems such as long-lasting (chronic) pain, a bowel obstruction, a fistula, or a pocket of infection (abscess).

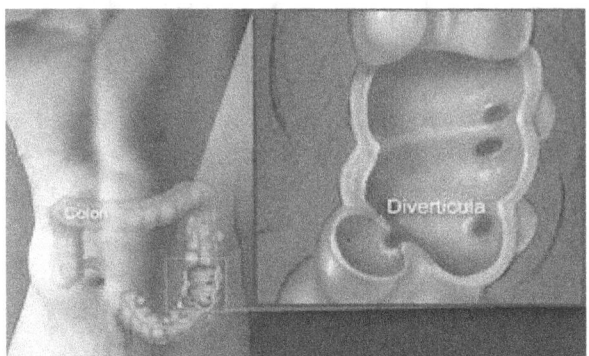

Fig: Diverticulitis

Prevention of diverticulitis

You may be able to prevent diverticulitis if you drink plenty of water, get regular exercise, and eat a high-fibre diet. A high-fibre diet includes whole grains, fresh fruits, and vegetables.

2.4.5 Ischemic colitis (colon inflammation) and treatment:

Ischemic colitis (IC) is an inflammatory condition of the large intestine, or colon that develops when there isn't enough blood flow to the colon. IC can occur at any age, but it's most common among those over the age of 60. A build up of plaque inside the arteries, which is called atherosclerosis, can cause chronic, or long-term, IC. This condition may also go away with mild treatment, such as a short-term liquid diet and antibiotics. Acute, or sudden and short-term, IC is usually caused by a blood clot. Acute IC is a medical emergency and must be treated quickly. The mortality rate is high if gangrene, or death of tissue, occurs in the colon. IC is also known as mesenteric artery ischemia, mesenteric vascular disease, or colonic ischemia.

Causes of Ischemic Colitis

IC occurs when there's a lack of blood flow to your colon. The hardening of one or more of the mesenteric arteries may cause a sudden reduction in blood flow, which is also called an infraction. These are the arteries that supply blood to your intestines. The arteries can harden when there's a build up of fatty deposits called plaque inside your artery walls. This condition is known as atherosclerosis. It's a common cause of IC among people who have a history of coronary artery disease or peripheral vascular disease.

A blood clot can also block the mesenteric arteries and stop or reduce blood flow. Clots are more common in people with an irregular heartbeat, or arrhythmia.

Risk Factors for Ischemic Colitis

- IC most often occurs in people who are over 60 years old. This may be because arteries tend to harden as you get older. As you age, your heart and blood vessels need to work harder to pump and receive blood. This causes your arteries to weaken, making them more prone to plaque build up. You also have a higher risk of developing IC if you:
- have congestive heart failure
- have diabetes
- have low blood pressure
- have a history of surgical procedures to the aorta
- take medications that can cause constipation

Symptoms of Ischemic Colitis

Most people with IC feel mild to moderate abdominal pain. This pain often occurs suddenly and feels like a stomach cramp. Some blood may also be present in the stool, but the bleeding shouldn't be severe. Excessive blood in the stool may be a sign of a different problem, such as Crohn's disease, which is an inflammatory bowel disease, or colon cancer. Other symptoms include:

- pain in your abdomen after eating
- an urgent need to have a bowel movement
- diarrhoea
- vomiting
- tenderness in the abdomen

Ischemic Colitis Diagnosis

IC can be hard to diagnose. It can easily be mistaken for inflammatory bowel disease, a group of diseases that includes Crohn's disease and ulcerative colitis.

Your doctor will ask you about your medical history and order several diagnostic tests. These tests can include the following:

An ultrasound or CT scan can create images of your blood vessels and intestines.

A mesenteric angiogram is an imaging test that uses X-rays to see inside your arteries and determine where the blockage has occurred.

A blood test can be used to check for a white blood cell count. If your white blood cell count is high, it may indicate acute IC.

Ischemic Colitis Treatment

Mild cases of IC are often treated with:

- antibiotics
- a liquid diet
- intravenous (IV) fluids
- pain medication

Acute IC is a medical emergency. It may require:

- thrombolytic, which are medicines that dissolve blot clots
- vasodilators, which are medicines that can widen your mesenteric arteries
- surgery to remove the blockage in your arteries
- People with chronic IC usually only need surgery if other treatments fail.

Potential Complications of Ischemic Colitis

The most dangerous complication of IC is gangrene, or tissue death. When blood flow to your colon is limited, the tissue can wither and die. Surgery may be needed to remove the dead tissue if this occurs.

Other complications associated with IC include:

Perforation, or hole, in your intestine

Peritonitis, which is an inflammation of the tissue lining your abdomen

Sepsis, which is a very serious and widespread bacterial infection

Prevention of Ischemic Colitis

A healthy lifestyle can reduce your risk of developing hardened arteries. The basics of a healthy lifestyle include:

- exercising regularly
- eating a healthy diet
- treating heart conditions that can lead to blood clots, such as an irregular heartbeat
- monitoring your blood cholesterol and blood pressure
- not smoking

Your doctor may also recommend that you stop taking any medication that can cause ischemic colitis. These drugs can include certain antibiotics or heart and migraine medications. Make sure you tell your doctor what medications you're currently taking.

2.4.6 Ganglion cyst (colon inflammation) and treatment:

A ganglion cyst is a tumour or swelling on top of a joint or the covering of a tendon (tissue that connects muscle to bone). It looks like a sac of liquid (cyst). Inside the cyst is a thick, sticky, clear, colourless, jellylike material. Depending on the size, cysts may feel firm or spongy. Ganglion cysts are noncancerous lumps that most commonly develop along the tendons or joints of your wrists or hands. They also may occur in the ankles and feet. Ganglion cysts are typically round or oval and are filled with a jellylike fluid. Small ganglion cysts can be pea-sized, while larger ones can be around an inch (2.5 centimetres) in diameter. Ganglion cysts can be painful if they press on a nearby nerve. Their location can sometimes interfere with joint movement.

If your ganglion cyst is causing you problems, your doctor may suggest trying to drain the cyst with a needle. Removing the cyst surgically also is an option. But if you have no symptoms, no treatment is necessary. In many cases, the cysts go away their own.

One large cyst or many smaller ones may develop. Multiple small cysts can give the appearance of more than one cyst, but a common stalk within the deeper tissue usually connects them. This type of cyst is not harmful and accounts for about half of all soft tissue tumours of the hand. Ganglion cysts, also known as Bible cysts, are more common in women, and 70% occur in people between the ages of 20-40. Rarely, ganglion cysts can occur in children younger than 10 years. Ganglion cysts most commonly occur on the back of the hand at the wrist joint but they can also develop on the palm side of the wrist. When found on the back of the wrist, they become more prominent when the wrist is flexed forward. Other sites, although less common, include these:

The base of the fingers on the palm, where they appear as small pea-sized bumps

The fingertip, just below the cuticle, where they are called mucous cysts

The outside of the knee and ankle

Symptoms of Ganglion cyst

The lumps associated with ganglion cysts can be characterized by:
Location: Ganglion cysts most commonly develop along the tendons or joints of your wrists or hands. The next most common locations are the ankles and feet. These cysts can occur near other joints as well.

Shape and size: Ganglion cysts are round or oval and usually measure less than an inch (2.5 centimetres) in diameter. Some are so small that they can't be felt. The size of a cyst can fluctuate, often getting larger when you use that joint for repetitive motions.

Pain: Ganglion cysts usually are painless. But if a cyst presses on a nerve — even if the cyst is too small to form a noticeable lump — it can cause pain, tingling, numbness or muscle weakness.

When you feel lump or pain in your wrist, hand, ankle or foot you must see a doctor. He or she can make a diagnosis and determine whether you need treatment.

Causes of Ganglion cyst

No one knows exactly what causes a ganglion cyst to develop. It grows out of a joint or the lining of a tendon, looking like a tiny water balloon on a stalk, and seems to occur when the tissue that surrounds a joint or a tendon bulges out of place. Inside the cyst is a thick lubricating fluid similar to that found in joints or around tendons.

Risk factors of Ganglion cyst

Factors that may increase your risk of ganglion cysts include:

Your sex and age: Ganglion cysts can develop in anyone, but they most commonly occur in women between the ages of 20 and 40.

Osteoarthritis: People who have wear-and-tear arthritis in the finger joints closest to their fingernails are at higher risk of developing ganglion cysts near those joints.

Joint or tendon injury: Joints or tendons that have been injured in the past are more likely to develop ganglion cysts.

2.4.7 Rectal Prolapsed and treatment

Rectal prolapsed is the protrusion of either the rectal mucosa or the entire wall of the rectum. Partial prolapsed involves only the mucosa and usually only protrudes by a few centimetres. Complete prolapsed involves all layers of the rectal wall. Prolepses of the rectum occur either with bowel movements or independently. In the elderly, rectal prolapsed initially only occurs with defecation and then retracts spontaneously. More advanced rectal prolepses may occur when standing and so greatly interfere with the patient's quality of life.

- It is most common in the elderly but can occur in all ages, including children. Complete prolapsed in adults is most common in elderly females. In children, rectal prolapsed occurs most often in patients between 1 and 3 years of age. Rectal prolapsed is caused by weakening of the ligaments and muscles that hold the rectum in place. In most people with a prolapsed rectum, the anal sphincter muscle is weak. The exact cause of this weakening is unknown; however, rectal prolapsed is usually associated with the following conditions:

- Advanced age
- Long-term constipation
- Long-term diarrhoea
- Long-term straining during defecation
- Pregnancy and the stresses of childbirth
- Previous surgery
- Cystic fibrosis
- Chronic obstructive pulmonary disease
- Whooping cough
- Multiple sclerosis
- Paralysis (Paraplegia)

Long-term haemorrhoidal disease is frequently associated with mucosal prolapsed that does not progress to complete rectal prolapsed.

Rectal Prolepses Symptoms

The symptoms of a prolapsed rectum are similar to those of haemorrhoids; however, rectal prolapsed originates higher in the body than haemorrhoids do. A person with a prolapsed rectum may feel tissue protruding from the anus and experience the following symptoms:

- Pain during bowel movements
- Mucus or blood discharge from the protruding tissue
- Faecal incontinence (inability to control bowel movements)
- Loss of urge to defecate (mostly with larger prolepses)
- Awareness of something protruding upon wiping
- Early in the development of a prolapsed rectum, the protrusion may occur during bowel movements and retract afterwards. The protrusion may become more frequent and appear when the person sneezes or coughs. Eventually, the protruding rectum may need to be manually replaced or may continually protrude.
- People with internal intussusceptions, in which the rectum is displaced but does not protrude from the body, often experience difficulty with bowel movements and a sense of incomplete bowel movements. Almost all cases of rectal prolapsed require medical care. Occasionally, successful treatment of the underlying cause

of a prolapsed rectum resolves the problem. However, these scenarios usually involve infants or children. In most people, surgery is necessary to treat a prolapsed rectum.

Rectal Prolepses Exams and Tests

To confirm the presence of a prolapsed rectum, the doctor may ask the person to sit on the toilet and strain. If the rectum does not protrude, the doctor may administer a phosphate enema to confirm the diagnosis. The main condition to distinguish rectal prolapsed from is protruding or prolapsed haemorrhoids.

A defecogram (a test that evaluates bowel control) may help distinguish between a mucosal prolapsed and a complete prolapsed.

Self-Care of Rectal Prolepses

For infants and children, reducing the need to strain during bowel movements with stool softeners may correct a prolapsed rectum. A doctor should always be consulted before any attempt to treat this condition at home.

Rectal Prolepses Treatment

Many cases of rectal prolapsed are caused by constipation or straining, but correcting these may not be enough to correct the prolapsed. Most prolapsed rectums worsen without surgery.

Medical treatment is normally used to ease the symptoms of a prolapsed rectum temporarily or to prepare the person for surgery. Bulking agents (such as bran or psyllium), stool softeners, and suppositories or enemas are used for these purposes.

Rectal Prolepses Medications

Stool softeners, such as sodium decussate (Colace) or calcium decussate (Surfak), may be used to reduce pain and straining during bowel movements. Bulk agents, such as psyllium (Metamucil or Fireball) or methylcellulose (Citrucel) may also be used.

Rectal Prolepses Surgery

The goal of all of the surgical techniques used to correct a prolapsed rectum is to attach or secure the rectum to the back side (or posterior) part of the inner pelvis. Surgery is performed through either the abdomen or the perineum. Surgery is done through the abdomen.

- Typically performed in younger or healthier people
- Type of abdominal surgery usually determined by severity of associated constipation

- Associated with higher morbidity rate than perineal approach but lower recurrence rate of prolapsed
- Performed under general anaesthesia
- Usually involves a hospital stay of 3-7 days
- Perinea approach
- Typically performed in elderly people or people in poor health
- Approach for people who cannot tolerate general anaesthesia
- Associated with higher recurrence rate than abdominal approach
- Usually involves a shorter hospital stay
- For people too weak for surgery, a doctor can prevent a prolapsed by inserting a wire or plastic loop to hold the sphincter closed.

Rectal Prolepses Prevention

A high-fibre diet and a daily intake of plenty of fluids can reduce a person's risk of developing constipation. Straining during bowel movements should be avoided. A person with long-term diarrhoea, constipation, or haemorrhoids should seek medical attention to treat these conditions in order to lessen the chance of developing a prolapsed rectum.

Risk factors of Rectal Prolepses

- Increased intra-abdominal pressure - e.g., constipation, diarrhoea, benign prostatic hypertrophy, pregnancy, severe or chronic cough (e.g., chronic obstructive pulmonary disease, cystic fibrosis, whooping cough).
- Previous surgery.
- Pelvic floor dysfunction.
- Parasitic infections - e.g., amoebiasis, schistosomiasis.
- Neurological disease - e.g., previous lower back or pelvic trauma, lumbar disc disease, cauda equine syndrome, spinal tumours, multiple sclerosis.
- Psychiatric disease.

- Presentation of Rectal Prolepses
- Mass protruding through the anus:
- Initially only after a bowel movement and usually retracts when the patient stands up.
- Later the mass protrudes more often, especially with straining and Valsalva manoeuvres such as sneezing or coughing.
- Finally, the rectum prolepses with daily activities such as walking and may progress to continual prolapsed.
- Patients may have to replace it manually.
- Pain, constipation, faecal incontinence, discharge of mucus or rectal bleeding may occur.
- If seen on examination, the protruding mass should show concentric rings of mucosa, which are classic signs of rectal prolapsed.
- Examination may also reveal a rectal ulcer and decreased anal sphincter tone.

Differential diagnosis

Rectal prolapsed must be differentiated from prolapsed of an intussusceptions or a rectal polyp.

Rectal prolapsed can usually be differentiated from a haemorrhoid by the presence of symmetrical circumferential folds occurring with a rectal prolapsed.

Investigations

Barium enema and/or colonoscopy: To evaluate the entire colon prior to surgery for rectal prolapsed to exclude any other colonic lesions.

Other investigations to assess underlying conditions include stool microscopy and cultures for gastrointestinal infection and sweat test for cystic fibrosis.

Anal physiology tests are sometimes used to distinguish between mucosal and full-thickness prolapsed and may be useful in patients about to undergo surgery. They include defecography, anal manometry, and continence tests, electromyography of the anal sphincter and the pelvic floor and nerve stimulation tests.

Rigid proctosigmoidoscopy should be performed to assess the rectum for additional lesions, especially solitary rectal ulcers. These ulcers are present in about 10-25% of patients with either internal or full-thickness prolapsed.

Associated diseases

Affected adult women may also have uterine or bladder prolapsed, or an associated cystocoele.

Management

Rectal prolapsed can usually be reduced with gentle digital pressure. Sedation and local perennial anaesthesia may help the reduction.

Contributing factors should be treated - e.g., constipation or diarrhoea.

Prompt surgical referral is recommended for an irreducible prolapsed and for strangulation or gangrene of the prolapsed tissue.

Partial prolapsed often responds to conservative measures but occasionally requires excision of prolapsed mucosa.

Conservative treatment

Children: gently replace using water-soluble lubricant. Advise parents on the need for a high-fibre diet and inadvisability of straining on stool. A mild laxative may be required. Very occasionally a sub mucosal injection of a sclerosant is also indicated.

Elderly: often well tolerated and concealed with the patient manually reducing the prolapsed. In those unfit for surgery, a subcutaneous circumanal rubber ring may be fitted. However, this often fails either because it is too tight or too loose, resulting in constipation or recurrent prolapsed.

Surgical treatment

Emergency rectosigmoidectomy is required if the prolapsed tissue is incarcerated and non-viable.

Mucosal prolapsed is treated with a haemorrhoidectomy. Stapled haemorrhoidopexy offers an alternative to conventional surgery.

Abdominal procedures:

Abdominal procedures are preferred for all patients fit for abdominal surgery.

Abdominal procedures include anterior resection (not often performed), Marlex rectopexy (Rip stein procedure), suture rectopexy and resection rectopexy (Frykman-Goldberg procedure).

In suture fixation rectopexy and resection rectopexy, the rectum is mobilised and the mesorectum sutured to the sacral promontory and the presacral fascia. In resection rectopexy, a sigmoid colectomy is also performed.

2.4.8 Solitary rectal ulcer syndrome and treatment:

Solitary rectal ulcer syndrome is an uncommon rectal disorder that can present with rectal bleeding, straining during defecation, and a sense of incomplete evacuation. The term solitary rectal ulcer syndrome is a misnomer. Solitary rectal ulcer syndrome is a condition that occurs when one or more open sores (ulcers) develop in the rectum. The rectum is a muscular tube that's connected to the end of your colon. Stool passes through the rectum on its way out of the body.

Solitary rectal ulcer syndrome is a rare and poorly understood disorder that often occurs in people with chronic constipation. Solitary rectal ulcer syndrome can cause rectal bleeding and straining during bowel movements. Despite its name, sometimes more than one rectal ulcer occurs in solitary rectal ulcer syndrome. Treatments for solitary rectal ulcer syndrome range from changing your diet along with fluid intake to surgery.

Symptoms of Solitary rectal ulcer syndrome

Signs and symptoms of solitary rectal ulcer syndrome include:

- Constipation
- Rectal bleeding
- Straining during bowel movements
- Pain or a feeling of fullness in your pelvis
- A feeling of incomplete passing of stool
- Passing mucus from your rectum
- Faecal incontinence
- Rectal pain

However, some people with solitary rectal ulcer syndrome may experience no symptoms. Make an appointment with your doctor if you notice any signs or symptoms that worry you.

Other diseases and conditions may cause signs and symptoms similar to those of solitary rectal ulcer syndrome. At your appointment, your doctor may recommend tests and procedures to rule out other causes of your signs and symptoms.

Causes of Solitary rectal ulcer syndrome

It's not always clear what causes solitary rectal ulcer syndrome. Doctors believe stress or injury to the rectum may cause rectal ulcers to form. Examples of situations that could injure the rectum include:

- Constipation or impacted stool
- Straining during bowel movements
- Rectal prolapsed, which occurs when the rectum protrudes from the anus

- Uncoordinated tightening of the pelvic floor muscles that slows blood flow to the rectum
- Attempts to manually remove impacted stool
- Intussusceptions, which occurs when part of the intestine slides inside another part
- Treatments for solitary rectal ulcer syndrome
- Treatment for solitary rectal ulcer syndrome depends on the severity of your condition. People with mild signs and symptoms may find relief through lifestyle changes, while people with more-severe signs and symptoms may require treatment.
- Lifestyle changes
- Dietary changes, including increasing fibre in your diet

Behaviour therapy is necessary to stop straining during bowel movements. Some people strain during bowel movements out of habit. Behaviour therapy can help you learn to relax your pelvic muscles during bowel movements. In one technique called biofeedback, a specialist teaches you to control certain involuntary body responses, such as tightening of your anus or pelvic floor muscles during defecation. Biofeedback may make you more aware of your straining and help you to control it.

Certain Medications such as topical steroids, sulfasalazine enemas and botulinum toxin (Botox) may help ease your rectal ulcer symptoms.

Rectal prolapsed surgery. If you have a rectal prolapsed that's causing symptoms, your doctor may recommend a rectopexy procedure. Rectopexy secures the rectum in its anatomically correct position.

Surgery to remove the rectum: An operation to remove the rectum may be an option for people with severe signs and symptoms who haven't been helped by other treatments. The surgeon may connect the colon to an opening in the abdomen for waste to leave the body (colostomy). If you have a colostomy, a pouch or bag is then attached to your abdomen to collect waste.

2.4.9 Ulcerative colitis and treatment:

If you or someone you love have recently been diagnosed with ulcerative colitis, it's important to begin learning as much as you can about what ulcerative colitis is. By developing a better understanding of ulcerative colitis, you will be more prepared to manage its symptoms and live a full life.

Ulcerative colitis is a chronic disease of the large intestine, also known as the colon, in which the lining of the colon becomes inflamed and develops tiny open sores, or ulcers, that produce pus and mucous. The combination of inflammation and ulceration can cause abdominal discomfort and frequent emptying of the colon.

Ulcerative colitis is the result of an abnormal response by your body's immune system. Normally, the cells and proteins that make up the immune system protect you from infection. In people with IBD, however, the immune system mistakes food, bacteria, and other materials in the intestine for foreign or invading substances. When this happens, the body sends white blood cells into the lining of the intestines, where they produce chronic inflammation and ulcerations.

It's important to understand the difference between ulcerative colitis and Crohn's disease. Crohn's disease can affect any part of the Gastrointestinal (GI) Tract, but ulcerative colitis affects only the colon. Additionally, while Crohn's disease can affect all layers of the bowel wall, ulcerative colitis only affects the lining of the colon.

While both ulcerative colitis and Crohn's disease are types of Inflammatory Bowel Diseases (IBD), they should not be confused with Irritable Bowel Syndrome (IBS), a disorder that affects the muscle contractions of the colon. IBS is not characterized by intestinal inflammation. Ulcerative colitis occurs when the lining of the large intestine (colon or bowel) and the rectum become inflamed. Ulcerative colitis is an inflammatory bowel disease (IBD). IBD comprises a group of diseases that affect the gastrointestinal tract. Ulcerative colitis occurs when the lining of the large intestine (colon or bowel) and the rectum become inflamed. This inflammation produces tiny sores called ulcers on the lining of the colon. It usually begins in the rectum and spreads upward. It rarely affects the small intestine beyond the lower portion.

The inflammation causes the bowel to move its contents rapidly and empty frequently. As cells on the surface of the lining of the bowel die, ulcers form. The ulcers may cause bleeding and discharge of mucus and pus. This disease affects people of all ages. Symptoms tend to develop when people are between the ages of 15 and 30, or between the ages of 50 and 70. UC is one of two conditions classified as inflammatory bowel disease. The other is Crohn's disease. UC is a long-lasting disease that produces inflammation and bleeding ulcers within the inner lining of your large intestine. It generally begins in your rectum and spreads to the colon. UC is the most commonly diagnosed type of colitis. It occurs when your immune system overreacts to bacteria in your digestive tract, but experts don't know why this happens.

Causes of Ulcerative Colitis:

Causes of colitis include:

- Infection from parasites, viruses, and food poisoning from bacteria. You may also develop the condition if your large intestine has been treated with radiation.
- The genes the person has inherited, the immune system, and something in the environment.
- Foreign substances (antigens) in the environment may be the direct cause of the inflammation, or they may stimulate the body's defences to produce an inflammation that continues without control.

Risk factors of colitis:

You're more at risk for UC if you fall into one of these categories:

You are between the ages of 15 and 30 (most common) or 60 and 80.

You are of Jewish or Caucasian descent.

You have a family member with UC. This type tends to run in families.

Certain abnormal genes are often present in those with UC.

You're more at risk for PC if you:

- are taking long-term antibiotics
- are hospitalized
- are receiving chemotherapy
- are taking immunosuppressant
- are older
- have had PC before
- You're more at risk for IC if:
- you're over age 50
- you have or are at risk for heart disease
- you have heart failure
- you have low blood pressure
- you have had an abdominal operation

Symptoms of Colitis

Depending on your condition, you may experience one or more of the following symptoms:

- Abdominal pain or cramping bloating in the abdomen weight loss diarrhoea blood in your stool urgent need to move your bowels chills and/or fever vomiting
- Bowel movements become looser and more urgent

- Persistent diarrhoea accompanied by abdominal pain and blood in the stool
- Stool is generally bloody
- Cramp abdominal pain
- Loss of appetite: People suffering from ulcerative colitis often experience loss of appetite and may lose weight as a result. A feeling of low energy and fatigue is also common. Among younger children, ulcerative colitis may delay growth and development.
- Colitis Treatment
- The primary goal in treating ulcerative colitis is to help patients regulate their immune system better. While there is no known cure for ulcerative colitis and flare ups may recur, a combination of treatment options can help you stay in control of your disease and lead a full and rewarding life.
- Treatment for ulcerative colitis and other IBD varieties is multifaceted and includes the use of medication, alterations in diet and nutrition, and sometimes surgical procedures to repair or remove affected portions of your GI tract.

Medication

Medication for ulcerative colitis can suppress the inflammation of the colon and allow for tissues to heal. Symptoms including diarrhoea, bleeding, and abdominal pain can also be reduced and controlled with effective medication.

In addition to controlling and suppressing symptoms (inducing remission), medication can also be used to decrease the frequency of symptom flare ups (maintaining remission). With proper treatment over time, periods of remission can be extended and periods of symptom flare ups can be reduced. Several types of medication are being used to treat ulcerative colitis today.

In some circumstances, a health care provider may recommend adding an additional therapy that will work in combination with the initial therapy to increase its effectiveness. For example, combination therapy could include the addition of a biologic to an immunomodulator. As with all therapy, there are risks and benefits of combination therapy. Combining therapies can increase the effectiveness of IBD treatment, but there may also be an increased risk of additional side effects and toxicity. Your health care provider will identify the treatment option that is most effective for your individual health care needs.

Diet & Nutrition: While ulcerative colitis is not caused by the foods you eat, you may find that once you have the disease, particular foods can aggravate the symptoms. It's important to maintain a healthy and soothing diet that helps reduce your symptoms, replace lost nutrients, and promote healing.

For people diagnosed with ulcerative colitis, it is essential to maintain good nutrition because the disease often reduces your appetite while increases your body's energy needs. Additionally, common symptoms like diarrhoea can reduce your body's ability to absorb protein, fat, carbohydrates, as well as water, vitamins, and minerals.

Many people with ulcerative colitis find that soft, bland foods cause less discomfort than spicy or high-fibre foods. While your diet can remain flexible and should include a variety of foods from all food groups, your doctor will likely recommend restricting your intake of dairy foods if you are found to be lactose-intolerant.

Surgery

In one-quarter to one-third of patients with ulcerative colitis, medical therapy is not completely successful or complications arise. Under these circumstances, surgery may be considered. This operation involves the removal of the colon (colectomy).

Depending on a number of factors, including the extent of the disease and the patient's age and overall health, one of two surgical approaches may be recommended. The first involves the removal of the entire colon and rectum, with the creation of an ileostomy or external stoma (an opening on the abdomen through which wastes are emptied into a pouch, which is attached to the skin with adhesive).

Today, many people are able to take advantage of new surgical techniques, which have been developed to offer another option. This procedure also calls for removal of the colon, but it avoids an ileostomy. By creating an internal pouch from the small bowel and attaching it to the anal sphincter muscle, the surgeon can preserve bowel integrity and eliminate the need for the patient to wear an external ostomy appliance.

2.4.10 Anal cancer:
Symptoms of Anal cancer

There are various forms of anal cancer, each defined by the type of tumour that develops. A tumour is an abnormal growth in the body. Tumours can either be benign or malignant. Malignant tumours can and will spread to other parts of the body over time. Anal cancer symptoms are similar to those of haemorrhoids, irritable bowel syndrome, and many gastrointestinal diseases. They include:

Changes in bowel habits
Thin stools
Bleeding from the rectum
Pain, pressure, or the formation of a lump near the anus
Discharge from the anus, or itching

Risk factors for Anal cancer:

Anal cancer often presents with rectal bleeding. People who experience bleeding, itching, or pain in the anus often goes to the doctor before anal cancer progresses past stage one. In other cases, anal cancer is diagnosed during routine exams or procedures. Anal cancer can occur in any person, but some people have a higher risk of developing it than others. Digital rectal exams can detect some cases of anal carcinoma. These are usually part of a prostate exam for men. Manual rectal exams, where the doctor inserts a finger into the anus to feel for lumps or growths, are common in pelvic exams for both genders. Anal Pap smears can also be used to test for anal cancer. This procedure is similar to a traditional Pap smear; a doctor will use a large cotton swab to collect cells from the anal lining. These cells are then studied for abnormalities. A doctor may also biopsy a set of cells or tissues to test for anal cancer if an abnormality is detected. Risk factors include:

Human papilloma virus infection (HPV): HPV is a group of viruses that are sexually transmitted and remain in the body after infection. HPV is present in most cases of anal cancer. It was also the leading cause of cervical cancer before the introduction of routine Pap smears.

Human immunodeficiency virus (HIV): HIV, the precursor to AIDS, puts people at a higher risk of anal cancer, because it compromises your immune system.

Sexual activity: Having multiple sex partners and having receptive anal sex can increase your risk of getting anal cancer. Not wearing barrier protection, like condoms, also increases the risk of anal cancer due to increased risk of contracting HPV.

Smoking: Smokers are more likely to develop cancer of the anus, even if they quit smoking.

Weak immune systems: This can leave your body defenceless against anal cancer and is most common in people with HIV and people who take immunosuppressant or who have had an organ transplant.

Old age: Most cases of anal cancer occur in people over the age of 50.

Causes of Anal cancer:

Anal cancer is caused by the development of abnormal cells in the body. These abnormal cells can grow uncontrollably and accumulate, forming masses known as tutors. Cancer cells can metastasize, or spread to other parts of the body and interfere with normal functions. Anal cancer is thought to be caused in part by the human papillomavirus (HPV), a sexually transmitted disease. It's prevalent in a majority of anal cancer cases.

Anal cancer may also be caused by other cancers in the body spreading to the anal canal. In other words, cancer develops somewhere else in the body first and then metastasizes to the anus.

Treatment of Anal cancer:

Depending on your age and the stage of the cancer, there are several treatment options that doctors may offer you, either by themselves or in combination:

Chemotherapy: Chemotherapy can be used to kill cancer cells and prevent them from growing. It can be injected into the body or taken orally. Pain relievers may also be used intermittently to control symptoms.

Surgery: Local resection surgery is often used to remove a tumour in the anus along with some healthy tissue around it. This procedure is most common with people whose cancer is in the lower part of the anus and has not spread to too many nearby structures. It is best performed in cancers that are early stage and for tumours that are small.

Abdominoperineal (AP) resection: Abdominoperineal (AP) resection is a more invasive surgery. This surgery is reserved for people who have not responded well to other treatments or who are late stage. It involves making an incision in the abdomen to remove the anus, rectum, or parts of the sigmoid colon. Because this surgery removes the entire lower portion of the GI tract, the surgeons create an ostomy, which is a connection from the GI tract to the skin. A patient who receives an ostomy will need to collect their stool in an ostomy bag.

Alternative therapy: Radiation therapies are common for many forms of cancer, including cancer of the anus. X-rays and other radiations are used to kill cancer cells in the body, though they may also kill surrounding healthy tissue. This treatment is non-invasive and is usually combined with other cancer treatments.

Outlook of anal cancer: Many people are able to live long, healthy lives after diagnosis. Early detection is the key to sustained health.

Preventing Anal cancer:

There is no guaranteed way to prevent anal cancer, but there are some ways to reduce your risk of getting it:

Practice safe sex by limiting the number of sex partners you have, using protection during sex, avoiding receptive anal sex, and getting tested regularly for sexually transmitted diseases.

Stop smoking and avoid second hand smoke.

Get vaccinated. A three-dose series HPV vaccination is approved for both females and males between the ages of 9 and 26. This vaccination will protect people from some HPV types that commonly Cause anal cancer: If you have a high risk of anal cancer due to other factors, such as family history or age, make sure to discuss your concerns with your doctor. Anal cancer is an uncommon type of cancer that occurs in the anal canal. The anal canal is a short tube at the end of your rectum through which stool leaves your body. Anal cancer can cause signs and symptoms such as rectal bleeding and anal pain. Most people with anal cancer are treated with a combination of chemotherapy and radiation. Though combining anal cancer treatments increases the chance of a cure, the combined treatments also increase the risk of side effects.

2.4.11   Rectal   bleeding   and treatment

Rectal bleeding is the passage of blood through the anus. Rectal bleeding can refer to any blood that passes from your anus, although rectal bleeding is usually assumed to refer to bleeding from your lower colon or rectum. Your rectum makes up the last few inches of your large intestine.

Rectal bleeding may show up as blood in your stool, on the toilet paper or in the toilet bowl. Blood that results from rectal bleeding can range in colour from bright red to dark maroon to a dark, tarry colour.

The bleeding may result in bright red blood in the stool as well as maroon colour or black stool. The bleeding also may be occulting (not visible with the human eye).

Rectal bleeding also may be seen with bleeding that is coming from higher in the intestinal tract, from the stomach, duodenum, or small intestine.

Rectal bleeding may not be painful; however, other symptoms that may accompany rectal bleeding are diarrhoea, and abdominal cramps due to the blood in the stool.

Rectal bleeding is commonly evaluated and treated by gastroenterologists and colorectal or general surgeons. The origin of rectal bleeding is determined by history and physical examination, anoscopy, flexible sigmoidoscopy, colonoscopy, radionuclide scans, visceral angiograms, flexible endoscopy or capsule endoscopy of the small intestine, and blood tests. Rectal bleeding may occur for many reasons. Common causes of rectal bleeding include:

- Anal fissure (tear in the skin of the anus)
- Chronic constipation
- Hard stools
- Haemorrhoids
- Less common causes of rectal bleeding:
- Anal cancer
- Angiodysplasia (abnormalities in the blood vessels near the intestines)
- Colon cancer
- Colon polyps
- Cholecystitis (gallbladder inflammation)
- Diarrhoea (causing anal irritation)
- Diverticulosis (a bulging pouch that forms on the wall of the intestine)
- Ischemic colitis (colon inflammation caused by reduced blood flow)
- Ganglion cyst (colon inflammation caused by an infection)
- Radiation therapy
- Rectal prolapsed (part of the rectum protrudes through the anus)
- Solitary rectal ulcer syndrome (a sore on the wall of the rectum)
- Ulcerative colitis

2.4.12 Chronic Constipation and treatment

However, the chronic constipation produces, gastric cancer, rectal cancer, and ischemic colitis were not expected. Stool is the end result of digestion, which starts in mouth. Imagine the body as a large reactor, which has a tube running from the top to the bottom of the container.

The inside tube that runs from top to bottom inside the body. This is a description of the digestive system that runs from mouth to anus, and never opens directly to the inside of the body.

In other words, while your digestive system is technically "inside" the body, it contains digestive juices and bacteria. The digestive tract plays a critical role in overall health. Digestion starts in mouth as one chew food and the food mixes with saliva.

Digestion ends in the large intestines, after the body has extracted nutrients and water, leaving only the waste products, which it can't use. The nutrients absorbed contain energy as calories.

The quality and source of foods are important factors in determining the overall health and wellness.

Another factor that impacts the overall health, and the risk of developing constipation, is the amount and type of bacteria living in the gut.

Chronic constipation can last for months or years. It's usually caused by poor diet, by some other disease, or by regularly ignoring the urge to go to the toilet. Low-fibre diets and insufficient water intake are the leading causes of constipation. While most otherwise healthy people will occasionally experience constipation, certain diseases or conditions can also be the cause, such as:

- bowel obstructions, such as a tumour or benign growth
- chronic kidney failure
- hypothyroidism
- irritable bowel syndrome
- neurologic disorders such as Parkinson's disease, multiple sclerosis, or spinal cord injury
- rectal or colon cancer

Acute constipation starts suddenly and lasts for a few days. It can be caused by a blockage, prolonged inactivity, medication, dehydration, or missing a bowel movement. Pregnant women can develop constipation when the womb presses on the intestine. Sometimes, general anaesthesia affects the bowel muscles for a few days after surgery. Lead poisoning and swallowing indigestible objects are other occasional causes. The following medications can slow the passage of faeces through the intestine, provoking acute constipation:

- anticonvulsants used for epilepsy
- antidepressants
- diuretics
- heart medications such as calcium-channel blockers
- iron supplements
- pain medications such as codeine* and morphine
- some cough and cold medications containing dextromethorphan
- some antacids

- Overuse of laxatives eventually makes the bowels less sensitive to the need to eliminate faeces and can cause chronic constipation. The bowels become dependent on laxatives to work, and this can lead to bowel distension and a condition called melanosis coli (dark brown colour inside the bowel).
- People who are bedridden can develop severe acute blockages called faecal impaction. The stools may have to be removed by their doctor.
- Constipation can cause complications. Very large, hard stools can stretch the anus, tearing the skin. These anal fissures can be very painful. Occasionally, a really tough bowel movement causes rectal prolapsed, in which a small section of intestinal lining pokes out of the anus and has to be pushed back in.
- Chronic constipation increases the risk of diverticulitis. This is when small pockets called diverticulitis are formed by the chronic increased pressure inside the bowel wall muscle and eventually get blocked and infected. Haemorrhoids can also be caused by the chronic pushing of constipation.

Making the Diagnosis

These microbes are responsible for the breakdown of food, how the calories or energy are processed, and can increase or decrease the risk of allergies, obesity, and more.

Researchers have also determined that while the gut responds to stress reactions from your brain, the brain also receives signals from the gut that can trigger feelings of sadness.

In other words, the digestive tract or gut is fundamentally related to more than just constipation, diarrhoea, and weight gain or loss. And, because of this interrelationship with the health of the rest of the body, it should not be surprising that the gut health will affect how one looks, feels, and acts.

2.4.13   Diarrhoea (Anal irritation):

Most people think of diarrhoea in terms of stool consistency, how watery it is. This may be the best concept also recognized by clinicians, who additionally define it in terms of stool frequency, consistency, volume or weight. Perhaps the simplest definition of diarrhoea is the passage of loose stools more frequently than is usual for the individual. The path physiology of diarrhoea further defines it.

There are five types of mechanisms by which the condition occurs, and there can be overlap between these in individual cases:

Chronic diarrhoea: Chronic diarrhoea lasts more than 4 weeks.

Osmotic diarrhoea: Osmotic diarrhoea occurs when the small intestine cannot absorb a soluble compound and fluid is drawn into the gut

Secretors diarrhoea: Secretors diarrhoea results from active chloride secretion into the bowel. Water follows the chloride ions, leading to a net loss of fluid due to:

- Inflammation of the intestinal lining
- Motility of the intestines is increased.

Acute diarrhoea: Acute diarrhoea is short-lasting, between several hours and a number of days, and for less than 2 weeks or 14 days. World guidelines further say that acute diarrhoea is the presence of 3 or more abnormally loose or watery stools in the preceding 24 hours. Acute diarrhoea includes cholera. If the acute diarrhoea is bloody, it is called dysentery.

Persistent diarrhoea: Persistent diarrhoea lasts for longer than 2 weeks but less than 4 weeks.

Causes of diarrhoea

Most cases of diarrhoea are the symptom of an infection in the gastrointestinal tract. The microbes causing gastrointestinal infection that leads to diarrhoea include:

- Bacteria
- Viruses
- Parasitic organisms.
- The most commonly identified causes of acute diarrhoea are the bacteria Salmonella, Campylobacter, Shigella and Shiga toxin-producing Escherichia coli.
- There are cases of chronic diarrhoea that are labelled "functional", because they cannot be explained by structural or biochemical abnormalities.
- In the developed world, irritable bowel syndrome (IBS) is the most common cause of functional diarrhoea.
- IBS is a complex of symptoms usually diagnosed by a process of elimination of other possible problems. There is cramping abdominal pain and altered bowel habit, either with diarrhoea or constipation.
- Inflammatory bowel disease (IBD) is another cause of chronic diarrhoea, in which case the diagnosis will be either ulcerative

colitis or Crohn's disease, and there is often blood and pus in the stool in both conditions.

Other major causes of chronic diarrhoea include:

- Microscopic colitis: This is secretory diarrhoea usually affecting older people. There is microscopic inflammation, with changes visible on microscopy of a colon biopsy. The persistent diarrhoea is often during the night.
- Malabsorptive and maldigestive diarrhoea: The first is caused by impaired nutrient absorption, the second by impaired digestive function. Celiac disease is one example.
- Chronic infections: These diarrhoeas are persistent whereas most infectious causes lead to acute diarrhoea. A numerous bacteria and parasites are culprits. These cases are primarily inflammatory, although malabsorption is caused by giardiasis, a parasitic infection
- Drug-induced diarrhoea: The obvious cause is laxatives, but a list of other drugs also leads to diarrhoea - check medications with a pharmacist or doctor
- Endocrine caused Diarrhoea: Chronic secretory diarrhoea can have a range of hormone system causes, including Addison disease, characinoid tumours. Meanwhile, hyperthyroidism can increase gut motility
- Cancer caused Diarrhoea: Neoplastic diarrhoea is associated with a number of gut cancers.

Symptoms and Diagnosis of Diarrhoea

Death may follow severe dehydration if treatment with rehydration therapy is not instituted urgently. Diarrhoea symptom may be accompanied by other symptoms as a result, including the following:

- Frequent and loose or watery stools
- Stomach pain
- Abdominal cramps
- Bloating
- Thirst
- Weight loss
- Fever.

Some symptoms are considered red flags for more serious illness: blood or pus, fever, signs of dehydration, persistent vomiting, chronic diarrhoea or weight loss - learn more about this in the next section covering diagnosis.

Diagnosis of diarrhoea:

Doctors start Diagnosis of diarrhoea by "taking a history", such as, asking questions about the problem, including about medicines received, past medical history and underlying conditions. Also established initially are:

- When the problem started
- Stool frequency, type (for example, watery, mucus-filled, pussy) and volume
- Whether blood is present in the stool
- Whether there has been vomiting.

Doctors will also be concerned about whether there is dehydration, and if so, its severity, the greatest danger to life with diarrhoea is created by dehydration, which has three stages:

- Early dehydration, which shows no signs or symptoms, or possibly light headedness and lassitude (lack of energy)
- Moderate dehydration, signs of this are thirst, restlessness or irritability, dizziness, reduced elasticity of the skin, pinched face, dry tongue and sunken eyes
- Severe dehydration, signs of this are increased severity of the above, and shock, with reduced consciousness, low urine output, cool, moist extremities, a rapid and feeble pulse, low or undetectable blood pressure, and pale skin; a coma can ensue.

Tests for diarrhoea

Because most cases of diarrhoea are self-limiting and resolve themselves, and because the diagnosis can be made clinically, tests are not usually required. But in more severe cases, for example, doctors may order further testing, which include:

- Acute cases, particularly if the patient is very young or old, that may require a stool sample to be tested (with microscopy, culture, faecal leukocyte testing, and, if recent antibiotics, Clostridium difficile testing), which include:
- A bacterial infection may cause white blood cells to appear in the stool, so WBC is tested in a sample. And a culture of the stool can check for pathogenic gastrointestinal bacteria
- Acute cases, particularly if the patient is very young or old, that may require a stool sample to be tested (with microscopy, culture, faecal leukocyte testing, and, if recent antibiotics, Clostridium difficile testing) include:

- Because most cases of diarrhoea are self-limiting and resolve themselves, and because the diagnosis can be made clinically, tests are not usually required. But in more severe cases, for example, doctors may order further testing.6
- Blood tests will also be needed for these patients to measure CBC (complete blood count) and electrolytes, BUN (blood urea nitrogen) and creatinine.
- Celiac disease testing - for antibodies.
- Chronic cases of diarrhoea will be tested according to the suspected underlying cause, and may include these investigations:
- Death may follow severe dehydration if treatment with rehydration therapy is not instituted urgently.
- Diarrhoea persisting for more than one week
- Doctors will also be concerned about whether there is dehydration, and if so, its severity - the greatest danger to life with diarrhoea is created by dehydration, which has three stages:1,4
- Early dehydration, which shows no signs or symptoms, or possibly light headedness and lassitude (lack of energy)
- ESR (erythrocyte sedimentation rate) and CRP (C-reactive protein) - with raised levels possibly pointing to inflammatory bowel disease (IBD)
- Full blood count - for anaemia or a raised platelet count suggesting inflammation
- Having bloody or pussy stools
- Liver function tests, including albumin level
- Low blood pressure
- Microscopy will evaluate the sample for parasites or their eggs.
- Moderate dehydration - signs of this are thirst, restlessness or irritability, dizziness, reduced elasticity of the skin, pinched face, dry tongue and sunken eyes
- Parasites or their eggs can be seen under a microscope.
- Severe dehydration - signs of this are increased severity of the above, and shock, with reduced consciousness, low urine output, cool, moist extremities, a rapid and feeble pulse, low or undetectable blood pressure, and pale skin; a coma can ensue.
- Stool frequency, type (for example, watery, mucus-filled, pussy) and volume
- Tests for malabsorption - calcium, vitamin B12 and red blood cell foliate, iron status (ferrites), thyroid function tests
- The person has recently received antibiotics or been in hospital

- The person is immune compromised
- There has been recent foreign travel to places outside Western Europe, North America, Australia and New Zealand
- There is a rapid test for Clostridium difficile toxin to pick up this bacterial infection, and labs can provide a number of other tests of the stool for numerous pathogens.
- Those showing signs of fever or dehydration
- Whether blood is present in the stool
- Whether there has been vomiting
- Whether there has been severe pain
- Nutrition
- Bananas are high in potassium.
- Sip on clear, still liquids such as fruit juice without added sugar, replacing lost water after each loose stool with at least one cup of liquid
- Do most of the drinking between, not during meals when they may otherwise increase passage of food in the gut
- Use high-potassium foods and liquids - examples include diluted fruit juices, potatoes (without the skin), bananas
- Use high-sodium foods and liquids - broths, soups, sports drinks, salted crackers, and so on.
- Eat foods high in soluble fibre to help thicken the stool - bananas, rice, oatmeal, for example
- Limit certain foods that may make the diarrhoea worse - such as creamy, fried and sugary foods
- Add a probiotic.
- The diet may make diarrhoea worse - avoid caffeine contained in coffee, tea, soft drinks such as cola, and some over-the-counter headache remedies. Other aggravating elements of the diet include:
- Sugar-free gum, mints, sweet cherries, prunes
- Fructose in high amounts, from fruit juices, grapes, honey, dates, nuts, figs, soft drinks and prunes
- Lactose in dairy products
- Magnesium
- Olestra (Olean), a fat substitute.

Roles of Probiotics in Diarrhoea

There is mixed evidence for the role of probiotics for people with diarrhoea, but there is thought to be an effect on the immune system.

In children, there is evidence of benefit in reducing diarrheal illness duration by one day.

Probiotics may have some prophylactic effect against traveller's diarrhoea

Antibiotic-associated diarrhoea may be reduced by the use of probiotics, as may diarrhoea related to Clostridium difficile, although the evidence is mixed. Advice from the doctor is recommended since there are numerous strains, but the most studied for antibiotic-associated diarrhoea are probiotics based on Lactobacillus rhamnosus and Saccharomyces boulardii.

Probiotics to help with Clostridium difficile and antibiotic diarrhoeas were subjected to a randomized, controlled trial published in The Lancet, which found "no evidence" that a multi strain preparation of the bacteria was effective in prevention of these conditions, calling for a better understanding of the development of antibiotic-associated diarrhoea.

Probiotics are available in capsules, tablets, powders and liquids.

Prevention of diarrhoea

In developing countries, prevention of diarrhoea may be more challenging; there may be dirty water and poor sanitation. The following practical measures help to prevent the condition:

- Safe drinking water
- Good sanitation (toilets and sewerage)
- Hand washing with soap after defecation, after cleaning a child who has defecated, after disposing of a child's stool, before preparing food, and before eating
- For mothers with young babies, breastfeeding for the first 6 months of life
- Good hygiene practices, both personal hygiene and in the kitchen
- Education on the spread of infections.
- There is evidence that interventions from public health bodies to simply promote hand washing can cut diarrhoea rates by about a third.
- Vaccine prevention
- Rotavirus vaccination helps to prevent diarrheal disease; in the US it is available for infants under the brand names RotaTeq and Rotarix.
- Giving children the measles immunization can substantially cut rates and severity of diarrheal diseases, and other vaccines have been researched against other infections.

Treatments for diarrhoea

- Antibiotic treatment is reserved for cases of diarrhoea that have been confirmed as caused by a bacterial infection. If the cause is medication, meanwhile, a review will be undertaken and switch to another drug if appropriate.
- Bismuth subsalicylate (for example, Pepto-Bismol) reduces diarrheal stool output in adults and children, and may be a safer alternative to loperamide. This drug can also be used as prophylaxis against traveller's diarrhea.2
- Correcting dehydration is the first priority of treatment.
- Correcting dehydration is the first priority of treatment. Replace lost fluids through measures ranging from drinking more fluids to receiving them intravenously in severe cases. Children and older people are more vulnerable to dehydration
- For all cases of diarrhoea, the first important step in treatment is to rehydrate:
- Loperamide (Imodium, for example) is an antimotility drug that reduces stool passage. Two tablets are taken after the first loose stool, one tablet after each subsequent loose stool.
- Mild cases of acute diarrhoea may be self-limiting and resolve without treatment. For underlying causes, particularly those leading to persistent or chronic diarrhoea, these will be diagnosed and treated in addition to the symptom of diarrhoea.
- Oral rehydration products are available commercially - for example, Oralyte, Rehydralyte.
- Oral rehydration solution/salts (ORS) - water containing salt and glucose absorbed by the small intestine to replace the water and electrolytes lost in the watery faeces. (In developing countries, ORS costs just a few cents, and the World Health Organization says ORS can safely and effectively treat over 90% of cases of non-severe diarrhoea.) The recommended preparation of the solution is 75 mEq/l of sodium and 75 mmol/l of glucose
- Over-the-counter ant diarrheal medicines are available:
- Replace lost fluids through measures ranging from drinking more fluids to receiving them intravenously in severe cases. Children and older people are more vulnerable to dehydration
- There is mixed advice that ant diarrheal medications could prolong bacterial infection by reducing excretion of pathogens via stools.
- Zinc supplementation with a daily dose of 10 to 20 milligrams may reduce the severity and duration of diarrhoea in children. The zinc

supplement is recommended for 10 to 14 days, and it can help to reduce subsequent episodes of diarrhoea in the child for 2 to 3 months.

2.4.14 Other Constipation side effects and treatment

Indeed, constipation is extremely dangerous for health and life, and one should do everything possible to reverse it while it is still possible. Chronic constipation as a lifestyle disorder doesn't lend itself to simple solutions along the lines of headache, pain reliever, or heartburn or antacid. Chronic constipation is a complex physiological, psychological, and social disorder to people in developed societies, specifically with respect to the following miscellaneous side effects of it as below:

"Toxins" Build Up in Bowel: Stool is made up of waste, and is meant to be exiting the body; but the colon is pretty good at containing it, even in cases of constipation, and its presence will cause discomfort and sicken you through the extended presence of "toxins". Their risk of bacterial infection is if waste products manage to get into any wounds in the colon or rectum.

Bad breath: Effects of constipation can create bad breath. Bad breath is also an indicator that we may be constipated. If you suffer from certain bowel disorders, constipation, or a sluggish digestive system, you are a prime candidate for developing bad breath.

Bowel incontinence (the leakage of liquid stools): Bowel incontinence is an inability to control bowel movements, resulting in involuntary soiling. It's also sometimes known as faecal incontinence. Bowel incontinence is a symptom of weakening of the muscle that controls the opening of the anus. Bowel incontinence isn't a normal part of ageing.

Bowel perforation: This is when the hardened faecal matter punctures through the intestinal wall and spills into the abdominal area. This cause's severe infection as waste products of the body comes into direct contact to other organs housed by the abdominal cavity. The severe infection caused by this overflow of faecal matter may even prove fatal when not treated immediately.

Cardiovascular, endocrine, and immune systems get affected: Constipation affects your quality of life, causes stress, and diminishes your overall sense of well-being. These things tend to self-perpetuate, and profoundly affect the cardiovascular, endocrine, and immune systems.

Celiac disease: People with celiac disease cannot tolerate gluten. Gluten is a protein found naturally in wheat, rye, and barley. When gluten is eaten, the immune system reacts by damaging the lining of the small intestine. As a result of this damage, nutrients cannot be absorbed properly. These disorders affect more women than men. They can last for weeks or months, although symptoms can come and go.

Chest Pain: When stomach acid backs up into your esophagus, a condition called acid reflux, you may feel a burning pain in the middle of your chest.

Colon breeding Harmful Bacteria: When your bowel is constipated and clogged with faeces, your colon becomes a breeding ground for harmful bacteria. Unclean bowels will lead to a whole host of problems throughout your body. Some of these problems include gall-bladder problems, varicose veins, arthritis, hernia, heart disorders, appendicitis and, in extreme cases, colon cancer.

Colorectal cancer: Colorectal cancer is cancer of the rectum and colon. Routine screening can help prevent colon cancer. Polyps that are found during routine screening can be removed easily before they become cancerous. Colorectal cancer usually shows no signs in the early stages of the disease. In the more advanced stages, signs and symptoms may include the following: A change in bowel habits; Bleeding from the rectum; and Blood in the stool. Stools is more narrow than usual; Abdominal discomfort (bloating, cramps, or frequent gas pains); A feeling that you need to have a bowel movement (that does not go away after a bowel movement); Loss of appetite; and Weakness and feeling tired. However, having these symptoms does not mean that you have cancer.

Crohn's Disease: Crohn's disease is part of a group of digestive conditions called inflammatory bowel disease (IBD). Crohn's most commonly affects the end of the small intestine called the ileum, but it can affect any part of the digestive tract. This chronic condition is an autoimmune disease, meaning that your immune system mistakenly attacks cells in your own body that it thinks are foreign invaders. The most common Crohn's symptoms are abdominal pain, diarrhoea, rectal bleeding, weight loss, and fever.

Urinary tract infections: The bladder and the colon are close together in the body. Large amounts of stool in the colon can put pressure on the bladder which can cause the bladder to not fill as much as it should, or cause the bladder to contract when the bladder is not supposed to contract. This large amount of stool can also cause the bladder to not empty well. All of these problems can lead to daytime wetting, night-time wetting, urinary tract infections, and in some cases vesicoureteral reflux.

Dehydration and imbalanced electrolytes: Constipation might be tempting to use over-the-counter remedies and laxatives, these remedies are not without risk. When too much is taken, too much water is drawn into the intestines, resulting in dehydration and an abnormal number of electrolytes in your blood. Both dehydration and imbalanced electrolytes can lead to kidney and heart damage.

Digestive disorders: Constipation is a serious health concern. The reality, however, is that if we are not having a minimum of 2 soft, easy to pass bowel movements daily then we are constipated and waste is accumulating in our system. Often times, people accept the condition of constipation because it's long been the way that they function, but constipation can be just the precursor to other more destructive disorders.

Diverticulitis: Long-term constipation has its own special brand of side effects. They aren't particularly nice, either. One is an increased risk of a phenomenon called diverticulitis, where diverticulitis (bulges or "pouches" that tend to form naturally on the lining of the colon as you get older) are formed by the pressure of straining to pass your stool, and may eventually become infected if any nastiest from the trapped stool get caught in them.

Dysbacteriosis: Constipation is one of the symptoms of dysbacteriosis, which is a condition where the normal, intestinal flora is dead and missing. When alive, this flora performs several, important functions. First, it protects the colon itself from any inflammation-causing pathogens. Second, it produces essential B-vitamins and vitamin K, responsible for blood clotting. Third, it governs primary immunity. And fourth, the bacteria form stools keep them soft and moist. When all of these functions are compromised, one cannot enjoy a long and healthy life.

Enlargement of Haemorrhoids: Constipation predisposes to all major colorectal disorders starting with enlarged haemorrhoids and ending up with colorectal cancer. The reasons are that the colon in digestive system is designed by nature to hold a few pounds of faeces in transit. When a person gets constipated, the colon may be holding 5, 10 or more Kgs. This much weight of faeces by itself isn't the problem, but the volume will be very large and the heavy stools enlarge and stretch out the colon, irritate the colon mucosa, harm the anal canal, and may produce toxins related to fermentation and rotting.

Faecal Impaction: Faecal impaction is another side effect of constipation that occurs when the stool becomes extremely impacted in the bowels, to the point that your body is unable to eliminate the collected waste. Symptoms of faecal impaction include abdominal pain (especially after meals), headache, nausea and vomiting just to name a few. Patients with faecal impaction may not have gastrointestinal symptoms. Instead, they may have circulation, heart, or breathing problems. Faecal incontinence includes the inability to hold a bowel movement until reaching a toilet as well as passing stool into one's underwear without being aware of it happening. Stool, also called faeces, is solid waste that is passed as a bowel movement and includes undigested food, bacteria, mucus, and dead cells. Mucus is a clear liquid that coats and protects tissues in the digestive system. Faecal incontinence can be upsetting and embarrassing. Faecal incontinence is slightly more common among women.

Fatal: The excretory system is a collection of organs whose main function is to rid the body of all its waste. These wastes may include solid, liquid or gaseous wastes that when kept inside the body for too long may prove fatal. Liquid wastes or urine is expelled from the body via the kidneys, the bladder and the tubes connected to these 2 organs. The process of eliminating liquid waste is called urination. Gaseous wastes are let out of the body by means of the mouth, nose, and the rectum. The process is called burping, when excess gas is released from the mouth; exhaling for when you let out carbon dioxide which is a by-product of respiration; and farting for release of toxic gases by way of the rectum. Solid and or semi-solid wastes are eliminated from the body through the anus in a process called defecation. Food passes the digestive system where nutrients and other nourishment is absorbed and processed. It then becomes faeces stored in the rectum until time of excretion. Food is pushed along the large intestine towards the rectum by waves of muscle contraction called peristalsis. Faecal matter should be expelled from the body at least on a daily basis to ensure that no waste materials are kept inside the body. However there are circumstances that the body

Flat lesions and polyps: Closer to the end of one's life, chronic constipation strips the large intestine from its thinning, mucosal membrane, and causes flat lesions and polyps that eventually transform into colon cancer.

Gallstones: Gallstones are hard deposits that form in your gallbladder — a small, pear-shaped sack that stores and secretes bile for digestion. Twenty million Americans are affected by gallstones, according to the NIDDK. Gallstones can form when there's too much cholesterol or waste in your bile or if your gallbladder doesn't empty properly. When gallstones block the ducts leading from your gallbladder to your intestines, they can cause sharp pain in your upper-right abdomen. Medications sometimes dissolve gallstones, but if that doesn't work, the next step is surgery to remove the gallbladder.

Genital and urinary: Chronic constipation can also affect the genital and urinary health of women.

Genitourinary health effects: Constipation affects genitourinary health, particularly for women, because the large intestine and the female reproductive organs reside in close proximity. These problems run the gamut from undue pressure on the uterus to rectal prolapsed inside the vagina, from faecal incontinence to miscarriage from straining, and numerous other, equally nasty problems.

Haemorrhoids: Haemorrhoids, also known as piles, are swellings containing enlarged blood vessels found inside or around the bottom (the rectum and anus). Haemorrhoids aren't usually painful, unless their blood supply slows down or is interrupted. The symptoms of haemorrhoids often clear up on their own, or by using simple treatments that can be bought from a pharmacy without a prescription. These are caused by too much strain on the anal sphincter while trying to force bowel movement. When you're constipated, and you find yourself straining to have a bowel movement, it is quite possible you may also be suffering from haemorrhoids and/or anal fissures. The NDDIC estimates that approximately half of the population will have developed haemorrhoids by the time they hit 50. Haemorrhoids are painful and can cause swelling in the rectal area. Haemorrhoids are enlarged veins in the anus or rectum that can rupture and bleed. Aside from constipation, other contributing factors to haemorrhoids include pregnancy, aging, chronic constipation, frequent diarrhoea, and anal intercourse. For instance, chronic pushing and painful stools may predispose you to large haemorrhoids which are irritating and painful. Your colon was designed to hold a few pounds of stool, but when constipated your colon may hold up to 10 pounds of dry, hard faeces.

Irritable bowel syndrome: Irritable bowel syndrome mainly affects women between the ages of 30 years and 50 years. Symptoms of irritable bowel syndrome may include the following: Cramps; Gas; and Bloating.

Itchy bottom, soreness, redness and swelling around your anus:

Kidney damage: This reflux causes permanent kidney damage and increases the risk of kidney infections.

Major colorectal disorders: Constipation predisposes you to all major colorectal disorders starting with enlarged haemorrhoids and ending up with colorectal cancer. The colon is designed by nature to hold a few pounds of faeces in transit. When a person gets constipated, the colon may be holding 10, 20 or more lbs. The weight by itself isn't the problem, but the volume is large, heavy stools enlarge and stretch out the colon, irritate the colon mucosa, harm the anal canal, and may produce toxins related to fermentation and rotting.

Medication can suppress the inflammation, and eliminating foods that cause discomfort may help as well. In severe cases, treatment for ulcerative colitis may involve surgery to remove the colon.

Miscarriage: Constipation affects genitourinary health, particularly for women, because the large intestine and the female reproductive organs reside in close proximity. These problems run the gamut from undue pressure on the uterus to rectal prolapsed inside the vagina, from faecal incontinence to miscarriage from straining, and numerous other, equally nasty problems.

Mucosal membrane thinning: Closer to the end of one's life, chronic constipation strips the large intestine from its thinning, mucosal membrane, and causes flat lesions and polyps that eventually transform into colon cancer.

Obesity: Obesity is a risk factor for multiple digestive problems, including haemorrhoids and diverticulitis.

Other Miscellaneous Side Effects: Obesity, Fatigue, Mood Swings, Sleep Disorders, Rheumatic Fever, Feeling of Lethargy, Lack of confidence, Feeling sluggish, Looking depressed, Bored, Bad health and Unsuccessful on a daily basis.

Pelvic floor muscles: Constipation can also affect your pelvic floor muscles. Pelvic floor muscle strength is important for both bladder and bowel control. These muscles stretch like a trampoline from the pubic bone at the front to the coccyx (tail-bone) at the back. They can be weakened by straining due to constipation, pregnancy and childbirth, or perhaps heavy lifting. Strong pelvic floor muscles are necessary for bladder and bowel control - to be able to 'hold on'.

Physical Health: Although the study presented at the American College of Gastroenterology Annual Meeting found links between chronic constipation and rectal cancer, gastric cancer, diverticulitis, and ischemic colitis, there are also other connections between suffering from constipation and your overall health.

Physiological, psychological, and social disorder: Chronic acquired constipation is a complex physiological, psychological, and social disorder specific to people and domesticated carnivorous pets in developed societies. Chronic constipation simply doesn't exist in indigenous societies and in the wild with the same degree of prevalence, or affects so many individuals and animals so early in life.

Protrusion of intestines: When people decide to postpone the surgery they risk stretching the anal sphincter even further, and increasing the amount of intestines that protrude from the body.

Quality of life effects: Constipation affects the quality of life, causes stress, and diminishes the overall sense of well-being. These things tend to self-perpetuate, and profoundly affect the cardiovascular, endocrine, and immune systems.

Rectal prolapsed: This is when a small amount of intestinal lining is pushed out of the anal opening while straining for bowel movement. Because the colon and female reproductive organs are structurally close in the body, pressure from large amounts of stool in the colon can lead to rectal prolapsed in the vagina, and increase the potential that the bladder will not empty completely or result in reflux of urine from the bladder back into the kidneys, called vesicoureteral reflux. Pushing large, hard stool from the rectum can result in some of your intestines protruding from the anus, called rectal prolapsed. Chronic constipation is a recurring problem in 30 to 67 percent of patients who suffer from rectal prolapsed. This requires surgery to repair.

Reflux of urine: Because the colon and female reproductive organs are structurally close in the body, pressure from large amounts of stool in the colon can lead to rectal prolapsed in the vagina, and increase the potential that the bladder will not empty completely or result in reflux of urine from the bladder back into the kidneys, called vesicoureteral reflux.

Scratching the surface: So, as it can be seen, the connections are plentiful, and it has been just.

Skin eruptions: Effects of constipation create skin eruptions. Skin eruptions can be caused or aggravated by colon toxicity. Skin is a major organ and one of its jobs is to help to eliminate waste usually through perspiration. The skin can't remove faecal matter, but it can show that our body is trying to get rid of toxins. Our body gives us indications when something is going wrong and it gives a hint.

Ulcerative Colitis: Ulcerative colitis is another inflammatory bowel disease that affects about 700,000 Americans. The symptoms of ulcerative colitis are very similar to those of Crohn's, but the part of the digestive tract affected is solely the large intestine, also known as the colon. If your immune system mistakes food or other materials for invaders, sores or ulcers develop in the colon's lining. If you experience frequent and urgent bowel movements, pain with diarrhoea, blood in your stool, or abdominal cramps, visit your doctor.

Urinary continence: Constipation can affect bladder control and urinary continence. If you sometimes leak urine or feel that you need to frequently visit the toilet to pass urine, it could be that constipation is involved. An over-full bowel (due to constipation) can press on the bladder, reducing the amount of urine it can hold or making you feel like to need to pass urine urgently.

Victim of medical error: Constipation significantly increases your risk of becoming a victim of medical error and/or of the side effects of drugs, all related to the treatment of any ensuing colorectal disorder.

Weakening of the Body's Immune System: When you're constipated, your immune system weakens thereby making you more prone to catch colds and other illnesses. As a result, there is great strain on other vital excretory organs like lymph, skin, liver, kidneys, and lungs. Because of this strain, these organs become overworked. When overworked, they are not functioning at full capacity and their ability to eliminate stool from the body gets hindered. Hence, this causes your cellular metabolism to slow down, which means your energy level drops.

3

Haemorrhoids (Piles)

3.1 Haemorrhoids (Piles)

The term haemorrhoids or piles refer to a condition in which the veins around the anus or lower rectum are swollen and inflamed. Haemorrhoids are very common in both men and women. About half of the population has haemorrhoids by age 50. Piles or Haemorrhoids (called Baw sir in Hindi language) is a disease affecting the anal region. In Piles, the veins in the rectal area swell due to stagnation of blood. The swollen veins cause pain, itching and discomfort while passing stool, sitting, standing or walking. The pain may last for a long time after passing stool. In some patients, there may be bleeding while passing stool. This is known as bleeding piles. The piles may be internal or external depending upon the location of the veins. When the problem is severe, the piles may protrude from the rectum and may have to be pushed back manually. Piles (haemorrhoids) are swellings that develop inside and around the back passage (anus). Occasionally, a clot may form in a haemorrhoid (thrombosis haemorrhoid). These are not dangerous but can be extremely painful and sometimes need to be lanced and drained. Fortunately, many effective options are available to treat haemorrhoids. Many people can get relief from symptoms with home treatments and lifestyle changes. Haemorrhoids are less common causes of rectal bleeding.

In many cases, piles are small and symptoms settle down without treatment. If required, treatment is usually effective. The anal canal is the last part of the large intestine and is about 4 cm long. At the lower end of the anal canal is the opening to the outside (usually referred to as the anus), through which faeces pass. At the upper end, the anal canal connects with the rectum (also part of the large intestine). There is a network of small veins (blood vessels) within the lining of the anal canal. These veins sometimes become wider and engorged with more blood than usual. The engorged veins and the overlying tissue may then form into one or more small swellings called piles.

3.2 Symptoms of piles (haemorrhoids):

Typical symptoms are pain, itching and bleeding around the anal area. Symptoms range from temporary and mild, to persistent and painful. The common symptoms that are seen in the majority of piles or haemorrhoids patients happen to be: There is pain while passing stool. The character of the pain may vary from one patient to the other. While some experience excruciating pain, others have only mild discomfort. Some patients describe the pain as if some splinter or a glass is pricking in the anal canal while others may feel burning pain. Often patients keep on feeling this pain for hours after passing stool. This pain can make sitting or standing difficult. Symptoms can vary. Sometimes no symptoms may be present and a person may not realise that they have piles (haemorrhoids).

- The most common symptom experienced is bleeding after going to the toilet after passing a stool (faeces) and the blood is usually bright red with the stools or separate. The blood is usually bright red and may be noticed on the toilet tissue, in the toilet pan or coating the stools.
- A haemorrhoid can hang down (prolapsed) and can be felt outside the anus. Often, it can be pushed back up after you have been to the toilet. However, more severe piles remain permanently prolapsed and cannot be pushed back up inside.
- Small internal piles are usually painless. Larger piles may cause a mucous discharge, some pain, irritation, and itch. The discharge may irritate the skin around the back passage (anus). You may have a sense of fullness in the anus, or a feeling of not fully emptying your back passage when you go to the toilet.
- A possible complication of piles that hang down is that they can 'strangulate' (the blood supply to the haemorrhoid can be cut off). This can be intensely painful. Another possible complication is a blood clot (thrombosis) which can form within the haemorrhoid. This is uncommon, but again causes intense pain if it occurs. The pain usually peaks after 48-72 hours, and then gradually goes away over 7-10 days.
- A lump hanging down outside of the anus, which may need to be pushed back in after passing a stool.
- A mucus discharge after passing a stool.
- Soreness, redness and swelling around your anus.

3.3 Types of piles (haemorrhoids):

Haemorrhoids may be located inside the rectum (internal haemorrhoids), or they may develop under the skin around the anus.

External piles: External piles are present on skin around anus and can be seen or felt from outside. External piles are those that form below that point, in the lower part of the anal canal. The main symptoms are Pain, swelling/lump around anus. Itching and bleeding may appear when they are irritated. Bleeding piles is mainly a feature of internal piles, while external piles may also bleed if irritated. External piles may be painful because the lower part of the anal canal has lots of pain nerve fibres. The external piles would mean outside of the anal canal (and so outside of the anus) but this is not always the case. There are external piles that are actually inside the anus. Internal piles can also enlarge and drop down (prolapsed), so that they hang outside of the anus. Some people develop internal and external piles at the same time.

Internal Piles: Internal piles lie deep inside the rectum and cannot be felt or seen from outside. Internal piles (haemorrhoids) are those that form above a point 2-3 cm inside the back passage (anus) in the upper part of the anal canal. They are painless owing to lack of pain receptors in the area in which they appear. The only symptom they cause is bleeding per anus while straining at stool. Internal piles are usually painless because the upper anal canal has no pain nerve fibres. Internal piles can be classified into grades 1 to 4 according to their severity and size:

Grade 1 are small swellings on the inside lining of the anal canal. They cannot be seen or felt from outside the anus. Grade 1 piles are common. In some people they enlarge further to grade 2 or more.

Grade 2 is larger and may be partly pushed out from the anus when you go to the toilet, but quickly spring back inside again.

Grade 3 hangs out from the anus when you go to the toilet. You may feel one or more as small, soft lumps that hang from the anus. However, you can push them back inside the anus with a finger.

Grade 4 permanently hangs down from within the anus, and you cannot push them back inside. They sometimes become quite large.

Protruding/Prolapsed piles: piles that while straining at stool are pushed on the anal verge are referred to as protruding/prolapsed piles. They lead to symptoms of pain, itching, and mucus discharge.

118

Blind Piles: Non-bleeding piles are referred to as blind piles.

3.4 Causes (the reasons) of piles (haemorrhoids):

There are various factors that predispose a person to develop piles include diet with less fibre content, lack of exercise, sedentary habits like prolonged sitting , increased straining during defecation, chronic constipation or diarrhoea, excessive alcohol intake, pregnancy, obesity . Genetic Factors also play a strong role in the development of piles. The most important cause or reason for the occurrence of piles is the changing lifestyle. While the food that we eat is becoming rich in fats and carbohydrates, our habits are becoming more and more sedentary. We do not move around. We do not walk enough or cycle. Even other physical activities while doing household chores have been taken over either by machines or helpers.

This leads to obesity and fat around the waist. Increased body weight and little physical activity can slow down the digestive system. In some parts of the world, people tend to eat lots of spices. Spicy food is a big contributor to the occurrence of piles. The exact reason why the changes in the veins within the lining of the anal canal occur and lead to piles (haemorrhoids) forming is not clear. Some piles seem to develop for no apparent reason. However, it is thought that an increased pressure in and around the back passage (anus) and anal canal can be a major factor in many cases. People develop one or more piles at some stage. Haemorrhoids have a number of causes, although often the cause is unknown. They may result from straining during bowel movements or from the increased pressure on these veins during pregnancy.

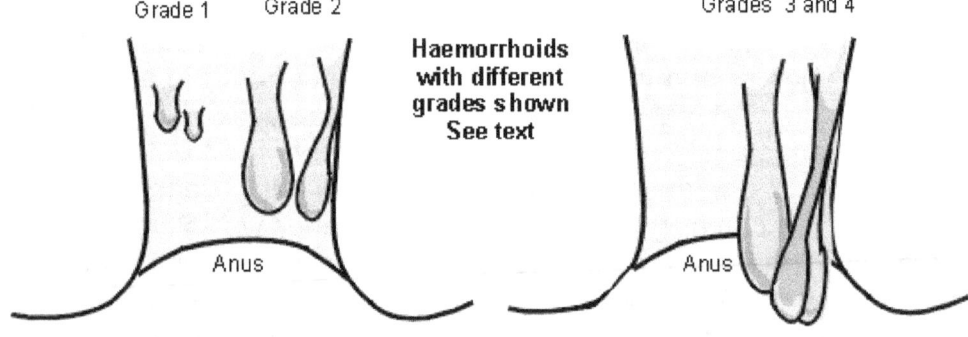

Grade 1 Grade 2 Haemorrhoids with different grades shown See text Grades 3 and 4

Anus Anus

When the fibre content is low, it makes it difficult to pass stool. Constipation results and one often has to strain to pass stool. As mentioned earlier, spices can also add to the already existing tendency of piles. Also, there is too much intake of aerated drinks in some parts of the world. These aerated drinks are not healthy and often are at the cost of normal intake of water. This replacing of water with aerated drinks is another contributory factor in causing piles. Also, non vegetarian food is a little harder on the digestive system and takes more time to digest. In some cultures, the predominant part of diet consists of non vegetarian food.

Certain situations increase the chance of piles developing:

- Constipation
- Increase in pressure in the lower rectum
- Straining during bowel movements
- Sitting for long periods of time, especially on the toilet
- Chronic (long lasting) constipation or diarrhoea
- Being overweight or obese
- Anal intercourse
- Low-fibre diet
- Spinal cord injury
- Poor posture.
- Passing large stools (faeces):
- Straining at the toilet: These increase the pressure in and around the veins in the anus and seem to be a common reason for piles to develop.
- Pregnancy: Piles are common during pregnancy. This is probably due to pressure effects of the baby lying above the rectum and anus, and the affect that the change in hormones during pregnancy can have on the veins.
- Ageing: The tissues in the lining of the anus may become less supportive as we get older.
- Hereditary factors: Some people may inherit a weakness of the wall of the veins in the anal region.
- Related discussions
- Symptoms of piles (haemorrhoids):
- Symptoms can vary. Sometimes no symptoms may be present and a person may not realise that they have piles (haemorrhoids). When irritated they can itch or bleed. Blood can pool inside an external haemorrhoid and form a clot, which causes severe pain, swelling, and inflammation. Signs and symptoms of haemorrhoids may include:

- Pain or discomfort, especially when sitting
- Pain during bowel movements
- Itching or irritation around the anal region
- Bright red blood on your stools, toilet paper or in the toilet bowl
- Swelling around the anus
- Lumps near the anus, which might be tender or painful.
- Bleed frequently or excessively
- Do not respond to self-treatment
- Obvious change in bowel habits
- Passing black or maroon-coloured stools
- Blood clots formed
- Blood is mixed in with the stool.
- Bleeding: The most common symptom experienced is bleeding after going to the toilet to pass stools (faeces). The blood is usually bright red and may be noticed on the toilet tissue, in the toilet pan or coating the stools. Bleeding during bowel movements is the most common sign of haemorrhoids. Rectal bleeding can, however, indicate a more serious condition, such as bowel cancer or anal cancer. You should consult your doctor if your haemorrhoids:
- Feeling: A haemorrhoid can hang down (prolapsed) and can be felt outside the anus. Often, it can be pushed back up after you have been to the toilet. However, more severe piles remain permanently prolapsed and cannot be pushed back up inside. Small internal piles are usually painless. Larger piles may cause a mucous discharge, some pain, irritation, and itch. The discharge may irritate the skin around the back passage (anus). You may have a sense of fullness in the anus, or a feeling of not fully emptying your back passage when you go to the toilet.
- A possible complication of piles that hang down is that they can 'strangulate' (the blood supply to the haemorrhoid can be cut off). This can be intensely painful. Another possible complication is a blood clot (thrombosis) which can form within the haemorrhoid. This is uncommon, but again causes intense pain if it occurs. The pain usually peaks after 48-72 hours, and then gradually goes away over 7-10 days.

Types and Symptoms of Piles:

External Piles: External piles are present on skin around anus and can be seen or felt from outside. The main symptoms are Pain, swelling/lump around anus. Itching and bleeding may appear when they are irritated. Bleeding piles is mainly a feature of internal piles, while external piles may also bleed if irritated.

Internal Piles: Internal piles lie deep inside the rectum and cannot be felt or seen from outside. They are painless owing to lack of pain receptors in the area in which they appear. The only symptom they cause is bleeding per anus while straining at stool.

Protruding/Prolapsed piles: piles that while straining at stool are pushed on the anal verge are referred to as protruding/prolapsed piles. They lead to symptoms of pain, itching, and mucus discharge.

Blind Piles: Non-bleeding piles are referred to as blind piles.

3.5   Piles   (haemorrhoids) diagnosis:

If you think that you may have piles (haemorrhoids), or have bleeding or pain from your back passage (anus), you should visit your doctor. Piles are usually diagnosed after your doctor asks you questions about your symptoms and performs a physical examination. The examination usually includes an examination of your back passage. Wearing gloves and using a lubricant, your doctor will examine your back passage with their finger to look for any signs of piles or other abnormalities.

Sometimes, if your piles are not obvious after an examination of your back passage, your doctor may suggest a further examination called a proctoscopy. This is where the inside of your back passage is examined using an instrument called a proctoscope. A proctoscope is a short, hollow tube that has a light at one end and allows the doctor to see the lining of your back passage, and any piles, more clearly.

In some cases, a more detailed examination of your bowel may be needed to help rule out other conditions.

Digital rectal examination in which your doctor inserts a lubricated gloved finger into your rectum to feel for anything unusual, such as growths

Visual inspection of the inside of your anal canal and rectum using a viewing device such as an anoscope, proctoscope or sigmoidscope

Colonoscopy may be performed to do a more extensive examination of your entire bowel (colon) if your signs and symptoms suggest that you might have another digestive system disease, or if you have risk factors for colorectal cancer

3.6 Treatment for piles (haemorrhoids):

Most cases of haemorrhoids can be self-treated. More serious or repeat cases may require medication or a surgical procedure. Haemorrhoids can recur after treatment; hence, they are controlled rather than cured. Avoid constipation and straining at the toilet. Keep the stools (faeces) soft, and don't strain on the toilet. You can do this by the following:

Eat plenty of fibre such as fruit, vegetables, cereals, wholegrain bread, etc.

Have lots of water or juice to drink. Adults should aim to drink at least two litres (6-8 glasses) per day. You will pass much of the fluid as urine, but some is passed out in the gut and softens faeces. Most sorts of drink will do, but alcoholic drinks can cause the body to lose fluids (they are dehydrating) and may not be good. Too much caffeine should also be avoided.

Fibre supplements. If a high-fibre diet is not helping, you can take fibre supplements (bulking agents) such as ispaghula, methylcellulose, bran or sterculia. You can buy these at pharmacies or get them on prescription. Methylcellulose also helps to soften faeces directly which makes them easier to pass.

Avoid painkillers that contain codeine such as co-codamol, as they are a common cause of constipation. However, simple painkillers such as paracetamol may help.

Go to the toilet as soon as possible after feeling the need. Some people suppress this feeling and plan to go to the toilet later. This may result in bigger and harder faeces forming which are then more difficult to pass. Do not strain on the toilet. Piles may cause a feeling of fullness in the rectum and it is tempting to strain at the end to try to empty the rectum further. Resist this. Do not spend too long on the toilet, which may encourage you to strain. Do not read whilst on the toilet.

The above measures will often ease symptoms such as bleeding and discomfort. It may be all that you need to treat small and non-prolapsed piles (grade 1). Small grade 1 piles often settle down over time.

Banding treatment: Banding is a common treatment for grade 2 and 3 piles. It may also be done to treat grade 1 piles which have not settled with the measures described above (such as an increase in fibre, etc). This procedure is usually done by a surgeon in an outpatient clinic. A haemorrhoid is grasped by the surgeon with forceps or a suction device. A rubber band is then placed at the base of the haemorrhoid. This cuts off the blood supply to the haemorrhoid which then dies and drops off after a few days. The tissue at the base of the haemorrhoid heals with some scar tissue. Banding of internal piles is usually painless, as the base of the haemorrhoid originates above the anal opening in the very last part of the gut where the gut lining is not sensitive to pain. Up to three piles may be treated at one time using this method. Banding does not work in a small number of cases. Piles are less likely to recur after banding if you do not become constipated and do not strain on the toilet. A small number of people have complications following banding, such as bleeding, urinary problems, or infection or ulcers forming at the site of a treated haemorrhoid.

Diathermy and electrotherapy: Use heat energy to destroy the piles. They appear to have similar success rates as infrared coagulation and the risk of any complications is low.

Stapled haemorrhoidopexy: A circular stapling gun is used to cut out a circular section of the lining of the anal canal above the piles. This has the effect of pulling the piles back up the anal canal. It also has the effect of reducing the blood supply to the piles and so they shrink as a consequence. Because the cutting is actually above the piles, it is usually a less painful procedure than the traditional operation to remove the piles. Haemorrhoid stapling is removal of a haemorrhoid with a special staple gun that also inserts a ring of staples to close the wound and prevent bleeding.

Haemorrhoidal artery ligation: The small arteries that supply blood to the piles are tied (ligated). This causes the haemorrhoid(s) to shrink.

Haemorrhoidectomy (the traditional operation): an operation to cut away the haemorrhoid(s) is an option to treat grade 3 or 4 piles or for piles not successfully treated by banding or other methods. The operation is done under general anaesthetic and is usually successful. However, it can be quite painful in the days following the operation.

Haemorrhoidectomy: - removal of a haemorrhoid with a scalpel or laser

Infrared coagulation/photocoagulation: This method uses infrared energy to burn and cut off the circulation to the haemorrhoid, which causes it to shrink in size. It seems to be as effective as banding treatment and injection sclera-therapy for first- and second-degree piles.

Injection (sclerotherapy): involves injecting a substance into the haemorrhoid to make it harden and shrink.

Laser or infrared coagulation: which is a type of heat treatment that causes the haemorrhoid to harden and shrivel. If non-surgical procedures are not successful or if the haemorrhoids are particularly large, one of the following surgical procedures may be necessary.

Ointments, creams and suppositories: Various preparations and brands are commonly used. They do not cure piles. However, they may ease symptoms such as discomfort and itch. A bland soothing cream, ointment, or suppository may ease discomfort. Several brands are available without a prescription. Ask a pharmacist to advice. Follow the instructions on the packet on how to use. One that contains an anaesthetic may ease pain better. You should only use one of these for short periods at a time (5-7 days). If you use it for longer, the anaesthetic may irritate or sensitise the skin around the back passage (anus). Piles of pregnancy usually settle after the birth of the child. Treatment is similar to the above.

Oral pain medication: Taking oral pain medication, such as paracetamol or ibuprofen, can help to relieve discomfort.

Other treatment options: Banding (described above) is perhaps the most common procedure done to treat piles. However, a variety of other surgical procedures are sometimes used. Some surgeons prefer one procedure over another. Your surgeon will advise of the pros and cons of the different procedures. Although each procedure is usually successful, as with any surgical procedure, there is some risk that complications or problems may occur during, or following, the procedure. Injection sclera-therapy: phenol in oil is injected into the tissues at the base of the piles. This causes a scarring (fibrotic) reaction which obliterates the blood vessels going to the piles. The piles then die and drop off, similar to after banding.

Self-treatment: Non-surgical and surgical procedures for an external haemorrhoid in which a clot has formed, prompt relief can be obtained from your doctor performing a simple incision to remove the clot. For persistent bleeding or painful haemorrhoids, the following non-surgical procedures to destroy the haemorrhoid can be performed in a doctor's office:

- Rubber band ligation, involves using a rubber band to cut off the blood supply to the haemorrhoid causing it to shrivel and die
- Home treatment is often all that is required to relieve mild pain, swelling, and inflammation associated with haemorrhoids. Home treatments include:

- Use of non-prescription haemorrhoid ointments, creams, suppositories, or pads containing a mild corticosteroid, e.g. hydrocortisone, or witch hazel extract
- Soak the anal area in warm water for 10 to 15 minutes two or three times a day
- Use stool softeners, which help stools to be passed more easily
- Ensure that the anal area is kept clean by bathing or showering daily – soap is not necessary and the affected area can be dried with a hair dryer
- Use moist towel or wet toilet paper (that do not contain perfume or alcohol) rather than dry toilet paper, to help keep the anal area clean after passing a stool
- Applying ice packs or cold compresses on the affected area can relieve swelling

3.7   Prevention of Piles:

Keeping your stools soft is the best way to prevent haemorrhoids from occurring. The following steps can help to prevent haemorrhoids from occurring and reduce symptoms of existing haemorrhoids:

- Eat high-fibre foods
- Drink plenty of fluids
- Consider using fibre supplements
- Avoid straining when on the toilet
- Go to the toilet as soon as you feel the urge
- Get plenty of exercise
- Avoid sitting for long periods.

3.8   Piles   (Haemorrhoids) Management:

- Making some changes to one's routine and lifestyle can go a long way in managing piles or haemorrhoids. Here are some tips to get rid of your piles or haemorrhoids: It is important that one should take care of what one eats. The daily diet should be rich in fibre or roughage. This roughage is present in large quantity in raw fruits and vegetables. Therefore taking raw fruits and salads daily is highly recommended.
- One should be cutting down on the intake of non-vegetarian food. As mentioned earlier, non-vegetarian food is difficult to digest and often contains a lot of spices which are added while cooking.

- Drinking lots of water are another important thing. Water hydrates the digestive system and makes it easy for the stool to be passed.
- Walking regularly or taking any form of exercise daily is also very helpful. It activates the sluggish digestive system and allows the bowels to be cleared easily without straining.
- Avoid straining while passing stool is the best for piles management.
- Abuse of laxatives is another important point here. The regular usage of laxatives can by itself cause piles and is often counterproductive.
- Avoid sitting in one position for long. In fact, one should not sit for long at all. It is better to get up and move around after some time.
- Sitz bath or sitting in a tub of hot water helps. It not only relieves the pain and inflammation but also helps in maintaining hygiene.

3.9   Diet's for piles disease:

Fibre content or roughage is very important to form the bulk of stool and helps in its easy evacuation. When the fibre content is low, it makes it difficult to pass stool. Constipation results and one often has to strain to pass stool. As mentioned earlier, spices can also add to the already existing tendency of piles. Also, there is too much intake of aerated drinks in some parts of the world. These aerated drinks are not healthy and often are at the cost of normal intake of water. This replacing of water with aerated drinks is another contributory factor in causing piles. Also, non vegetarian food is a little harder on the digestive system and takes more time to digest. In some cultures, the predominant part of diet consists of non vegetarian food.

4

Anal fissures

4.1 General:

An anal fissure is a shallow ulceration or a small tear in the tissue or crack in the lining of the anus (the opening through which stool passes out of the body) that extends upwards into the anal canal or ulcer in the lining of the anal canal that extends into the anal canal. Anal fissure are tears in the skin or crack in the lining around the anus brought about by over-stretching while trying to pass hard stool. Chronic constipation can also lead to tearing of the anus, called an anal fissure. These fissures are caused by trauma to the inner lining of the anus, often before a large, dry stool. Fissures, or ulcers, are cuts or tears in the skin, or around the anal area. An anal fissure can affect people of all ages, but it's most often seen in infants and young children. An anal fissure usually isn't a serious condition. In most cases, the tear heals on its own within four to six weeks. Certain treatments can promote healing and help relieve discomfort, including stool softeners and topical pain relievers. If an anal fissure doesn't improve with these treatments, surgery may be required or your doctor may need to look for other underlying disorders that can cause anal fissures.

It is a common cause of red blood in the stool (faeces) and toilet paper. It may occur when passing large or hard stools, straining during childbirth, or experiencing bouts of diarrhoea. Fissures are a common condition of the anus and anal canal and are responsible for 6% to 15% of the visits to a colon and rectal (colorectal) surgeon. They affect men and women equally and both the young and the old. Fissures usually cause pain during bowel movements that often is severe. Anal fissure is the most common cause of rectal bleeding in infancy. An anal fissure can cause sharp pain and bleeding during and after bowel movements. It may also cause itching and burning in the anal area. An anal fissure is usually a minor condition that goes away within six weeks. Anal fissures occur in the specialized tissue that lines the anus and anal canal, called anoderm. At a line just inside the anus (referred to as the anal verge or intersphincteric groove) the skin (dermis) of the inner buttocks changes to anoderm.

Unlike skin, anoderm has no hairs, sweat glands, or sebaceous (oil) glands and contains a larger number of sensory nerves that sense light touch and pain. (The abundance of nerves explains why anal fissures are so painful.) The hairless, gland-less, extremely sensitive anoderm continues for the entire length of the anal canal until it meets the demarcating line for the rectum, called the dentate line.

The crack in the skin exposes the muscle tissue underneath, causing severe pain and bleeding during and after bowel movements. An anal fissure can affect people of all ages, but it's most often seen in infants and young children. An anal fissure usually isn't a serious condition. In most cases, the tear heals on its own within four to six weeks. Certain treatments can promote healing and help relieve discomfort, including stool softeners and topical pain relievers. If an anal fissure doesn't improve with these treatments, surgery may be required or your doctor may need to look for other underlying disorders that can cause anal fissures. An anal fissure that fails to heal within six weeks is considered chronic and may need further treatment. Once you've experienced an anal fissure, you are prone to having another one. A tear extends to surrounding muscles. An anal fissure may extend into the ring of muscle that holds your anus closed (internal anal sphincter), making it more difficult for your anal fissure to heal. An unhealed fissure can trigger a cycle of discomfort that may require medications or surgery to reduce the pain and to repair or remove the fissure.

These are known as chronic anal fissures. These require treatment. Anal fissures mainly result from straining while passing hard or large stool. In some persons, chronic diarrhoea may also lead to anal fissures. Anal fissures may arise in women from trauma caused to the anal canal during childbirth. Anal fissures are very common in infants (children aged 1 month to 12 months). The main symptoms of anal fissure are pain during defecation and anal bleeding. The pain from anal fissures may last for hours after passing stool. The pain is often accompanied by marked burning in the anal area. Anal fissures can be quite painful. Passing the stool becomes a difficult and painful exercise and the result can be nothing short of traumatic for the patient. Itching around the anus and malodorous discharge from the anal fissure are other symptoms that present themselves. Anal Fissure is a result of the trauma caused by the passage of hard, long stool (constipation) and repeated episodes of diarrhoea. Anal Fissure actually refers to a tear in the anus. Anus, of course, is the opening that marks the lower end of the gastro-intestinal system of the body or the opening through which stool are passed out of the body.

Homeopathic remedies can be quite beneficial in the treatment of Anal Fissures. The typical symptoms of an anal fissure are extreme pain during defecation and red blood streaking the stool. Patients may try to avoid defecation because of the pain. The pain is usually felt while passing stool and may remain for a long time afterwards. The pain may be burning or stinging in character. There may be discharge of pus or some foul matter too. An anal fissure is just a cut or a crack in the mucous membrane lining the anal canal. It may occur due to hard stools. When one is constipated, one has to strain to pass stool. This can also cause a break or a crack in the mucous membrane. At times, diarrhoea can also cause anal fissures. In females, anal fissures occur commonly after a vaginal delivery. Homeopathic remedies for fissure promote the natural healing of anal fissure. Homoeopathic treatment mainly improves the entire process of digestion thus helps patient to get relief from constipation and straining from stools which is the main causative factor for fissure in anus. Homeopathic remedies commonly used for the treatment of anal fissures are capable of completely curing the problem. You can easily get yourself cured and that too without any surgery

4.1   Symptoms of Anal Fissure:

The symptoms of anal fissure are in many ways similar to piles. In some cases it may be difficult for the patient to understand whether he or she is suffering from anal fissure or piles. An experienced doctor or a surgeon is the best person to diagnose it properly. The common symptoms of anal fissure are as follows-Onset of acute anal fissure is characterized by tearing, cutting, or burning pain during or immediately after bowel movement. A few drops of blood may streak toilet paper or underclothes. Painful anal sphincter spasms result from ulceration of "sential pile" (swelling at the lower end of the fissure).

A fissure may heal spontaneously and completely or it may partially heal and break open again. Chronic fissure produces scar tissue that hampers normal bowel evacuation. Because of the crack or cut in the anal fissure, as mentioned earlier, the anal mucosa is rich in nerve endings and this makes the area sensitive to any touch or injury. There is a lot of pain which is worse while passing stool. The pain may be burning or stinging in character. The pain may last for a long time after passing stool. This can make sitting or walking difficult. At times, the pain is so severe that the patient dreads bowel movements and desists from passing stool. Itching in the anal and perinea region may also be present. This is another common symptom observed in patients with anal fissures. Some patients may describe it as irritation.

Bleeding is also commonly seen in patients with anal fissures. The blood may be bright red in colour.

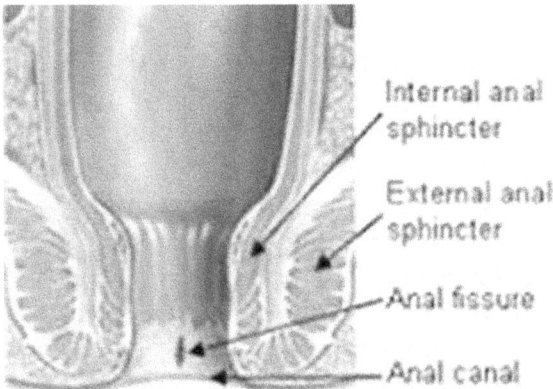

Internal anal sphincter

External anal sphincter

Anal fissure

Anal canal

Usually the bleeding is not profuse. A crack or a wound like feeling may be experienced by patients. The pain may continue even after passing stool, which is accompanied by bleeding too. The other symptoms include hard stool, itching in the anus and in a few longstanding fissure cases, offensive discharge from the anus. This pain is aggravated while passing stool. In some cases, the pain may be only while passing stools. Some other patients may experience the pain throughout the day. But passing stool is the most difficult part. The aggravation of pain at that time may last for hours afterwards. The pain may be sharp or stinging in character. The other most common or important symptom of an anal fissure is the presence of bleeding while passing stool. The quantity of blood may again vary from one patient to the other. But bleeding is a common symptom of anal fissures. The blood is bright red and not mixed with stool. Blackish stools or blood mixed with stool may be due to some other cause and not anal fissure. A crack or a Rhagae or a wound is felt in the anal region. This is quite often differentiated by the patient himself that he has a crack in the skin. Itching or irritation in the anal region is also present. In case of chronic constipation, the stools are large, knotty and difficult. Cutting pain during stools followed by constriction that lasts several hours after stool. Bleeding from the fissure and marked itching at the anus. An anal fissure may cause one or more of the symptoms. The main signs and symptoms of an anal fissure include:

- A skin tag or small lump of skin, next to the tear
- A visible tear in the skin around the anus
- Blood flow- because the blood is fresh, it will be bright red and may be noticed on the stools or the toilet paper. Anal fissures in infants commonly bleed. Children may be alarmed at the sight of bright-red blood in their stools or toilet paper.
- Bright red blood in stool or bloody streaks on toilet paper or underwear.
- Burning or itching in the anal area

- Diarrhoea or constipation
- Dysuria - discomfort when urinating (less common). Some patients may urinate more frequently.
- Fear of pain may put some patients off going to the toilet,
- Headache
- Itching in the anal area
- Pain, especially when going to the toilet (passing stools). During the passing of a stool the pain is sharp, and then afterwards there may be a longer deep burning sensation.
- Pain, sometimes severe, during bowel movements
- Pus - a malodorous (bad smelling) discharge of pus may come from the anal fissure.
- Rectal itching
- Sensation may be intermittent or persistent
- Sharp or burning rectal pain during and immediately after bowel movements, especially when the stool is hard or bulky
- Sharp pain in the anal area during bowel movements. Some people may experience a sharp pain when they clean themselves with toilet paper.
- Streaks of blood on stools or on tissue paper after wiping

4.2   Causes of Anal Fissures:

The smooth lining of the anal canal is soft and elastic in nature so as to allow stool to pass. It is hairless and full of small nerve endings. Therefore it is quite sensitive to touch and pain. That is precisely why fissures are quite painful. Anal fissures are caused by injury or trauma to the anal mucosa. This trauma may result from hard or large stools. It may also occur due to repeated diarrhoea or constipation when one has to strain a lot to pass stool. It may also occur during labour when there may be a tear in the perinea region. It may also occur during occasionally insertion of rectal thermometer or a colonoscopy or during enema. In other cases HIV, anal cancer, syphilis, leukaemia or TB may cause an anal fissure. There is also the possibility of anal fissure being caused by the presence of inflammatory bowel diseases like Ulcerative Colitis or Crohn's disease. As mentioned earlier, an anal fissure is a crack in the anal canal. It is more in the form of an injury to the anal canal. The common causes of this could be Constipation, which is a prominent cause of anal fissures. If you have to strain a lot to pass stool or the stool is quite hard, it can damage the anal canal. A large and dry stool can also result in an anal fissure. Frequent stools can also result in anal fissure. This happens in chronic diarrhoea cases or in some other diseases like ulcerative colitis or crohn's disease. Damage to the anal canal can also occur during delivery in the case of females. A prolonged labour or difficult labour can sometimes result in an anal fissure. It is also common in infants in the first year of their life. The precise reason for this incidence at this stage of life is poorly understood. The exact cause is unknown. They're caused by trauma or injury that stretches your anal canal. Common causes of anal fissure include:

- Anal cancer.
- Anorectic scarring and decreased blood flow to the rectum or anus also can cause fissures.
- Childbirth
- Chronic diarrhoea
- Chronic poor bowel habits,
- Constipation and straining during bowel movements
- Crohn's disease or another inflammatory bowel disease
- Explosive or ongoing diarrhoea
- Failure to heal constipation
- Fissures may also occur as a secondary complication to anal surgery,
- Hard stools tear the lining of the anal canal as they pass.
- Having anal sex or putting things into your anus can overstretch the skin and cause a fissure.
- Herpes
- HIV
- Immune system disorders.
- Inflammation of the anorectic area,
- Insertion of recto scope, endoscope.
- Large, hard faeces (stools) are more likely to cause lesions in the anal area during a bowel movement than soft and smaller ones.
- Multiple pregnancies.
- Muscle spasms may increase the risk of developing an anal fissure. A spasm is a brief, automatic jerking muscle movement, when the muscle can suddenly tighten. Muscle spasms may also undermine the healing process.
- Obesity may lead to increased sweating, which may be an aggravating factor.
- Owing to age-related changes in the skin as well as increased frequency of constipation.
- Passing large and hard stools

- People who frequently experience constipation are at an increased risk for anal fissures as well.
- People with an inflammatory bowel disease, such as Crohn's disease,
- Pregnancy and childbirth - pregnant women have a higher risk of developing an anal fissure towards the end of their pregnancy. The lining of the anus may also tear during childbirth.
- Proctitis (inflammation of the rectum) or other disorders
- Repeated use of enema nozzles
- Sexually transmitted diseases (e.g., gonorrhea, cancroids, syphilis, Chlamydia and HIV) can cause anal fissure.
- Straining and passing large, hard stools are the most common causes of anal fissures.
- Straining during delivery
- Syphilis
- The inflammation that occurs in the intestinal lining makes the tissue around the anus more prone to tearing.
- Tight or spastic anal sphincter muscles (muscles that control the closing of the anus),
- Too much pressure, tight anal sphincter muscles, and poor blood supply to your anus may lead to their development and poor healing.
- Trauma to the inner lining of the anus can cause a fissure.
- Tuberculosis.
- Underlying medical conditions such as Crohn's disease and ulcerative colitis, anal cancer, leukaemia; infectious diseases (e.g., tuberculosis),

4.3   Diagnosis of anal fissure:

A doctor can usually diagnose an anal fissure simply by examining the area around the anus.

They may want to perform a digital rectal exam to confirm the diagnosis. During this exam, the doctor will insert an endoscope or anoscope into your rectum to make it easier to see the tear. These medical instruments are thin tubes with attached cameras and lights that allow doctors to inspect the anal canal.

Using an anoscope may also help your doctor find other causes of anal or rectal pain such as haemorrhoids.

Patient history and physical examination are needed.

Examination with sigmoidoscope is required to detect the fissure and to rule out other causes of rectal bleeding.

The doctor will perform visual inspection of the anus or gently examine the anus with the tip of the finger.

4.4   Management   of   Anal Fissures:

A few precautions can help in managing anal fissures. All these things are easy to perform and involve minor changes in one's routine. Eat lots of fresh fruits and vegetables. Nuts are also helpful. This allows a lot of roughage in diet and prevents constipation. When the stool is soft, it does not cause any injury to the anal mucosa while passing. At the same time, this allows sufficient time for the fissure to heal. Take lots of water every day. Staying hydrated is very important. It again allows the stool to remain soft and prevents constipation.

Walk or exercise daily. This keeps the digestive system in good condition and also improves blood circulation. 30-40 minutes of walk every day is advisable. Avoid constipation by all means. If the stool remains constipated despite all efforts, one can take a little bit of laxative like psyllium husk or isabhagol. This keeps the stool soft by adding fibre. Taking Sitz bath is also very helpful. Sitz bath means sitting in a bath tub with some warm water in it. This allows the hardened tissue to soften, keeps the area clean and promotes healing. Preventing constipation is an important thing that one has to take care of so as to allow the fissure to heal. This can be done by drinking lots of water and eating enough fruits, vegetables and cereals that are rich in fibre. One should avoid smoking and drinking alcohol. Junk food is also best avoided. Junk food only provides empty calories and leads to weight gain. Walking regularly can help improve digestion as well as blood circulation. Sitting in a tub full of hot water is also quite helpful as it softens the hard tissues and takes care of hygiene. Homeopathy is one of the most popular holistic systems of medicine. The selection of remedy is based upon the theory of individualization and symptoms similarity by using holistic approach. This is the only way through which a state of complete health can be regained by removing all the sign and symptoms from which the patient is suffering. The aim of homeopathy is not only to treat anal fissure but to address its underlying cause and individual susceptibility. As far as therapeutic medication is concerned, several remedies are available to treat anal fissure that can be selected on the basis of cause, sensations and modalities of the complaints. For individualized remedy selection and treatment, the patient should consult a qualified homeopathic doctor in person. Homoeopathy is a good choice over temporary pain killers and soothing ointments suggested for short term relief of anal fissure. Homoeopathic treatment can even prevent surgery (fissurectomy) to remove anal fissures. Homeopathic remedies for anal fissures can be beneficial and of great help in providing relief and working as a remedy for the treatment of Anal Fissures. Homeopathic treatment for anal fissures works by using body's own restorative processes and is considered very safe. It can only help, never harm.

Homeopathy is a natural mode of treatment that assures permanent cure of anal fissure. Homeopathic medicines for anal fissure first help to manage the most troublesome symptoms of pain, bleeding and itching from anal fissures. They then help heal cuts and tears in the anal canal, thus effecting permanent cure. Homeopathy is a great alternative treatment method for anal fissure and can be safely used among persons of all age groups. In my clinical practice, Doctors have seen many cases of anal fissure recover completely from use of Homeopathic medicines. The medicines are selected as per the symptoms that present themselves in each case. All the Homeopathic medicines described here are equally effective in treating anal fissures, irrespective of the order in which they are mentioned.

A common belief, which is actually completely misplaced, is that there is hardly any treatment for anal fissures. Most of the people believe that surgery is the only possible option when it comes to anal fissure treatment. This is completely wrong. While there is no treatment of anal fissures in allopathic except surgery, Homeopathic remedies can easily cure anal fissures. There is no need to get a surgery done if you are suffering from anal fissures. Just improve your lifestyle as has been mentioned. Follow the diet and exercise patterns that have been given here.

4.5 Side Effects (Risk factors) of anal fissures:

- Side Effects (Risk factors) of anal fissures include:
- Chronic inflammation of the intestinal tract, which may make the lining of the anal canal more vulnerable to tearing.
- Pain after bowel movements that can last up to several hours.
- Bright red blood on the stool or toilet paper after a bowel movement.
- Itching or irritation around the anus.
- A visible crack in the skin around the anus.
- A small lump or skin tag on the skin near the anal fissure.

4.6 Management of Anal fissures:

Several lifestyle changes may help relieve discomfort and promote healing of an anal fissure, as well as prevent recurrences:

- Add fibre to your diet. Eating about 25 to 30 grams of fibre a day can help keep stools soft and improve fissure healing. Fibre-rich foods include fruits, vegetables, nuts and whole grains. You also can take a fibre supplement. Adding fibre may cause gas and bloating, so increase your intake gradually.
- Drink adequate fluids. Fluids help prevent constipation.
- Exercise regularly: Engage in 30 minutes or more of moderate physical activity, such as walking, most days of the week. Exercise promotes regular bowel movements and increases blood flow to all parts of your body, which may promote healing of an anal fissure.
- Avoid straining during bowel movements. Straining creates pressure, which can open a healing tear or cause a new tear.
- If your infant has an anal fissure, be sure to change diapers frequently, wash the area gently and discuss the problem with your child's doctor.

4.7 Fissure treatment without surgery:

A commonly held belief which is mostly propagated by surgeons is that surgery is the one and only treatment for anal fissures. The reality is far from this. An anal fissure is easily treatable without surgery. It is only those patients who do not know about this reality that end up getting laid on the surgeon's table for the treatment of an anal fissure. Anyone who knows better will never do that. This is because a painless and very easy treatment option exists to cure the anal fissures. In my opinion, surgery offers no cure as I have seen many cases where the problem recurs after some time. Most anal fissures don't require extensive treatment. Most anal fissures heal naturally within a few days (although spasms of the sphincter may aggravate the condition and delay healing). However, certain home remedies can help promote healing and relieve uncomfortable symptoms. Trauma or injury can stretch the anal canal and create a tear in the lining of the anus. These tears, known as anal fissures, usually come from passing large or hard stools. They can cause pain and bleeding during and after bowel movements. The goal of treatment is to relieve pain and discomfort, and heal the torn lining. Acute anal fissures -- the ones that don't last longer than 6 weeks -- are common and usually heal on their own with self-care. Chronic anal fissures -- those that last longer than 6 weeks -- may need medicine or surgery to help them heal. If your fissures are caused by constipation or diarrhoea, you can change a few habits to help lessen the strain on the anal canal. These steps can help relieve symptoms and encourage healing in most cases.

Therefore it is better that one should treat the problem in a holistic manner so that once cured, it does not recur. There may be many claims about the possibility of alternative or complementary treatment of anal fissures. Ayurvedic or herbal remedies are often suggested as being a possible cure for the treatment of anal fissures. Many home remedies are often touted as the cure for anal fissures. Some of this work on some of the patients but the results is not consistent. Having practiced for almost two decades, Doctors say with surety and certainty that of all the possible alternative, natural or complementary treatments available for anal fissures, homeopathy is the best option for the treatment of an anal fissure.

When one opts for Homeopathy for anal fissures, one is able to avoid surgery. Homeopathy aims at curing anal fissures in this holistic manner. It improves the digestive system along with curing the immediate symptoms of anal fissures. Homeopathy not only treats and cures the acute anal fissure; it is able to cure the chronic form of anal fissures too. Moreover, the Homeopathic medicines for anal fissures are able to eradicate the tendency to have fissures. This means that recurrence of anal fissures is avoided. That is why Homeopathy is known to have the best treatment of anal fissures. As mentioned earlier, taking Homeopathy for anal fissures is a better bet because it completely eradicates the fissure as well as the tendency to form fissures. There is an added advantage that it does not have any adverse or side effects. This is because the Homeopathic medicines are completely natural medicines. They are sourced from plants, fruits, vegetables or natural minerals. There is no chemical or synthetic material present in the homeopathic medicines. Even further, while preparing the medicines, the medicines are serially diluted which leaves no scope for any material presence in the ultimate medicine. That is why there are no side effects of the Homeopathic remedies or any homeopathic treatment. You can treat an anal fissure at home by:

- Apply a non-prescription topical cream, such as zinc oxide or a nitro-glycerine ointment, such as "Cortisone-10" or Nitro-glycerine ointment (0.2%) to promote healing.
- Applying topical pain relievers, such as Anusol-HC and Lidocaine, to the anus to ease discomfort.
- Avoid constipating foods and ask your doctor whether any drugs you take may be the cause of constipation.
- Avoid irritating the area.
- Don't strain during bowel movements.
- Drink plenty of liquids (at least fifteen glasses of water a day) to soften the stool and help prevent constipation.
- Drink plenty of caffeine-free fluids throughout the day. (Too much alcohol and caffeine can lead to dehydration.)
- Eat a fibre-rich diet, 20 to 35 grams of fibre, every day, such as, Wheat bran, Oat bran, Whole grains, including brown rice, oatmeal, and whole-grain pastas, cereals, and breads, Peas and beans, Citrus fruits, Prunes and prune juice.
- Don't strain or sit on the toilet too long. This can increase pressure in the anal canal.
- Gently clean and dry your anal area after each bowel movement.
- Avoid irritants to the skin, such as scented soaps or bubble baths.
- Eat lots of high-fibre fresh fruits and dry fruits, legumes and whole-grain products.
- Get treatment for chronic constipation or ongoing diarrhoea.
- Lubricate the anorectic area using petroleum jelly.
- Maintain good hygiene in the anal area.
- Promptly treat all occurrences of constipation and diarrhoea.
- Sitz baths, or hip baths, can promote healing of an anal fissure. Stay hydrated.
- Take Stool softeners prescribed by your doctor
- Taking fibre supplements and increasing intake of fibrous foods, such as raw fruits and vegetables.
- These habits are usually enough to heal most anal fissures within a few weeks to a few months. But when they aren't enough, ask your doctor about other treatments.
- Using over-the-counter stool softeners.

5

Perfect Home Remedies & Treatment for Constipation, Piles & Anal Fissures

Constipation is most common digestive problems which is a by product of modern dietary habits and sedentary lifestyle. When the waste matter stays for more time in the colon, toxins and fluids are absorbed in the colon and the faecal matter becomes hard. In this condition, bowel movement is irregular, painful or bowels are not emptied completely when it moves. When we sleep our body keeps working to eliminate waste products from our body. Early dinner coupled with stress free sleep of 7 to 8 hours will help our body in proper elimination of these waste products.

Most of the persons suffering from constipation have mild symptoms which are not attributed to any digestive system abnormality or systemic disease. Simple constipation can get cured by healthy eating, taking proper sleep and yoga. Yoga practice can provide an effective remedy for constipation. Yoga will be more effective if it is supplemented with healthy eating and lifestyle changes. You can also start yoga for constipation in addition to other methods of treatment you are following. The benefit of yoga is you get the cure naturally and gradually.

It must be remembered that effect of a given asana is not limited to treating a particular disease. Therefore choose a yoga sequence of asanas which you are comfortable and can practice regularly. The Yoga for constipation poses listed here exercises the abdominal organs and restores their normal function. The muscles of large intestine also become stronger and help in easy waste elimination.

Constipation is supposed to be the main cause of all diseases. Therefore, it should be treated thoroughly. Several other diseases and disorders also crop up if the bowel is constipated. Causes like unbalanced food habits, irregular sleeping pattern, inadequate intake of water, and low physical exercise are few of them. In elderly population, about 70% people are affecting or complaining about it.

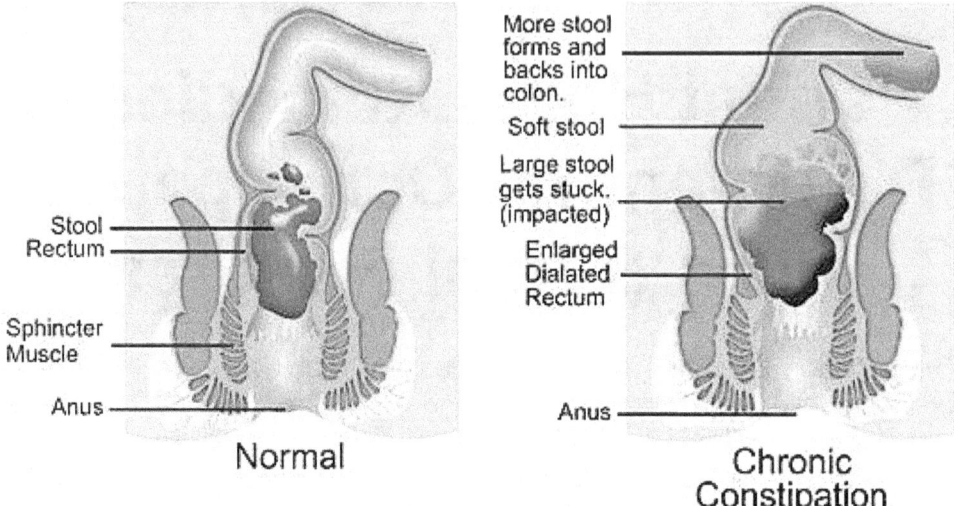

Normal

Chronic Constipation

Home Remedies to prevent constipation:

If you are suffering from constipation, followings are the safe, effective, and natural Home Remedies recommended keeping your bowel in good condition and to treat and relieve constipation are as follow:

- One cup lime juice water could be taken early morning.
- A Spoon of Ginger juice boiled with water taken regularly helps to overcome Constipation.
- Add high fibre foods such as whole grain food, dried fruit, raisins, fresh fruit and vegetables to your diet.
- Avoid alcohol, caffeine, processed and junk food if you are suffering from constipation.
- Avoid regular use of laxatives or enemas.
- Add Bitter gourd (karalla) juice taken regularly or eating Bitter gourd helps to overcome constipation problem.
- Add Buttermilk taken with Carrom seeds (Ajwain) helps to overcome Constipation.
- Drink Juice made of Neem leaves now and then to fight with Constipation. The Tickt rasa in the leaves is proved beneficial for indigestion.
- Drink plenty of liquids such as water, fresh fruit juices and lemon water to stimulate the bowels.

- Drinking 2-3 drops of Castor oil (Errand) with Milk in the night helps to overcome Constipation.
- Drinking at least 12 glasses of water per day preferably hot water in the morning and evening, which helps to cure Constipation.
- Drinking hot milk with Lemon juice or Flea seeds (Isabhagol) in the night to help to overcome Constipation.
- Drinking raw Spinach juice (palak) for few days, which gives permanent relief from Constipation.
- Drinking wheat grass juice regularly helps to overcome constipation problem.
- Dry the leaves of Peepal tree in the shade and powder them. Make pills using adequate amount jiggery and anise solutions with water. Take this pill with warm milk at bed time.
- Eat one ripe Banana before going to bed every day to avoid constipation.
- Eating 250 grams of Fresh Carrot (Gajar) everyday helps to increase appetite and reduce Constipation.
- Eating a Harad (Terminally chebula, hartaki) everyday helps to overcome Constipation.
- Eating a ripe Fig (Anjeeer) in the night or 5 dried figs boiled with Milk or water taken before going to bed helps to overcome Constipation.
- Eating a ripe Mango after meals helps to get relief from Constipation.
- Eating a ripe papita (papaya) before going to bed gives relief from Constipation problem.
- Eating a spoon of powdered Aniseed (Sauf) with hot water in the night helps to cure Constipation.
- Eating Bale fruit or drinking Bale juice everyday helps to overcome Constipation as Bale is a good laxative and having more cooling effect on the body.
- Eating Grapes everyday also helps to overcome Constipation.
- Eating Lentil (Masoor dal) regularly helps to clear the stomach and cures Constipation problem.
- Eating one raw Onion with every meals helps to cure Constipation problem.
- Eating raw Beetroot everyday helps to overcome Constipation.
- Eating raw Cabbage (Patta Gobi) everyday helps to overcome Constipation.
- Eating Watermelon (Tarbooj) regularly for few days helps to cure Constipation problem.

- Exercise
- Few drops of Castor oil mixed with a spoon of Lemon juice taken in the night helps to cure constipation.
- Add Flax seeds in your diet
- Food must be properly chewed. Hurried meals and meals at odd times must be avoided.
- Ginger tea is an effective home remedy for constipation (for babies opt for homeopathic remedies instead of herbal ones).
- Grapes have proved very helpful in overcoming constipation. The combination of the properties of the cellulose, sugar, and organic acid in grapes build them a laxative food.
- High Fibre Diet, like Oats, Wheat, Gram, Mung, Cereals etc.
- Hot water with Lemon juice taken in the night gives relief from Constipation.
- Increase your intake of magnesium by taking supplements or eating foods such as nuts, seeds or green leafy vegetables.
- Massaging the stomach everyday night with Mustard (Sarson) oil helps to cure Constipation problem.
- Normally all fruits, except banana and jackfruit, are useful in the treatment of constipation. Certain fruits are, however, more useful. Bale fruit is regarded as the finest of all laxatives. It cleans and tones up the bowels. Its normal use for two or three months throws out even the old accumulated faecal matter. It must be rather taken in its original form and before dinner. About sixty grams of the fruit are enough for an adult. One of the good home remedies for constipation.
- Opening of the Ileocecal Valve
- Orange is also beneficial in the constipation treatment. Taking one or two oranges at bedtime and again on increasing in the morning is an excellent way of stimulating the bowels.
- Pears are useful in the treatment of constipation. Patients suffering from chronic constipation must accept an exclusive diet of this fruit or its juice for a few days.
- Practice regular bowel habits by visiting the toilet for at least ten minutes after breakfast even if you are unable to have a bowel movement. The best time is usually the first hour after breakfast. Done regularly this will help to set up a healthy bowel routine.
- Radish (Muli) taken with Salt and Black pepper (kali mirch) clears the stomach and gives relief from constipation.
- Regular exercise such as walking or swimming everyday can help to both prevent and relieve constipation.

- Ripe Banana pulp mixed with Curd taken everyday helps to get relief from Constipation.
- Senna is a good remedy to relieve from constipation.
- Sprouted Green gram (Mung) is a good remedy to relieve from constipation.
- Stool softeners taken daily may also prevent constipation.
- Taking a spoon of Triphala (Triphala is composed of Hard (Haritaki), Indian gooseberries (Amla) and Behada (Bibhitaki) every night before going to bed helps to clear the stomach next morning and cures Constipation problem.
- Taking Guava (Amrud) with seeds provides roughage to diet and it acts as a laxative in the intestine. It should be taken only before meals to get relief from Constipation.
- Taking half spoon of Black pepper powder mixed with pure Ghee which helps the stick stool to loosen. Later drink hot milk which helps to clear and stomach and cure Constipation.
- Tomato is also said to be very good for constipation which helps in cleaning the stools which are sticking in the intestine.
- Using Amaranth (Cholayi) regularly in meals also helps to overcome Constipation.
- Using Fenugreek leaves (Methi) in meals also helps to reduce Constipation.
- Using Garlic (Lehsun) regularly in cooking helps to get relief from Constipation.
- Yoga

5.1 Exercise to prevent Constipation:

Here are some exercises you should try out every morning if you want to prevent constipation. Exercise in the morning can do wonders for your health. Constipation may be annoying, but curing constipation is not at all a problem. Exercise is a natural way to relieve and cure chronic constipation. Doing simple but useful exercise can help you in curing constipation easily. Here are the top benefits of performing exercise early in the morning.

Benefit 1 - It regulates your sleep rhythm and balances your hormones.

Benefit 2 - It increases your metabolism and allows you to eat more throughout the day.

Benefit 3 - It stretches your stiff muscles which you haven't used all night and revs up your circulation.

After waking up in the morning, one can do exercise. You don't need a gap between sleep and exercise. After completing your all Kriya, start exercise gently. Exercise is done empty stomach. Early morning exercise is very healthy. Exercise is extremely beneficial remedy in removing constipation, gas and flatulence.

No physical inactivity may cause Constipation. Pregnancy (About 1 in 5 pregnant women will become constipated). It is due to the hormonal changes of pregnancy that slow down the gut movements. In later pregnancy, it can simply be due to the baby taking up a lot of room in the tummy and the bowels being pushed to one side. Problems with the nerves and muscles in the digestive system may cause Constipation. Regular exercise is one of the best ways to get your bowels moving. Walking and other rhythmic exercise massages the intestinal tract and stimulates peristalsis. Pregnant women must do walking everyday to prevent constipation. Regular exercise also helps alleviate the stress that can contribute to constipation. The National Institutes of Health, NIH, says that exercising regularly helps keep your digestion system, including your intestines, healthy and active. The NIH recommends getting about 20 to 30 minutes of exercise every day to help prevent constipation. Stress is also a risk factor for constipation, so try activities like yoga or tai chi that combine exercise and stress reduction. If your bowel habits are sluggish and you suffer constipation, maybe some exercise can help speed things up. According to experts, exercise does more than tone your heart and other muscles. Exercise is essential for regular bowel movements. In fact, one of the key risk factors for constipation is inactivity. Exercise helps constipation by decreasing the time it takes food to move through the large intestine, thus limiting the amount of water absorbed from the stool into the body. Hard, dry stools are harder to pass. In addition, aerobic exercise accelerates your breathing and heart rate. This helps to stimulate the natural contraction of intestinal muscles. Intestinal muscles that contract efficiently help move stools out quickly.

Best Time to Exercise:

Morning is the best time for exercise when your stomach is empty or two hour after a big meal before engaging in any rigorous physical activity. After eating, blood flow increases to the stomach and intestines to help the body digest the food. However, if you exercise right after eating, the blood flows toward the heart and muscles instead. Since the strength of the gut's muscle contractions directly relate to the quantity of blood flowing in the area, less blood in the GI tract means weaker intestinal contractions, fewer digestive enzymes, and the food waste moving sluggishly through the intestine. One of the best choices of exercise for constipation relief is a brisk 10- to 20-minute walk. Make walking a habit by taking a stroll after dinner and before bedtime. This can lead to bloating, excess gas, and constipation. So after a big meal, give your body a chance to digest it before you start on that nature hike. The Best Exercises for Constipation is simply getting up and moving in ground. A regular walking regimen, even 10 to 15 minutes several times a day, can help the body and digestive system function optimally. If you are already fit, you might opt for aerobic exercise: running, jogging, swimming, or swing dancing. All these exercises can help keep the digestive tract healthy. Stretching may also help alleviate constipation, as might certain yoga positions. The slowing down of you bowel movements causes your intestines to swell up having an adverse effect on your health. The result is your stomach sticking out leaving only bloated feelings behind as you worry about how you are going to deal with the problem. This bulge in your stomach is different than the fat you shed while dieting. However, that doesn't mean you can exercise and eat healthy to make it go away. In fact, there are ways you can send constipation away fast and easy with very little effort.

People who need to go on a diet and people who are often constipated are in the same boat. One reason why many people suffer from constipation is that they lack exercise. When your stomach muscles are weak your body can't send food through your bowels as swiftly, or not at all, hence the symptoms of constipation. The first step to fixing constipation is exercise. For pregnant women not able to push their bodies as much as they used to, and people lacking exercise because of sitting at the desk all day are said to be develop constipation easier than most. Exercises and healthy foods that can help rid constipation from your body.

In order to treat constipation by exercising, you need to train the muscles around your stomach, i.e. your abs that work to make your intestines function better, producing smoother bowel movements. Although strength training would work the same way; but we all know how hard that would be.

Best Exercises for Constipation

One of the best choices of exercise for constipation relief is a brisk 10 to 20 minute walk. Make walking a habit by taking a stroll after dinner and before bedtime. If you've eaten a large meal, you may want to wait an hour or so before walking. After you eat, blood flows to the intestines to help you digest your food. If you exercise immediately following a meal, blood will be diverted toward your heart and muscles and away from your digestive tract.

If walking doesn't appeal to you, try yoga. Yoga masters believe that certain yoga positions and breathing exercises aid digestion and strengthen stomach muscles, thus helping to relieve constipation. Whatever exercise you choose, make sure not to overdo it. Extreme exercise might cause diarrhoea, so all things in moderation," he advises. Remember, the key is to get your heart rate going, and you'll get your digestive system going, too. "Really, any exercise, as long as it is not to the extreme, will increase intestinal contractions and improve your digestive health,"

When it comes to constipation, aerobic exercise is the key. While any type of movement will help, exercises that have a slight impact are best. Think running or rebounding. This type of exercise will get things moving simply because of the force it puts on the intestines. With that said, let's start out with some light exercise to ease constipation away. Start from a position lying on the floor similarly to the way you would do flutter kicks while swimming. Extend your legs outward and flutter your legs up and down without losing balance. Next, slightly bend at your knees performing the same flutter kick movements again. Does each portion of the exercise 10 times each? It is very easy.

If your bowel habits are sluggish and you suffer constipation, maybe some exercise can help speed things up. According to experts, exercise does more than tone your heart and other muscles. Exercise is essential for regular healthy bowel movements. In fact, one of the key risk factors for constipation is inactivity.

Exercise helps constipation by decreasing the time it takes food to move through the large intestine, thus limiting the amount of water absorbed from the stool into the body. Hard, dry stools are harder to pass. In addition, aerobic exercise accelerates your breathing and heart rate. This helps to stimulate the natural contraction of intestinal muscles. Intestinal muscles that contract

If you are already fit, you might opt for aerobic exercise: running, jogging, swimming, or swing dancing, for example. All these exercises can help keep the digestive tract healthy. Stretching may also help alleviate constipation, as might certain yoga positions.

Doing simple but useful exercises can help you in curing constipation easily. In this complete course, exercise will help you to recover from the underlying factors of constipation. Choose a time of day you can stick with, so that exercise becomes a habit. No matter what time of day you choose to exercise, make sure to plan your workout two to three hours after your meal.

1. Marching: Stand straight. Raise your both hands up above the shoulders. Now start marching raising your legs simultaneously. While raising your legs pull your abdomen inside. Counting will be right 1 and left 2. Do this for 20 times. Benefits: Marching helps in making more oxygen available for absorption and utilization within the body.

2. Leg crossing: Lie down straight. Place the palms under hips or beside your body. Now lift both legs above the ground by about two feet without bending your knees. In this position, alternatively lift both legs i.e. when we lift the right leg, the left leg will go down. After completing rest your legs on ground. Do this for 10 times. Benefits: Abdominal movement exercise makes easier to pass the stools.

3. Leg flying: Lie down straight on back. Place both hands under hips. Now, lift both the legs together from the ground by about one foot. In this position, stretch right leg to the right side and left leg to the left side. Then return back and again stretch your legs. Do this for 10 times. After completing rest your legs on ground. Benefits: Massages the organs of the abdomen.

4. Leg press and push: Lie down straight on your back. Bend your both legs and put it on the abdomen. With the help of your hands press your legs on abdomen. Then remove your hands and stretch your legs outward without touching the ground. Do this for 10 times. Then put your feet on the ground. Benefits: The pressure on the abdominal muscles helps in bowel movement.

5. Sit up: Lie down straight on back. Place both the hands above the head and keep them on both sides of the ears. Now keeping both the hands straight sit up and touch the toes with your fingers. Head should touch the knees. Again lie down straight with hands straight. Do this for 10 times. Benefits: Sit up strengthens and tones underlying core muscles.

6. Flutter Kicks: Lie flat on your stomach on flat floor sticking your legs together facing downward. Straighten your legs and raise your feet at least 1 foot off the floor one at a time and then put down that raised foot down and lift another leg. Put down this raised leg down and lift

another leg again. Do this lifting of legs alternatively for a period of 10 minutes. Repeat doing 3 full sets. Hand position is fixed by the side of the body.

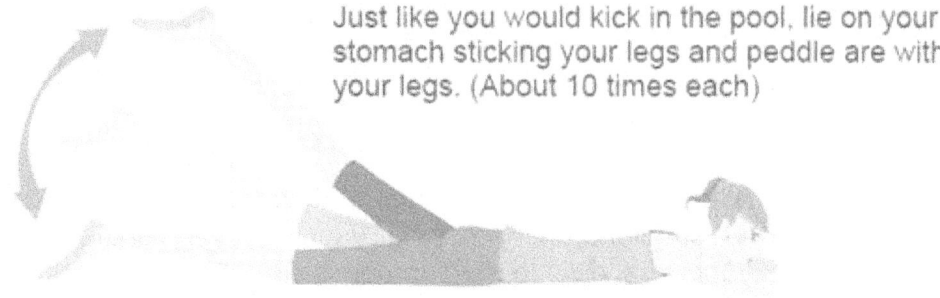

Just like you would kick in the pool, lie on your stomach sticking your legs and peddle are with your legs. (About 10 times each)

6. Leg Lift: Lay flat on the floor facing upward. Straighten your legs and raise your feet at least 1 foot off the floor and hold that position for a period of 10 seconds. Repeat doing 3 full sets. Hand position is fixed by the side of the body.

Lying flat on the floor facing the ceiling, from a straight leg position raise your feet off the floor at least 1 foot and hold for 10 seconds.

Repeat doing 3 sets.

At least 1 foot

7. L-Shaped Tilt: Lay on the floor making an L shaped with your legs. Raise your arms above your chest. Slowly exhaling, tilt your body up to the sitting position. Returning back to a laying position, repeat 5 times.

Lying on the floor, using your legs make an L shape with your body and extend your arms upward. Breathing slowly, tilt your body up to a sitting position. Do this 5 times.

Slowly exhaling lift your body upward

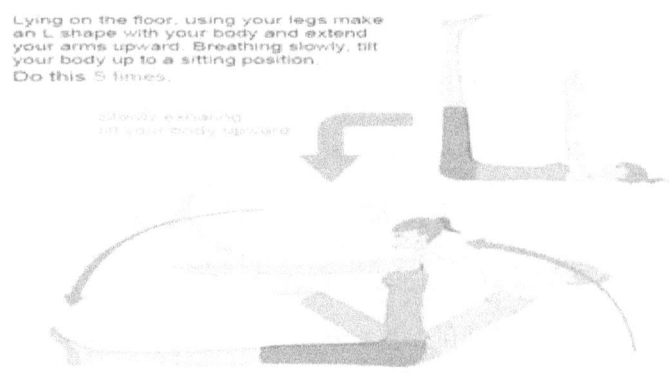

The exercises presented in this article, flutter kicks, leg lifts, and the L-shaped tilt, are best done in the morning right after waking up in bed every day. Brief exercise right after getting out of bed not only helps you wake up; it also gives your abdominal muscles a nice clean stretch before you start your day. Constipation can be permanently cured with the help of yoga and exercise. Lifestyle changes like a good amount of exercise can be really effective. Remember to include a lot of insoluble fibre in your diet by way of whole grains and drinking plenty of water to tackle constipation. Take light meals till you deal with constipation permanently.

5.2 Yoga to prevent Constipation:

Yoga helps constipation to go away permanently. In yoga, there are some exercises and poses that help get rid of constipation. Simple poses include Surya namaskars or sun salutations, Pawanmuktasana or the wind pose, or the tree pose, Shalabhasana or the locust pose, Paschimottansana or the head to knee pose, Dhanurasana or the bow pose, Vajrasana or the diamond pose and Bhujangasana or the cobra pose. There are even some complicated poses like Sarvangasana or the shoulder stand, Maurasana or the peacock pose, Halasana or the plough pose and ardha matsyendra or the half spinal twist. In the different Pranayama, Anulom Vilom and Bhastrika are very effective in dealing with constipation. The Uddiyana Bandha and the Mula Bandha are also two important practices of yoga that help deal with constipation.

Acidity is usually caused by the stomach generating more acids than needed for digestion. Eating well and healthy food is usually the only long term cure for acidity. Eat more roughage and fibre and avoid too many refined foods and stimulants like tea and coffee. Chew food slowly so that you break it down before the food enters the digestive tract. If you suffer from a bad bout of acidity, you can also try yoga as a cure for acidity. Yoga helps the balance in your body get restored. This helps the digestive system return to normal. There are some poses that especially help out in acidity. Meditation and breathing exercises are very good to increase the flow of oxygen to the organs, including the stomach.

Treat Constipation by Yoga and Pranayama:

Most of the persons suffering from constipation have mild symptoms which are not attributed to any digestive system abnormality or systemic disease. Simple constipation can get cured by healthy eating, taking proper sleep and yoga. Yoga practice can provide an effective remedy for constipation. Yoga will be more effective if it is supplemented with healthy eating and lifestyle changes. You can also start yoga for constipation in addition to other methods of treatment you are following. The benefit of yoga is you get the cure naturally and gradually you can get rid of any medication or laxatives.

Yoga Asanas for Constipation

It must be remembered that effect of a given asana is not limited to treating a particular disease. Therefore choose a yoga sequence of asanas which you are comfortable and can practice regularly. The Yoga for constipation poses listed here exercises the abdominal organs and restores their normal function. The muscle of large intestine also become stronger and helps in easy waste elimination.

Simple Poses for Constipation Cure: Surya Namaskara (Sun Salutation Pose), Tada Asana, Trikonasana, Pawanamuktasana, Bhujangasana (Cobra Pose), Shalabhasana (Locust Pose), Dhanurasana (Bow Pose), Yoga Mudra, Paschimottansana (Head to Knee Pose), Vajrasana (Diamond Pose)

Advanced Poses For Constipation Cure. Sarvanghasana (Shoulder Stand), Hal asana (Plough Pose), Mayurasana (Peacock Pose), Ardha Matsyendrasana (Half Spinal Twist)

Yoga Pranayama for Constipation

Yoga breathing exercises help stimulate bowel action. If you suffer from high blood pressure do not attempt Bhastrika and Kapalabhati Pranayama. Agnisar Pranayama (Abdominal Lifts) is an excellent exercise for getting relief from chronic constipation and indigestion. It also strengthens flabby abdominal muscles. Effective Pranayama for constipation cure are Alom Vilom, Agnisar, Bhastrika and Kapalabhati.

Yoga Bandha for Constipation

For constipation relief, Uddiyana Bandha and Mulabandha, done early in the morning are most effective.

Asanas

Asana means 'sitting down', or means a sitting position. The word asana in Sanskrit does appear in many contexts denoting a static physical position, although traditional usage is specific to the practice of yoga. Traditional usage defines asana as both singular and plural. In the context of yoga practice sometimes asana is specified as Yogasana or yoga asana, particularly with regard to the system of the Ashtanga Vinyasa Yoga.

However, Yogasana is also the name of a particular posture that is referred to the eight limbs of Yoga. Yoga first originated in India. In the Yoga Sutras, Patanjali describes asana as the third of the eight limbs of classical, or Raja Yoga. Asanas are the physical movements of yoga practice and, in combination with Pranayama or breathing techniques, constitute the style of yoga referred to as Hatha Yoga. In the Yoga Sutra, Patanjali describes asana as a "steady and comfortable posture", referring specifically to the seated, meditative postures used for meditation practices. He further suggests that meditation is the path to Samadhi; transpersonal self-realization.

In the Yoga Sutras, the only rule Patanjali suggests for practicing asana is that it should be "steady and comfortable". The body is held poised with the practitioner experiencing no discomfort. When control of the body is mastered, practitioners are believed to free themselves from the duality of heat/cold, hunger/satiety, joy/grief, which is the first step toward the no attachment that relieves suffering.

Traditional Rules for Performing Asanas:

Listed below are traditional rules for performing asanas:

- The stomach should be empty.
- Force or pressure should not be used, and the body should not tremble.
- Lower the head and other parts of the body slowly; in particular, raised heels should be lowered slowly.
- The breathing should be controlled. The benefits of asanas increase if the specific Pranayama is performed.
- The body is not stressed,
- Perform Corpse Pose or Child Pose after each Asana.
- Sukhasana or Shavasana help to reduce headaches.

Asana Benefits: The physical aspect of the practice of asanas is considered to:

- improve flexibility
- improve strength

- improve balance
- reduce stress and anxiety
- reduce symptoms of lower back pain be beneficial for asthma and chronic obstructive pulmonary disease (COPD)
- increase energy and decrease fatigue
- shorten labour and improve birth outcomes
- improve physical health and quality of life measures in the elderly
- improve diabetes management
- reduce sleep disturbances
- reduce hypertension
- improve blood circulation
- reduce weight

Guide lines for Asana:

It is advisable to follow the following points to take the full advantage of Yoga asanas:

(1) For practising Yogasana, early morning is the ideal time. Before starting Yoga practices, the bowels and the bladder should be emptied. It is better to do Yogasana after a bath because it makes the body light and active and one can practise Yogasana with greater ease. If one wishes to take a bath again after practising Yogasana, one should use warm water instead of cold water.

(2) The ground for practising asanas should be level, clean and free from noise. Asanas should be practised on a mat or a carpet.

(3) Clothing should be in accordance with the season. Men should wear a loincloth or shorts. Women should wear a loose blouse and stretch pants.

(4) One should remain silent while practising asanas. While practising asanas, concentration should be on breathing and on the limbs which have a stress or strain. Concentration in the practice of Yoga asanas is necessary for the all round progress of the body and the mind.

(5) Before one begins to practise other asanas, one should perform Shavasana in order to make breathing normal, the body and the mind tranquil.

(6) Yogasana is a non-violent activity and therefore no force or jerk should be exerted in the practice of Yogasana.

(7) There should be a gradual increase in the time duration in the practice of Yogasana. By this process, the body becomes flexible and in a short time, it will easily accomplish a perfect state in each asana.

(8) Yoga asana is a scientific process which deals with the internal and external parts of the body. A beginner should start practising

Yogasana after having learnt all their techniques under proper guidance.

(9) The performer of asanas should take light food in order to keep the body light.

(10) If one is suffering from complicated diseases or severe fever, one should not practise asanas. Women should not practise asanas four months after conception, for three months after delivery and during menstruation. A woman aspirant should not as far as possible perform, without proper guidance asanas which involve lifting up the weight of the whole body on her hands.

(11) The number of asanas and the duration for each of them should be increased gradually. Practising many asanas on the first day should be avoided.

(12) Haste or quickness in coming to the final position from the initial position and vice versa should be avoided.

(13) After practising Yogasana, Shavasana should be performed. Shavasana is a perfect asana. By Shavasana, the body gets speedy relaxation and becomes energetic.

(14) Yogasana are supposed to be performed advantageously in the right direction if the aspirant, after practising Yogasana, feels no tiredness and has an increased capacity to work with his light and refreshed body.

Science, Benefits and Insights of Asana:

The science of asanas is known as Hatha Yoga. "Ha" means sun, "ta" means moon. The first process of yoga is to bring balance between the masculine and feminine in you. Otherwise there will be no scaling of consciousness. An asana is a posture. There are innumerable postures your body can take. The Hatha yoga of the sun and the moon is bringing balance between the masculine and the feminine. That is the first step to take.

Among these, certain postures have been identified as "yoga asanas" or also called Yogasana. "Yoga" means that it takes you on to a higher dimension or higher perception of life and the kind of posture which leads you to a higher possibility is called a "Yogasana." Yogasana are not exercises. They are very subtle processes of manipulating your energy in a certain direction. It needs to be done with a certain level of awareness. There are various levels of doing asanas. You can practice asanas just physically, or more deeply, being aware of the breath, sensations, reverberations, being aware of the Nadi, or with appropriate mantras and without moving a limb.

Asana Siddhi: People generally take up one asana for their life's sadhana for Hatha yoga as their way of life. This is known as Asana Siddhi. Asana Siddhi means one is able to sit in a particular way with absolute ease. When you give your body to the process of yoga, slowly the body becomes at ease. When you sit like this, it is absolutely at ease and this is your Asana Siddhi.

Yogasana is just to get your body geometrically in line with the cosmic geometry by having mastery over a single physical posture. When you learn to just hold it rightly, you can download the whole cosmos and this is yoga.

Ease and stability in Asana: Patanjali describes asana as the third limb of yoga, which is "Sthira, Sukhasana". If you are comfortable and stable, that is all the asana is about. When your body is at ease, your mind is at ease, and your energy is at full vibrancy and balance and so you are naturally meditative. You will find full potential to your life.

No Talk during asanas: An asana is a dynamic way of meditating. Patanjali said Sthira Sukhasana. That which is absolutely stable and comfortable is an asana. This means your body is at ease, your mind is at ease, and your energy is vibrant and balanced. Asanas are a preparatory step to come to a state of being naturally meditative. In a way, asanas are a dynamic way of meditating. Talking during asana triggers a number of changes in your system. Speaking not only changes the physiological parameters, but even the energy parameters change dramatically. Above all, you need to focus during an asana. Asanas are a preliminary meditative state and so one cannot talk in meditation. Speaking can cause serious imbalance. There should be no talking while doing an asana. If you speak while doing an asana, you will disturb the breath, the mental focus, and the stability of your energy system.

Air temperature and mixture: If you breathe in hot air, even though there is enough oxygen, you will gasp as if you were in high altitude. The human body is comfortable at a certain temperature and it needs a certain air mixture. Even a small change in the air temperature will affect it, but the body has correction measures if you are breathing properly. It will correct itself for the rareness of air and for even a small change in the air temperature. Creating ease to explore other dimensions is yoga. To bring the body to such ease, you must breathe slightly deeper than normal, and over time, in any asana with the perfect posture. When body comes to a state of ease, there will be no disease.

Closing the eyes: The world disappears, if you close the eyes. Your imagination is running wild because you have no control over it, and if you close your eyes, the world is gone for you. When you do an asana, you want to internalize everything. One basic step towards any internalization is to close your eyes. Best way to shut off the world is to lose your vision. For a human being, vision is the most dominant sense and once you close your eyes, half the world is shut off. So, internalization works best when your eyes are closed.

Control of negative emotions (anger): The physical body and the mind are the two basic vehicles without which you cannot go through this life. The whole system of yoga is about exploring and controlling the nature of your body and your mind. When you get up in the morning and do asanas, it is not because it is a stretching exercise, but because, it is an exploration of your body and your mind.

Understanding the Life vehicle: For the life journey to be comfortable, the life vehicle has to be good, and you must understand the vehicle also, that how it behaves, what it does, and why it does. How comfortably you travel through your life depends on how deeply you have grasped your body and your mind. That is why the yogic system is an experiential exploration without trying to go into it intellectually. When you do your asanas, you explore the nature of your body and your mind. If you move your fingers in a certain way, your mind will function accordingly. Everything that you do with your body does something with your mind. You will not come to this understanding by reading a book. It will come to you only by exploration. If you close your eyes and try to forcefully remove something from your mind, you will never be successful. This is the most basic and at the same time the most important realization that everyone needs to come to. Without this realization, you will make a complete mess out of yourself. If you are not so sharp in your head, it will be okay. But if you are sharp, you will cut yourself all over, and before anyone can save you, you will be mutilated, because you have a very sharp knife.

Fundamentals of Asana:

Understanding the fundamentals of Yogasana, we need to do it, hold the body in one posture, and see how mind functions in a certain way. Hold the body in another posture, and see the mind functions in a different way. So do asana and explore the nature of your body and your mind. Hatha Yoga is a preparatory work. If you stay in an asana and breathe properly, as you go through this process, the mind will go into various states. The exploration is the most fundamental aspect of yoga. Some amount of physical preparation is needed, because body and mind are not two separate things. Those who want to benefit from the technology should simply learn to use it.

1. Padmasana: Position (Sanskrit: Padmasana) is a cross legged sitting asana originating in meditative practices of ancient India, in which the feet are placed on the opposing thighs. It is an established asana, commonly used for meditation, in the Hindu, Jain and Buddhist Yoga contemplative traditions. Padmasana is the asanas traditionally used for dhyana (meditation) and Pranayama. The asana is said to resemble a lotus, (Lotus Pose) to encourage breathing proper to associated meditative practice, and to foster physical stability. Padmasana means "Lotus throne" and is also a term for actual thrones, often decorated with lotus foliage motifs, on which figures in art sit. This is the easiest asana which can be done by all the age group of men and women they can get benefits of all asana. Padmasana is much suited for the Pranayama. It provides a good workout for body and is good for mind and breathing. It conditions the body and core, and increases flexibility. When you first start doing Padmasana, your muscles quickly adapt. Padma Means Lotus position. Asana indicates the seat which in turn indicates sitting in a position without any movement (Lotus Pose). Practice of Padmasana: Sit on mat on the floor and stretch the legs. Now hold the right leg in both the hands, fold the legs slowly and place it on the left thigh. Make sure that its sole is facing upward and heel is close to the abdomen. Likewise fold the left leg, hold it with both the hands and place it on the right thigh in a symmetrical way. At this point both the knees should touch the floor and the foot should face upwardly. The torso is placed in balance and alignment such that the spinal column supports it with minimal muscular effort. The torso is cantered above the hips. To relax the head and neck, the jaw is allowed to fall towards the neck and the back of the neck to lengthen. The spinal cord should be straight. The shoulders move backwards and the ribcage lifts. The tongue rests on the roof of the mouth. The hands may rest on the knees in chin or Janna mudra. The arms are relaxed with the elbows slightly bent. The eyes may be closed, the body relaxed, with awareness of the overall asana. Adjustments are made until balance and alignment are experienced. Alignment that creates relaxation is indicative of a suitable position for the asana. The asana should be natural and comfortable, without any sharp pains. In most cases, a cushion or mat is necessary in order to achieve this balance. One sits on the forward edge of the cushion or mat in order to incline one's pelvis forward, making it possible to centre the spine and provide the necessary support. Only the most flexible people can achieve this asana without a support under their pelvis. If you feel difficulty in sitting in the posture for a long time you can change the legs and then sit on the same position. Spinal cord should be erect, both the hands should be either together one above the other; or put the palms on the knee joints facing upside and the thumb must touch the index finger and the other fingers should be straight facing upward. Do this Padmasana for one minute then open the eyes slowly, open the palm then release the left leg first then release the right leg. Stretch the legs and relax. Do this asana for 15 to 30 minutes. Precautions: Should not bend the body while doing this asana. Health Benefits: Padmasana is the highly preferred asanas by yoga practitioner for increase the focus of mind and concentration. It helps Calms the brain. It increases the hunger. It helps to relax the body. The Lotus position is adopted to allow the body to be held completely steady for long periods of time. This allows the mind to calm the first step towards meditation. The asana applies pressure to the lower spine which may facilitate relaxation. The breath can slow down, muscular tension can decrease and blood pressure may subside. The coccygeal and sacral nerves are toned as the normally large blood flow to the legs is redirected to the abdominal region, which may help to improve digestion. The practice of this asana leads to a straight spinal cord. It is believed that sitting in this posture causes good thoughts to come to the mind and thoughts of anger and lust to subside. The practice of this asana with repetition of OM leads to reduction in stress. It stretches the ankles and knees and helps to stimulate the abdomen, spine and bladder. This asana is the base for all asanas and it strengthens the hip and knee joints of the female and can get painless peaceful mind. The unwanted fat will be reduced in hip and the thigh. It stretches the spine.

2. Shavasana (Corpse Pose): The name comes from the Sanskrit words Sava meaning "corpse", and Asana meaning "posture" or "seat". Shavasana is known as the corpse pose or Mritasana (death pose). Shavasana is designed to give your body the opportunity to relax and recover from the exertion of other yoga poses. This pose also offers wonderful meditative benefits; completing this pose has been shown to help reduce stress and improve academic performance in its practitioners. Relaxation and meditation are the key components. Shavasana and sitting postures maintain the balance by their equal input of physical stimuli. Yoga Nidra is a deep mental relaxation approach. Shavasana is perhaps the most important part of yoga practice. Preparation for Pose: Pick the fully ventilated location with quietness. Keeping a peaceful mind perform Shavasana correctly and focus on your breathing and meditation. Make sure the room has a comfortable temperature and a comfortable surface to lie on. Extreme temperatures in heat or cold could distract you from the mental calmness of the pose. You will have to lie down fully in the Shavasana pose and so you must have enough space to complete the pose. This means your legs will extend past your mat. You must have a yoga mat or towels to give you a buffer on hardwood floors. Avoid practicing this pose on concrete or tile floors without a mat. Maintain your space. The Shavasana pose has wonderful benefits for the back and abdominal muscles. Mental benefits of Shavasana give you the power to control and minimize negative thoughts, which can lead to stress, anxiety or depression. Practice: Lie down on your back. As you recline on your yoga mat, place your feet spread slightly (one and half foot) apart from each other. Put your arms straight at your side spread slightly (one foot) apart from your body with your palms facing up. The arms and legs are spread at about 30 to 40 degrees, the eyes are closed and the breath is normal. Your fingers should be curled up in natural way. Close your eyes and focus on the centre point of eye brows and your breathing. Breathe from your diaphragm generously. Relax your body. Take out any anxiety, stress or negative thoughts while you are performing this pose. Imagine your mind emptying all these into the sky. The whole body is relaxed onto the floor with an awareness of the chest and abdomen rising and falling with each breath. Try to relax your body all at once and don't feel pressure to rush into relaxation. Gradually breathe in and out to feel your body is relaxing on the floor. All parts of the body are scanned for muscular tension of any kind, which is consciously released as it is found, optionally with a small repetitive movement of the area. All control of the breath, the mind, and the body is then released for the duration of the asana, typically 20–30 minutes. Shavasana then becomes the beginning of deeper, meditative yogic practices and in state of sensory withdrawal it becomes easier to be aware of the breath and of the state of the mind itself. There is no time limit for this pose. If you have completed 45-60 minutes of yoga exercises, try relaxing in the Shavasana pose for 10 minutes to fully appreciate your session. It is not unusual to fall asleep in this pose, but doesn't sleep, but feel that your body is lying on floor without any movement in the body like a corpse. Make sure that you do not have an important meeting or event afterward. Recovering from the corpse Pose: Awaken your sense and body. Begin by wiggling your toes and fingers, then ankles, knees, heaps, elbow, shoulder joints and finally your neck. Then cover your eyes with both palms and open your eyes slowly at last by chanting the Mantra, "OM BRAHMA – BISHNU – MAHESHWARAI NAMAHA";

OR "OM LAXAMI – SRSWATI – GOVINDAI NAMAHA". Imagine that you are opening up to a new body as you come out of the pose. Shavasana should give you a sense of renewal and rebirth. Roll out your pose. Turn onto your right side. Then, slowly push yourself to an upright position using your right elbow. Maintain your breathing so you exhale as you push up onto your right elbow. Benefit: It is intended to rejuvenate body, mind, and spirit. Shavasana allows the body a chance to regroup and reset itself. The muscles will have the opportunity to let go and shed their regular habits. It helps the body to regulate with respect to, a decrease in heart rate and the rate of respiration, a decrease in blood pressure, a decrease in muscle tension, a decrease in metabolic rate and the consumption of oxygen, a reduction in general anxiety, a reduction in the number and frequency of anxiety attacks, an increase in energy levels and in general productivity, an improvement in concentration and in memory, an increase in focus, and Integration. Shavasana practice will furnish the nervous system with a host of new neuromuscular information and gives the nervous system a chance to integrate that in what can be thought of as a brief pause before it is forced once again to deal with all the usual stresses of daily life. Precautions: Comfort is essential in the asana and the slightest point of discomfort can be endlessly distracting. Shavasana is a good way to reduce stress and tension. On the other hand, yoga-Nidra ("yogic sleep") meditation is often practiced in a lying position. Drowsiness or restlessness of the mind while in Shavasana may be counteracted by increasing the rate and depth of breathing. Shavasana is a relaxation asana which may involve cooling after exertion.

3. Sarvangasana (Candle Pose): Lie down on your back. Keep your feet together and let your hands be by your side. Put pressure on your hands and raise your legs slowly to an angle of 90°. Then raise your spine to the same angle. Keep this position for 10 seconds. Then slowly lower your body to the ground and rest. Repeat this four times.

4. Siddhasana: The name Siddhasana comes from the Sanskrit words Siddha meaning both "perfect" and "adept", and asana meaning "posture" or "seat". Siddhasana. Siddhasana means a posture for uncovering hidden powers. The Siddhasana posture is the first step towards the yogic practice of 'Samadhi'. One, who masters the Siddhasana pose, can easily conquer himself. The pose teaches disciplining of the senses and improves concentration. The Accomplished Pose for men and women is the same, and both can reap the benefits of this pose if they continue to perform it regularly. Practice: It is a seated position and is considered one of the most satisfying in the seated postures. The Siddhasana pose is considered a purification pose, helping you cleanse about 72,000 of the body's energy paths or Nadi. The pose is helpful in attaining spiritual uplifting. In Siddhasana pose, sit straight on the floor, with both your legs outstretched right in front of you. Keep your feet vertical and parallel to each other, with the balls of your heels firmly planted on the ground. Bend the left leg at the knee, bringing the left heel to your perineum. Once your heel begins to touch the perineum, fold your right leg from the knee and let the right heel rest against the area of the pubic bone. One heel is brought to press on the perineum with the sole of the foot flat against the inner thigh. The body sits on the side of this heel. Adjustments are made until the body is comfortable and the pressure is firmly applied. Allow the right foot to stay in a downward angle. Then the opposite ankle is placed over the first, so the ankle bones are touching and the heels are above one another with the top heel pressing the pubis directly above the genitals. The genitals will then lie in between the two heels. Place one ankle on top of the other so that there is no pressure on the genitals. The gentle downwards angle of the right foot should be able to help you with that. Allow both your knees to touch the floor along with your left heel. Lengthen your spine and sit straight. Stretch your arms forward and place both your hands on each of the knees. Let the tip of your thumb meet the index finger on each of the hands with the rest of the fingers straight. The toes and outer edge of the top foot are pushed down into the space between the calf and thigh muscles. The toes of the bottom foot are pulled up into the similar space on the opposite side. The spine is held erect. A small meditation cushion or mat is used to aid vertical back alignment. Siddhasana Pose for women is accomplished in which heel is placed firmly against or inside the labia majora of the vagina and the top heel is placed so it presses the clitoris. Close your eyes and meditate. Try to clear your head and fix your attention on one point in space. Keep breathing normally and stay in the pose for a few seconds, or possibly minutes if you are an advanced practitioner. You can repeat the pose again after reversing the order in which you folded your legs earlier. Continue breathing normally and remain in the pose for around the same time you did the previous cycle. Siddhasana is the asanas is used for dhyana or meditation and Pranayama. Sukhasana (Pleasant Pose) is a substitute that is easier on the knees. Many people are not able to practice Padmasana for them Siddhasana is highly recommended. It can be done in another way to with slight variations like: In the first variation, the practitioner is advised to place the two feet in a manner that the penis is clamped between them. In the second variation, both the heels should be placed above the penis to redirect the blood forcefully to the genitals. Benefits: Siddhasana has a lot of benefits, such as, the impetus to a healthy circulation system, and stimulates the Muladhara Chakra that is located in the pelvic region, the Swadishtana Chakra, which located slightly north of the Muladhara Chakra; stimulation of chakras can further redirect the nervous impulses of sexuality, and therefore control the reproductive hormones in the body. The Siddhasana pose reduces the strain on the knees, ankles and hips by strengthening them and making more nourishment available to them; the stimulation of the blood flow to the genitals further helps to improve continence; to improve sexual disorders, cardiac function and blood pressure and other health conditions like piles and haemorrhoids. In men, Siddhasana helps regulate the flow of the hormone testes and controls masculine emotions as well as sexual metabolism and also prevents problems such as nocturnal emissions. The posture is useful in redirecting the blood circulation to the abdomen and lower spine and thus makes a lot of blood available to the pelvis, abdominal region and reproductive system. This pose helps to reduce weight and to treat asthma and insomnia. Precautions: It is best to avoid performing it when you have certain physical ailments and problems like having any surgeries, especially on their back or hip; those who suffer from pain in the lower back and sciatica and People with knee pain, arthritis or recent knee injuries.

5. Sukhasana: Sukhasana is (soo – kah – sah - nah) an easy Pose, decent Pose, or Pleasant Pose and is practised in Yoga, Buddhism and Hinduism. Sukhasana or the easy sitting pose is one of the simplest pose for meditation suited for all beginners. Sukhasana comes from the Sanskrit work 'Sukha' which can mean 'comfort' , 'easy', 'joyful' and 'pleasure'. Sukhasana can be done by all age groups. Sukhasana is part of the daily routine. Traditionally people would take their meals sitting on the floor in Sukhasana. Hence for them, Sukhasana is simple. Sukhasana is the simplest of the sitting postures in yoga. It is easy to perform and can be done even by elderly people. Practice: This is a seated position, which brings your knees into a simple cross legged pose. Sit on the floor with legs stretched out. Always use a yoga mat or a cushion or a carpet while sitting on the floor. Fold the left leg and tug it inside the right thigh. Then fold the right leg and tug in inside the left thigh. Keep the hands on the knees and rest it on the knees or the lap with the palms facing up. Janna mudra or Chin mudra can be used if you are using this posture for meditation. Sit with erect spine straight. Relax your whole body and breathe normally. Maintain this position for as long a comfortable. Both knees should be below the hips. Place the hands on the thighs or knees and keep the spine straight. Benefits: It opens the hips and stretches the knees and ankles; strengthens the back; calms the mind, reduces stress and anxiety and improves circulation and blood flow to the pelvis. Sukhasana is the most suited sitting posture for beginners. It opens your hips; lengthens spine; promotes grounding and inner calm; amplifies the state of serenity, tranquillity, and eliminates anxiety; relieves physical and mental exhaustion and tiredness and is good for practice of meditation and Pranayama. This is good for those who have tight hips cannot sit in advanced postures like Padmasana. For them Sukhasana is the easiest alternative. Once you are comfortable with Sukhasana, you should move on to more advanced sitting postures like Padmasana or Siddhasana for meditation. If you are meditating for less than 30 minutes per session, Sukhasana may be sufficient. But to hold the body steady for longer durations, one needs to adopt more advanced sitting postures. Precautions: Those with serious knee or hip injuries should avoid this posture. It is similar to sitting in a simple cross legged position while opening the hips and lengthening the spine, vertical erect. The asanas relative ease on the knees makes it easier than Siddhasana or Padmasana for people with physical difficulties. For meditation or Pranayama, it is important that the spine is straight and aligned with the head and neck. But if the practitioner steadies the Sukhasana pose by putting pillows or blankets under the knees to create a steadiness, it may be easier to sit longer in Sukhasana for meditation without slumping forward. An additional blanket or pillow under the buttocks may also be beneficial and steadying. This Asana is suitable for attaining Enlightenment. The name comes from the Sanskrit words Sukha meaning pleasure", and Asana (Asana) meaning "posture" or "seat".

6. Simhasana: Simhasana is a Lion Pose. The name comes from the Sanskrit words Simha meaning "lion", and asana meaning "posture" or "seat". The asana resembles a seated lion; hence the name Simha (lion in Sanskrit) came for this asana. The practitioner's facial expressions are modified to resemble a lion. The Lion Face Gesture (Simha Mudra) is performed. Practice: The lion pose is pretty simple to execute. Although there may be a number of steps, this pose really requires very little effort. For the lion pose, sit with your legs folded under you so that your toes are pointing straight behind and you are sitting on your heels. Keep your spine straight and erect but as relaxed as possible. Close your eyes and look to your third eye. (The third eye is a symbolic eye in the centre of the forehead). Closing your mouth, touch your palette with your tongue. Inhale a deep breath through your nose while your tongue is still touching your palette. Exhale in one violent move while sticking out your tongue and opening your jaws as much as possible. Put your arms thrown out, straight and stretched with your fingers splayed downward on your knee. Roar at the top of your voice while exhaling. The roar should be with a "Haa" sound and should not be a long drawn out one. Rather, it should be one violent explosion of breath that empties your lungs in the shortest time possible. Hold this pose for 20 to 30 seconds. Does not inhale immediately after this pose; inhale after the specified 20 to 30 seconds. Repeat this process 5 or 6 times. This asana (posture) gets its name from the way you stick your tongue out as far as possible and the way you hold your fingers splayed out, resembling a roaring lion. The pose can be repeated as many times as you wish, although if properly done, 5 to 6 times are sufficient. Variations: Since the Simhasana is such an easy pose, there are not too many variations. However, since the focus is on relaxation, different people make slight variations to the way they perform the pose. Listed below are some of the variations for lion pose. Variation 1: Some people like to sit with their ankles crossed, so that you sit on one heel instead of two. Variation 2: As you are supposed to sit completely relaxed and because the most relaxed position while holding this sitting position is to have your hands on your knees, many people do that and just splay their fingers while exhaling. Variation 3: Some use the same pose, but laugh instead of roar in order to reduce stress. Variation 4: Instead of closing the eyes and looking to the third eye, this pose is sometimes held with the eyes open and looking to the tip of the nose. The Simhasana has to be a violent release of tension. Benefits: The stretching of the tongue helps with voice related difficulties e.g., stammering and throat related problems e.g., hoarseness and tonsillitis. The asana has been claimed to aid better functioning of the carotid sinus, the sinus nerves, the larynx, and the thyroid and parathyroid glands. The carotid bodies assist in maintaining normal blood pressure and heartbeats. The breathing exercise is claimed to help the chest and abdomen. The Lion Pose effectively gives an outlet for the negative energy. Physically the lion pose benefits the Face and the Throat, Eyes, Respiratory tract, Tongue, Vocal chords, Abdomen, Chest, Diaphragm, Fingers and Hands. The violent stretching of the muscles of the face and the throat relieve tension; any infection of the throat and the respiratory tract. The tongue also receives unaccustomed exercise because it is stretched out fully outside the mouth. Therapeutic usages of the lion pose include: Curing bad breadth; Curing stutters; Curing teeth grinding; Curing clenched jaws; removing wrinkles; Helping in decreased burning in eyes; Reliving back pain; Relaxing tensed up neck muscles; improving the tone of the voice; stimulates the platysma, which is a flat thin muscle in the front of the throat. This is the muscle that pulls down the corners of the mouth and also wrinkles the throat. It is believed that this exercise will help to prevent the sagging of the throat with age. Additionally, this pose helps promote good posture and in turn increases confidence levels. Precautions: The Lion Pose is basically a stress reliever and can be practiced at anytime and by anybody. There are usually no problems associated with practicing this pose because it does not require any complicated manoeuvring of the body. However, if you suffer from any chronic illnesses or physical problems, it is best that you have a discussion with your doctor before you attempt any yoga posture.

7. Vajrasana: Vajrasana or the kneeling yoga pose is also called the diamond pose or the thunderbolt pose. The name comes from the Sanskrit word 'Vajra' which can mean thunderbolt or diamond. Normally, Asanas should be performed on an empty stomach. But, Vajrasana is one of the few exceptions. This asana can be done immediately after the meal. In fact, it is most effective after the meal and aids in proper digestion. Vajrasana is a "Vajra Pose", and is a sitting asana in yoga. It is position sitting on the knees. The name comes from the Sanskrit words Vajra meaning "thunderbolt" or "diamond like", asana (meaning "posture" or "seat". Practice: Sit on your heels. Your buttocks will be resting on the heels and the thighs on the calf muscles with the calves beneath the thighs. Keep your hands on your knees and keep the head straight. Concentrate on the breath and observe the process of inhalation and exhalation. Close the eyes to get good concentration and to calm the mind. Remain in this position for at least 5 to 10 minutes. In the initial stages, there may be pain in the legs when you sit in this position. When that happens, undo the asana and stretch your legs. Massage the ankles, knees and calf muscles with your hand. With practice one can go up to 30 minutes sitting in this position. There is a four finger gap between the knee-caps, and the first toe of both the feet touch each other and sit erect. Benefits: Benefits of Vajrasana (The Thunderbolt Pose) is that it modifies the blood flow in the lower pelvic region. It's considered the best to do Vajrasana just after having food but you can do it at any time of the day. The blood flow to the legs is reduced and the blood flow to the digestive organs is increased. This increases the efficiency of the digestive system and helps those with weak digestion to digest a full meal easily. It helps to prevent acidity and ulcers by improving the digestion. It is a good meditative pose for those suffering from sciatica and severe lower back problems. Slow and rhythmic breathing in this position can induce a meditative state. This asana helps in digestive issues like constipation. It also strengthens the muscles of the legs and back; helps in digestion; in reduction of the hips; getting rid of constipation; fight stomach disorder; mind calming and relaxing; increasing the blood circulation in the body; weight loss; curing urinary problem; making the lower body flexible; in combating acidity; in strengthening the sexual organs; in toning of body muscles like the hips, thighs and the calf muscles; in curing various body ailments like varicose veins and joint pains and is a magic pose for people suffering from arthritis as it acts as a painkiller. Precautions: Don't do this asana if you have a knee problem; or leg injury, please do not do this without expert guidance or if had a recent knee surgery, as it may put additional strain on the knee. Also, pregnant women should try this asana with their knees apart to avoid stress on the abdomen. Vajrasana may be harmful to knees. It has also been linked to damage to the common fibular nerve resulting in foot drop, where dorsiflexion of the foot is compromised and the foot drags (the toe points) during walking; and in sensory loss to the dorsal surface of the foot and portions of the anterior, lower lateral leg. In this context it has been called "yoga foot drop".

8. Swastikasana: Swastikasana (Auspicious Pose) is an easy meditation pose for those who cannot attempt the more difficult asanas like Padmasana and Siddhasana. In Swastikasana, the position of the legs resembles the symbol of the Swastika. The word Swastika comes from the Sanskrit root words 'Su' meaning good, 'Asti' means 'to be' or 'existence' and 'Ka' means to make. Svastikasana when split into "Su-asti-ka" also means "being well and healthy". Hence, among the meditative postures, Svastikasana is considered as an auspicious sign. This asana can be described as one that helps to realize the unity of existence. Swastikasana is relatively easy to perform and can be used for meditative purposes and for prolonged sitting. Practice: Sit on the floor with legs spread out in front of you. Fold the left leg and place the sole of the left leg against the inner thigh of the right leg. Bend the right leg and place the right foot in the space between the left thigh and calf muscles. Grasp the left foot by the toes and pull it up and place it between the right calf and thigh. The knees should firmly touch the floor. Adjust the pose so that you feel comfortable. Keep the body and trunk straight. The hands can be placed on the knees in any of the classical meditation mudra like Chin mudra or Jnana mudra. Awareness can be maintained on the breath. One may also concentrate on the tip of the nose or the eye brow centre. Benefits: Swatikasana is a good meditation pose for those who find it difficult to sit in more classical poses like Padmasana and Siddhasana. Swastikasana is a healthy position to sit in, especially for those suffering from varicose veins, tired and aching muscles or fluid retention in the legs. It increases balance in body and mind. It helps to maintain normal body temperature. It tones the abdominal muscles. It improves the strength of the backbone. It tones the sciatic nerve. Precautions: Swastikasana should not be done by those suffering from sciatica and sacral infections. You should sit straight and your supine should be erect to avoid back injury. The soles of the feet should be between the thigh and the calf muscles to avoid calf and hamstring injury.

9. Shirshasana: This posture may look imposing to those who haven't attempted it. Nevertheless, it is an extremely powerful asana. It is called the "king of asanas" because of its overall effect on the whole body. For beginners, it is better to ask a friend to help you with this in the beginning. Shirshasana Technique: 1. Start by kneeling down on your yoga mat. Interlock the fingers of your hands and place them and your forearms on the yoga mat. Keep the elbows fairly close together. 2. Then place the back of your head into the hollow of the palms (not on the palms or fingers). 3. Now rise up off your knees and take a step or two towards your head. Inhale, and slowly raise the legs until they are vertical. Keep your back straight and try to relax. Breathe slowly and deeply from the abdomen. 4. Concentrate on the brain or the pineal gland between the eyebrows. Bend your knees and lower one leg and then the other and then come down slowly. Benefits: 1. Headstand increases circulation to the brain, which causes improved brain function (intelligence and memory) and increased vitality and confidence. It improves many ailments, such as nervousness, tension, fatigue, sleeplessness, dullness, fear, poor blood circulation, bad memory, asthma, headaches, constipation, congested throat and liver or spleen. 2. Adding to the benefits list this asana stimulates four of the most important endocrine glands - the pituitary, the pineal, the thyroid, and the parathyroid glands that are responsible for our very existence. They also keep the body mechanism in good working order. The pituitary gland is called the master gland of the body. 3. If you are losing hair and worried about getting bald soon or later then this asana might help - The headstand promotes hair growth by increasing circulation to the scalp. 4. The headstand or Shirshasana can help you out to cure sleeping disorder. The headstand causes an increase in circulation to the neck, which stimulates the bar receptors in the neck. This calms the reticular formation down, causing reduced nerve impulses to the cerebral cortex. As a result, you sleep well. Caution: Don't do the headstand if you have high or low blood pressure. Atherosclerosis (blocked blood vessels) and any history of strokes is also a deterrent to doing the headstand. You must improve your circulatory system first, before attempting it. If you have any serious eye diseases, ask your eye specialist's first before doing the headstand. If you suffer from a neck injury or advanced arthritis in your neck, then doing this exercise should be a strict no-no.

10.   Matsya Asana (Fish Pose): Lie on your back and keep your hands at your side. Bend your knees completely. With the help of your head, hands and legs, raise your chest. Keep this position in place for about 30 seconds and then release it. Practice this four times in a day. You can also practice this position without bending your knee. Some other asanas are Shirsha Asana (Headstand), Chakrasana (Wheel Pose), Uttanasana (Standing Forward Bend pose), Sarvanga Asana (The Shoulder stand), Tada Asana (The Mountain Pose), Padahasta Asana (Hand to Foot Pose), Surya Namaskara (Sun Salutation), Pavanamukta Asana (The Wind Releasing Pose), and Pranayama (Breathing Control). As you can see, piles and yoga go hand in hand.

11. Dhanurasana (Bow Pose): Dhanurasana Bow Pose strengthens total abdominal organs. It strengthens ankles, thighs, groins, chest and abdominal organs and spinal cord. Those suffering from digestion problems should practice Dhanurasana for 3 to 4 minutes.

Vajrasana	Dhanurasana	Suryanamaskar

12.   Suryanamaskar (Sun   salutation): Suryanamaskar (Sun salutation) consists of 12 different poses which gives total exercise to whole body. Suryanamaskar improves the digestive system and cures constipation. It helps to reduce weight.

13. Bhujangasana (Cobra Pose): Bhujangasana (Cobra Pose) is effective and beneficial for improving the function of digestion. This yoga pose strengthens the abdominal muscles, clean digestive tract and cures constipation and indigestion problems naturally.

Bhujangasana	Halasana	Pavanamuktasana

14. Halasana (Plough Pose): Hal asana is known as Plough pose which strengthens the back muscles and gives flexibility. It cures indigestion and constipation as well as reduces stress. It stimulates the abdominal organs and digestion problems.

15. Pavanamuktasana (Wind Removing Pose): Pavanamuktasana is really effective in removing gases from the stomach and improving the digestive system. It is one of the best yoga poses for constipation and indigestion which increases your bowel movement. It strengthens the abdominal organs, cures acidity, eases digestion problems and reduces fat.

Ardha Hal asana	Paschimottansana	Uttanpadasana

16. Ardha Hal asana (Half Plough Pose): Half Plough Pose is similar to Uttanpadasana which is good for improving the function of abdominal organs. Stimulates abdominal organs very fast and cures constipation and indigestion.

17. Paschimottansana (Forward Bend Pose): Excellent for constipation and digestive disorder: This asana is recommended especially for women after delivery to reduce belly fat. Strengthens the back muscles as well as stimulate the abdominal organs.

18. Uttanpadasana, Leg Raised Yoga Pose: Raised leg pose is beneficial for those having back pain and stomach disorder. Uttanpadasana is highly recommended for stomach ABS. Cures stomach disorders like acidity, indigestion and constipation. It improves digestive system.

Yoga Bandha

Bandha in Sanskrit means to lock, to hold, or to tighten. Bandha is a term for the "body locks" in Hatha Yoga. Uddiyana Bandha and Mulabandha are done early in the morning and are most effective for constipation relief. If you are doing yoga for constipation, diet control and lifestyle change are a must which will add up to the benefits of yoga for curing constipation. There are three (3) main Bandha in the body, and a fourth that ties them all together in Hatha Yoga practice. The ancient yogi said that when you concur or master the locks, you master the yoga practice. The Bandha help you to regulate and control all your internal systems, hormonal, sexual, metabolic, digestive, and much more. The Bandha are a critical factor to you and to yoga.

Precautions: Bandha should not be practiced while pregnant. There are three specific Bandha, such as, (i) Mula Bandha (Anal Lock) / (Muladhara Chakra -Brahma Loka); (2) Uddiyana Bandha (Throat lock) / (Manipura Chakra - Vishnu Loka); and (3) Jalandhara Bandha (Chin Lock) / (Vishuddha Chakra - Rudra Loka). (i) Mula Bandha is contraction of the perineum; (ii) Uddiyana Bandha is contraction of the abdomen into the rib cage; (iii) Jalandhara Bandha is tucking the chin close to the chest; and (iv) Maha Bandha is the combining all three Bandha of the above three. In Bandha, generally, the breath is held during practice of the Bandha. Mula Bandha and Jalandhara Bandha can be performed after the inhalation as well as after the exhalation. Uddiyana Bandha and Maha Bandha are only performed after the exhalation.

Benefits: As the Bandha momentarily stop the flow of blood, there is an increased flow of fresh blood with the release of the Bandha, which flushes away old, dead cells. In this way all the organs are strengthened, renewed and rejuvenated and circulation is improved. Bandha are also beneficial for the brain centres, the Nadi and the Chakras. The energy channels are purified, blockages released and the exchange of energy is improved. Bandha alleviate stress and mental restlessness and bring about inner harmony and balance. Caution: Before attempting to perform the Bandha, the breathing techniques of the previous levels must have been practiced regularly for a long period of time. Before proceeding with the breath exercise in this and the following levels, first read and study the explanation given for the relevant Bandha and Mudra as they are incorporated into the breathing techniques.

1. **Mula Bandha (Root Lock):** Mula Bandha is compound term, which denotes "root", "base", "beginning", "foundation", "origin or cause", and denotes a posture where the body from the anus to the navel is contracted towards the spine and lifted up. Mula Bandha is your "Root Lock". The root refers here is the root of the spine, the pelvic floor or more precisely, the centre of the pelvic floor, the perineum. The perineum is the muscular body between the anus and the genitals. By slightly contracting it, we create an energetic seal that locks prana into the body and so prevents it from leaking out at the base of the spine. Mula Bandha is said to move prana into the central channel, called Sushumna, which is the subtle equivalent of the spine. Mula Bandha is the principal, key and primary Bandha of the Yogic traditions and is endemic to all safe, grounded workings of body mind disciplines. Mula Bandha should be held as a restraint only after Kumbhaka, which in this instance is where the breath is expressed in its entirety and held outside the body. The function of the Bandha, especially Mula Bandha, is like a "safety Valve" which is kept shut during the practice of Kumbhaka and the energetic prana of Vayu engaged through Mula Bandha as "Apana Vayu" (the prana in the lower abdomen), whose course is downwards, is made to flow up to unite with Prana Vayu, which has its seat within the region of the chest. The region of the lower abdomen between the navel and the anus is contracted towards the spine and pulled up to the diaphragm. Practice: Sit in any position of Meditation Pose. Inhale deeply and hold the breath. Place the hands on the knees, raise the shoulders and tilt the upper body slightly forward. Concentrate on the Muladhara Chakra and firmly contract the anal muscles. Hold the muscular contraction and the breath as long as possible and comfortable with a long exhalation and return to the starting position. Breathing normally remains in this position for some time. Repeat 3 to 5 rounds. The truth is that Mula Bandha should be held throughout your entire yoga practice. There are countless reasons, but quite simply think of it as the lock that allows your energy to flow up, not down and out through anus. Your energy is forced to flow up and stay inside you. Mula Bandha allows you to be lighter on your limbs, and thus lighter on your asana. This lightness prevents you from becoming fatigued. Mula Bandha stimulates the pelvic nerves, the genital system, the endocrine system, and the excretory system. It has also been seen to relieve constipation and depression. Activating and engaging these pelvic floor muscles tones and supports the internal organs of the lower abdominal cavity and brings much needed awareness to the space between the pubis (front) and the

coccyx (back). Continuous awareness of this in yoga poses and transitions can help alleviate already existing tightness, tension and/or lower back pain and can counteract any future possibility of lower back injury. Energetically, bringing our awareness to Mula Bandha brings awareness to the dormant energy of Shakti Kundalini at the base of the Sushumna Nadi. By continuously working with and activating Mula Bandha we can begin the slow process of awakening Shakti Kundalini, allowing this feminine creative force to rise up through the lower chakras, healing specific areas of our psycho-spiritual development. The three chakras most affected are, (i) Muladhara (root chakra), survival, safety, trust; (ii) Svadhishthana (sacral chakra), sensuality, sexuality, creativity; (iii) Manipura (solar plexus chakra), self-worth, power, will. Benefits: It strengthens the pelvic floor, relieves haemorrhoids and congestion in the pelvic area, calms the autonomic nervous system, calms and relaxes the mind. On the spiritual level, Mula Bandha activates and purifies the Muladhara Chakra. It awakens dormant consciousness and the Kundalini Shakti.

Caution: A longer and more intensive practice of Mula Bandha should only be undertaken with the guidance of an experienced instructor for "Yoga in Daily Life".

2.   Uddiyana Bandha (Throat Lock): Uddiyana Bandha (U-dhiyana mean out flying from pot) is the abdominal Bandha described and employed in Hatha yoga. Moving up from Mula Bandha we have the second Bandha, Uddiyana. In Sanskrit, Uddiyana means to fly up, or to rise up. This 'flying up lock' is thus all about your insides flying upwards, intangibly meaning your energy, tangibly meaning your diaphragm, stomach, and abdominal organs. It involves, after having exhaled all the air out, pulling the abdomen under the rib cage by taking a false inhale while holding the breath and then releases the abdomen after a pause. The process is repeated many times before letting the air into the lungs, resuming normal breath. Uddiyana Bandha is to be practiced after the practice of asana and Pranayama and before starting any meditation practices.

Practice: Sit in Padmasana/Siddhasana with the spine straight. Place the palms on the knees, breathe normally and relax the whole body. Inhale deeply and then exhale fully. Hold the breath outside. Slightly bend the shoulders and lean forward. Perform Jalandhara Bandha or the chin lock and press down the knees with the palm. Contract the abdominal muscles and pull it inside and upwards. Feel as if there is suction from a point just behind the sternum. This will enable the abdomen to go fully inside pressing all the abdominal organs against the back wall of the spine. Hold the lock with the breath outside for as long as you are comfortable. One can start with few seconds and then gradually increase it to a minute over a period of time. Experts can hold the breath outside for even two minutes or more. To release the lock, first release the abdominal muscles. Then bring the shoulders back to normal position, release the chin lock and inhale slowly and fully. Wait till the breathing process comes back to normal. This process can be repeated as many times as you are comfortable. Uddiyana Bandha (the Abdominal Lock) is one of the three main Bandha is described in the yogic texts Hatha Yoga Pradipika Uddiyana Bandha moves the energy upwards Uddiyana Bandha is the ultimate remedy for abdominal and stomach ailments, from constipation to indigestion. It stimulates your digestive juices, thus increasing your metabolism, and tones your overworked abdominal organs. It also balances the adrenal system, relieving stress, lethargy and tension. Uddiyana Bandha is the active.

Benefits: Uddiyana Bandha massages all the organs in the abdomen. It tones the adrenal glands and balances its function. It improves digestion by increasing the digestive fire. It helps to remove stress and tension. It improves the function of the liver and pancreas. In Uddiyana Bandha, the air is held outside. The upward movement of the abdominal muscles also massages the respiratory system. Practicing Kumbhaka (external holding of breath) systematically improve the lung capacity. It also has effect on the heart and improves circulation of blood throughout the body. Uddiyana Bandha activates the Manipura Chakra, the solar plexus and improves all functions related to that nerve centre. It activates the Manipura Chakra and solar plexus. Stimulates intestinal activity and helps relieve constipation. Stimulates the pancreas and is helpful for diabetes. It strengthens the immune system. Balances the mind, soothes irritability and anger and dispels a depressive mood. Precaution: Perform only on an empty stomach! Do not practice this Bandha with high blood pressure. Repeat 3 to 5 rounds.

Yoga Mudra

Hand Mudra works according to the principles of Ayurveda. According to Ayurveda, all the diseases are caused due to an imbalance in the Constitutions (Vata, Pitta and Kapha). Hand Mudra is useful to manipulate and balance Vata, Pitta and Kapha. In this post, you will get information about the mudra for a particular disease. The 'Mudra', a Sanskrit word means 'closure' or 'seal'. Mudra being hand positions are physical gestures that have an effect on the energy flow of the body. The ancient practice of yoga links the hand Mudra to the changing spiritual and mental aspects of a person. The Mudra is usually finger positions. This is a Yoga Mudra, which are used in conjunction with Pranayama (yogic breathing exercises), generally while seated in Siddhasana, Padmasana, Vajrasana, or Sukhasana pose. It stimulates different parts of the body and mind, and to affect the flow of Prana in the body. Mudra is a natural and non medical way of treatment which had no harmful side effects. According to Ayurveda, all the diseases are caused due to an imbalance in constitutions (Vata, Pitta and Kapha). Hand Mudra are useful to manipulate (such as, increase or decrease) these Dosha. Hand mudra is various postures using all the fingers. You can heal various diseases through hand mudra. Hand mudra has an extraordinary power to balance your health condition and improve resistance power. With improved resistance power, you can easily overcome any disease. Mudra is the most simple in all non medical and alternative treatments. Mudra has no side effects, and anyone can do it with some basic knowledge. Mudra is safe and a no cost natural treatment. It is a self-treatment, and you can use as a defensive move towards illness. Any person who analyzes and understands his temperament and his bodily constitution can realize what ailments he is susceptible to and can, then regularly practice certain mudra to prevent those susceptibilities from manifesting into overt illness. Mudra enjoys a universal application. They can help all types of disorders; sub-acute, acute or chronic; they can help all kind of people, young or old, men or women. Mudra therapy can use as advantageously combined with other forms of treatment, non-medical as well as medical. Being a part of Ayurveda, it goes especially well with Ayurvedic medicine. Even though Mudra help in many diseases, but somewhere it has no role in the treatment of the following disorders, such as, purely mechanical disorders like mature cataract, a big hole in the eardrum, deviated nasal septum, cleft palate, hare lip, valvular heart disease, varicose veins, hernia, big stones in the gall bladders / urinary tract, prolapsed uterus / rectum / inter vertebral disc, fracture, etc. These disorders will, of course, need surgical intervention. Ailments caused by deficiencies of nutrients, vitamins, minerals disorders are a part and parcel of old age (senile degeneration). Life threatening ailments like cancer, AIDS, encephalitis, diphtheria, heart failure, kidney failure, cirrhosis of the live, septicaemia, gangrene call for active, extreme measures rather than gentle mudra. So what I say that mudra therapy is an excellent key to try in the lock of illness. More often than not, it succeeds in opening up the lock. This key should, undoubtedly, be tried when other keys (e.g., modern medicines) have either failed or are undesirable / inapplicable. You may say that mudra therapy seems too simple to be effective. Our fingers have the characteristics of these elements and each of these five elements serve a specific and important function within the body. The fingers are essentially electrical circuits. The use of Mudra adjusts the flow of energy - affecting the balance of air, fire, water, earth, ether and accommodating healing. There are many interpretations of the various finger positions. Whether they are represented as aspects of the self, the three energies inherent in the gunas, the mind, intellect, ego, illusion or karma, remains a mystery. The main point being that they introduce a non-intellectual sensibility. There are five types of Mudra, such as, Hasta (hand mudra); Manna (head mudra); Kaya (postural mudra); Bandha (lock mudra); and Adhara (perinea mudra). There are 10 important Hasta Mudra (Hand Mudra) as explained below:

- Apana Mudra
- Apana Vayu Mudra
- Chin Mudra
- Ganesha Mudra
- Gyan Mudra
- Hakini Mudra
- Jnana Mudra
- Khechari Mudra
- Kundalini Mudra
- Linga Mudra
- Mandala Mudra
- Pran Mudra
- Prithvi Mudra
- Rudra Mudra
- Shankh Mudra
- Shunya Mudra
- Surahi Mudra
- Surya Mudra
- Varun Mudra
- Vayu Mudra
- Yoni Mudra

Among all the above Mudra, Prithvi Mudra, Apana Mudra, Varuna Mudra; Vayu shaamak Mudra, Vata naashak Mudra, Vayu Mudra/Vata Nashak are very good for cure of Constipation.

1. Prithvi Mudra (the Mudra of Earth): Prithvi Mudra is one of the important Mudra in healing Mudra. Prithvi Mudra is very useful to increase earth element and decrease fire element in the body. Other names of Prithvi Mudra are Vayu Shaamak Mudra, Vata Nashak Mudra, Agni shamak Mudra and Prithvi vardhak Mudra, which is very useful to decrease Vata-dosha. It is a set of hand gestures that help to focus and balance the five elements that exist within the human body. The Prithvi Mudra helps to equalize the element of Prithvi or earth within the body. This Mudra is also said to activate the Root Chakra. Prithvi Mudra is very effective to gain weight and strengthen the body. You may practice Prithvi mudra while travelling or watching T.V or anywhere and anytime. Prithvi Mudra and healing properties: This Mudra is very useful to increase the earth element and decrease fire element in the body. Earth is the major component of bones, cartilage moleskin hair, nails, flesh, muscles, tendons, internal organs, etc and practice of Prithvi Mudra strengthens these tissues. Prithvi Mudra reduces body temperature and strengthens your body. Prithvi mudra has the healing power to heal following illness, such as, Chronic fatigue; Debility; Convalescence, Endurance or lack of stamina, Loss of weight; Emaciation; Inexplicable; Osteoporosis; Fracture, Degeneration of articular cartilage, Weakness atrophied muscles; Myopathies; Paresis; Paralysis; Poliomyelitis; Dry, cracked, burning, mature skin; Brittle nails; Hair loss, premature greying of hair; Burning in eyes; Acidity, Burning sensation of urinating, Burning in anus, Burning in hands, feet, and head; Aphthous; Ulcers in the mouth and stomach; Inflammatory diseases; Jaundice; Fever and Hyperthyroidism. Sit down in a meditative pose such as the Sukha Asana (Easy Pose), Vajra Asana (Diamond Pose), or Padma Asana (Lotus Pose). Ensure that your back is held straight and your chest and head held up high. Close your eyes and focus on your breath and to enhance the effectiveness of the Prithvi Mudra, chant the word Om (Aum) in conjunction with every exhale. Rest your hands on your knees with your palms facing upwards or downward. In this Mudra, the tips of the thumb and the ring finger are touched together. The other fingers are kept straight and parallel. Thirty to forty-five minutes of regular practice is enough to get good results. You can do it anytime or in any place but the morning hour or when you are in meditation is the best choice to get best results. To get the outcome in a quick pace, please practice it regularly. Keeping a healthy diet plan is also beneficial. Precaution for Prithvi-Vardhak mudra: If you are a

Prithvi Mudra

Kapha dosha person, then do it in moderation only.

Benefits: Regular practice of this Mudra is helpful in body weakness, thinness and also obesity. It improves the functioning of the digestive system and reduces the deficiency of vitamins. It gives energy and lustre to the body.

2. Apana Mudra (the Mudra of Digestion): Apana Mudra is also known as gesture of Yoga of the hands. These hand gestures help to channel the flow of energy through the body. They also help in balancing the five elements inside the body. The Apana Mudra is also known as the purification mudra. It helps to increase the balance of the elements of space and earth within the body. Apana mudra is an important mudra that is beneficial to detoxify and energize the body. Apana mudra is a combination of both Prithvi and Aakaash mudra. The practice of Apana mudra increases both Kapha and Vata humour and reduces Pita humour. Sit down in a meditative pose such as the Sukha Asana (Easy Pose), Vajra Asana (Diamond Pose), or Padmasana (Lotus Pose). Ensure that your back is held straight and your chest and head held up high. Close your eyes and focus on your breath and to enhance the effectiveness of the Apana Mudra, chant the word Om (Aum) in conjunction with every exhale. Rest your hands on your knees with your palms facing upwards or downward. This Mudra is made by joining the tips of the thumb, the middle finger and the ring finger, without exerting any pressure and keeping the other fingers straight. Apana Mudra and healing properties: Apana Mudra is combined form of Prithvi and Aakash mudra. This Mudra increases Vata and Kapha and decreases pita humour. Apana mudra is useful in the treatment of following conditions, such as, Piles, Flatulence, and Constipation. 2. Anuria and absence of sweat. 3. Burning sensation in body or body parts.

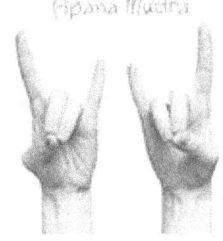

Apana Mudra

4. Delayed delivery of a child. 5. All the diseases caused due to deficiency of Vata. 6. All the disorders caused due to deficiency of Kapha. 7. All the diseases caused due to an excess of Pita. Forty five minutes of regular practice is enough to get good results of Apana Mudra. Benefits: Toxins are removed from the body and the body becomes pure. It also relieves constipation, piles, diseases caused by Vayu or air, is helpful in diabetes, stoppage of urine, kidney defects and dental problems. It is beneficial in stomach and heart diseases and brings out perspiration

3. Varuna Mudra (Mudra of Water): Varuna mudra is very effective to increase water element in the body. Due its impact on a Jal (water)

element in the body, it is also called as a Jal vardhak mudra. Varuna mudra or Jal vardhak Mudra is very easy to do. Sit down in a meditative pose such as the Sukha Asana (Easy Pose), Vajra Asana (Diamond Pose), or Padma Asana (Lotus Pose). Ensure that your back is held straight and your chest and head held up high. Close your eyes and focus on your breath and to enhance the effectiveness of the Varuna Mudra, chant the word Om (Aum) in conjunction with every exhale. Rest your hands on your knees with your palms facing upwards or downward. This Mudra is made by touching the tips of the thumb and the little finger, without exerting any pressure. Impact of Varuna Mudra and healing properties: Varuna Mudra helps to increase water element in the body.

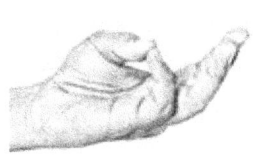
Varun mudra
Gesture of water

Our body has 75 percent water. Water is plays major role in every activity of our health system. Water is present in protoplasm of cells, extracellular fluid, lymph, blood, tears, saliva, and mucus, digestive juices, enzymes, hormones, semen, cerebrospinal fluid, etc. Any slight decrease in the percentage of water would result too many disturbances like dehydration. Practising Varuna Mudra helps to increase water element in the body and restore the balance in the system. The element of water has a major role in taste and tongue. Jal vardhak Mudra is very useful to treat the disorders related to the tongue, taste, senses, and dryness of the mouth. Jal is the main part of pita and Kapha Prakriti. If you are a Pitta or Kapha Prakriti person then you should practice this Mudra moderately, this Mudra increases pita and Kapha dosha. If you are a Vata dosha person then practising this Mudra regularly will be greatly beneficial to prevent illness. Varuna Mudra is useful in the treatment of; Dryness of eyes and mouth, throat and intestines; Indigestion constipation; Constipation; Dryness of skin and moister skin in the winter; Degeneration of joint cartilage osteoarthritis; Dry eczema; Psoriasis; Osteoarthritis; Cramps; Dehydration; Deficiency of hormones; Scanty urination; Scanty menses; Loss of taste; Tongues disorders. All the diseases cause due to an excess of Vata dosha can be healed by practising Varuna Mudra. 30 minutes of regular practice is enough to get the benefits of Varuna Mudra or Jal vardhak Mudra. You can do this Mudra at any time or in any place, but early hours of the morning or in meditation are preferable. If you are a Pitta or Kapha Prakriti person then practice this Mudra moderate only. Benefits: It reduces dryness of the skin and improves skin lustre and softness. It is useful in skin diseases, acne and blood defects. It improves facial beauty.

178

Precautions: Persons suffering from Asthma and respiratory problems should do this Mudra for a short duration only.

4. Jal Vardhak Mudra: Varuna mudra is very effective to increase water element in the body and is known as Jal Vardhaka Mudra. Due its impact on a Jal (water) element in the body, it is also called as a Jal vardhak mudra. Varuna mudra or Jal vardhak mudra is very easy to do.

Practice: Sit in any Asana and Just place the tip of the thumb on the tip of the little finger and applying the little pressure. Impact of Varuna mudra on health: Varuna mudra helps to increase water element in the body. Our body has 75 percent water. Water is plays major role in every activity of our health system.

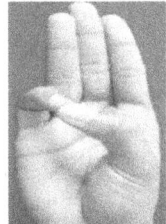

Water is present in protoplasm of cells, extracellular fluid, lymph, blood, tears, saliva, mucus, digestive juices, enzymes, hormones, semen, cerebrospinal fluid, etc. Any slight decrease in the percentage of water would result too many disturbances like dehydration. Practicing Varuna mudra helps to increase water element in the body and restore the balance in the system. The element of water has a major role in taste and tongue. Jal vardhak mudra is very useful to treat the disorders related to the tongue, taste, senses, and dryness of the mouth. Jal is the main part of pita and Kapha Prakriti. If you are a Pitta or Kapha Prakriti person then you should practice this mudra moderately, this mudra increases pita and Kapha dosha. If you are a Vata dosha person then practising this mudra regularly will be greatly beneficial to prevent illness. Benefits: Jal vardhak Mudra / Varuna Mudra is useful in the treatment of; Dryness of eyes and mouth, throat and intestines; Indigestion constipation; Constipation; Dryness of skin and moister skin in the winter; Degeneration of joint cartilage osteoarthritis; Dry eczema; Psoriasis; Osteoarthritis; Cramps; Dehydration; Deficiency of hormones; Scanty urination; Scanty menses; Loss of taste; Tongues disorders, and all the diseases caused due to an excess of Vata dosha and they can be healed by practicing Varuna mudra or Jalvardhaka Mudra. 30 minutes of regular practice is enough to get the benefits of Varuna mudra or Jal vardhak mudra. You can do this mudra at any time or in any place, but early hours of the morning or in meditation are preferable. Precautions for Varuna Mudra: If you are a Pitta or Kapha Prakriti person then practice this mudra moderate only.

Vata Nashak/Vayu Mudra (the Mudra of Air): Vayu means air and the Vayu Mudra helps to regulate the element of air inside the body, which enables various health benefits. Yoga mudra

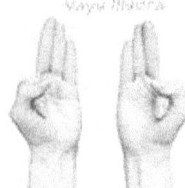
Vayu Mudra

is specific hand gestures that help to channel the flow and balance off the different elements inside the body. Yoga mudra is specific hand gestures that help to channel the flow and balance off the different elements inside the body. Vayu mudra is very useful to decrease air element in the body. This mudra is called as Vayu shaamak Mudra also because of its impact on Vayu element. Vayu Mudra and healing properties: This mudra is very easy to do. Thus, the benefits of the Vayu Mudra extend to problems such as flatulence and joint pain related to rheumatism, sciatica, arthritis, or gout and helps with the uncontrollable tremors experienced by those suffering from Parkinson's disease. If you feel uneasy after a meal, you should practice the Vayu Mudra while seated in the Vajra Asana (Diamond Pose). It can also be used for pain management for the victims of polio. If your mind is anxious and restless or over excited, then Vayu shamak mudra is best natural remedy to overcome and calm down your nervous system and you can feel relaxation. Hormone imbalance of endocrine glands can be overcome through practicing Vayu mudra. Other benefits of Vayu shamak mudra are useful in case of Clears voice problems, allows re-hydration of skin and articular cartilage; Hormone imbalance of endocrine glands can be overcome through practicing Vayu mudra. Other benefits of Vayu shamak mudra are, Clears voice problems, allows re-hydration of skin and articular cartilage.

Vayu is the important component of Vata Prakriti. Decreasing Vayu element in the body enables to overcome Vata dosha. If you are Vata Prakriti daily practising of Vayu shaamak mudra helps to live a disease free life. Daily practice of 30 to forty five minutes is enough to get best results. You can do Vayu mudra any time or in any pose. It is recommended those early hours in the morning or in meditation to get quick results. Sit down in a meditative pose such as the Sukha Asana (Easy Pose), Vajra Asana (Diamond Pose), or Padma Asana (Lotus Pose). Ensure that your back is held straight and your chest and head held up high. Close your eyes and focus on your breath and to enhance the effectiveness of the Vayu Mudra, chant the word Om (Aum) in conjunction with every exhale. Rest your hands on your knees with your palms facing upwards, without exerting any pressure. Press the tip of each index finger onto the mound of your thumb. Fold your thumb so that it presses down lightly on the bent index finger. The other fingers should be held straight and parallel. Perform this Mudra for as long as the problem persists. Benefits: It prevents problems relating to the imbalance of the air element inside the body from cropping up. It helps in treating the problems such as flatulence and joint pain related to rheumatism, sciatica, arthritis, or gout, uncontrollable tremors experienced by those suffering from Parkinson's disease. If you feel uneasy after a meal, you should practice the Vayu Mudra while seated in the Vajra Asana (Diamond Pose). It can also be used for pain management for the victims of polio. It helps to regulate the element of air inside the body. Yoga Mudra is specific hand gestures that help to channel the flow and balance off the different elements inside the body. Benefits: By the practice of this Mudra, all Vayu related afflictions, like Arthritis, Gout, Sciatica, Knee pain, Constipation and Gas are relieved. It especially benefits in neck pain and spinal pain.

Pranayama

There are many asanas or poses in yoga for constipation and to give relief from constipation. Along with yoga, you can also try some natural constipation remedies to feel better quickly. One of the best and most effective natural remedy is increasing your intake of fibre. Fibre includes fruits and raw vegetables and whole grains. These items contain large amounts of insoluble fibre which help constipation. Eating fibre every day gradually can help people deal with constipation on a daily basis. Increasing the amount of fluid you consume can also help deal with constipation. Avoiding carbonated drinks, tea and coffee will also decrease your chances of constipation. Avoiding refined flours is also recommended. Magnesium remedies are known to benefit constipation. Seeds like fenugreek are also very good for constipation. Probiotics are also considered a natural remedy for constipation. Probiotics are good bacteria that can be found yogurt and buttermilk. These bacteria work well in the intestines, preventing constipation. Exercise is also a good natural remedy for constipation.

Regular practice of yoga is known to balance out all systems of the body. Therefore yoga is good for acidity too. Acidity and gas form due bad eating habits and bad digestion. Both these habits lead to an accumulation of excess stomach acids. In extreme cases this stomach acid can cause an acid reflux which is also acidity. Eating a balanced diet, especially one with fruits and vegetables is good to contain acidity. A salad of watermelon and cucumber can be very cooling for the stomach. Holy basil leaves, muddled and had with water can relieve symptoms of acidity and provide relief. Tender coconut water is also good for the stomach. Two- three tablespoons of apple cider vinegar is also considered a quick remedy.

If you suffer from acidity take care of the food which you eat as food has a major influence on acidity. Keep the following points in mind for the same:

- Have small divided meals; avoid having a heavy fatty meal especially in dinner to avoid acidity.
- Avoid fatty oily foods, junk foods, coffee, tea (don't drink tea or coffee alone, always have a piece of cracker or toast along with it), caffeinated drinks, chocolates, and sodas.
- Avoid clubbing fruits with your major meals.
- Do not lie down immediately after a meal; keep at least a minimum gap of 2-3 hours.

Certain yoga poses increase blood flow to the digestive tract and stimulate the intestines to contract. This can make digestion more efficient and help relieve constipation. Virasana, known as the hero's pose, is done by kneeling on the ground, knees apart, and feet together with the toes pointing behind you. Keeping your back straight, slowly sink your hips down until they are resting between your feet.

Place your hands on your knees and breathe normally. Next, move into Adho Mukha Virasana, or down facing hero's pose, by bending forward and resting your forehead on the ground. Your arms should be straight out in front of your head with your palms together. Hold for 30 to 60 seconds. Another pose that might help is Pavanmuktasana, or the gas releasing pose. Lying on your back, bring both knees up to your chest, breathing out as you pull them up. Gently add pressure, bringing your thighs into your belly. Roll your head up, touching your knees with your forehead. Hold for 30 to 60 seconds breathing normally.

If you get your heart and lungs going, your gut will get going, too. Constipation is a common digestive problem. Fortunately, there are several natural cures, like eating a diet rich in fibre and drinking plenty of fluids. Most importantly, exercise may be just what you need to give you constipation relief if your bowel movements aren't running on schedule. Exercise that accelerates your breathing and gets your heart pumping can help get everything else going, too. Exercise can tone and strengthen your colon walls. So, once you get going, your colon will follow suit.

Aerobic exercise increase blood flow. Aerobic activities are probably the best exercises for relieving constipation, Aerobic exercise increases blood flow to our organs, and bringing more blood to the gastrointestinal tract results in stronger intestinal contractions and more digestive enzymes. The stronger the contractions and the more those juices flow, the more quickly and easily food waste will move through the colon and out of the body. Aerobic exercise can include walking, running, swimming, biking, and many other similar activities. The benefits of cardiovascular exercises are better than static exercises, such as weightlifting, for alleviating constipation. Weightlifting has its own benefits in terms of stronger bones and more effective use of calories, but something that involves true movement is probably best in terms of getting the gut going."

Stop Stressing Out. Stress plays a big role in constipation. I mean, they don't call it anal retentive for nothing! Relax, forgive people, focus on the positive and let things go. If you do these things, it's not only good for your digestion but also for your mind and spirit. We have seen how yoga helps to relieve ulcerative colitis constipation, irritable bowel syndrome (IBS) and heartburn. Yoga poses to relieve constipation include:

- Ardha Matsyendrasana (Half spinal twist): Yoga posture like this improves digestion helps from chronic situation.
- Bhujangasana
- Dhanurasana (Bow pose): helpful for its remedies and makes stool to pass easily.
- Hal asana (Plough pose): Relieves it and keep the spine supple. It keeps healthy thyroid and parathyroid glands and helps in preventing diabetes mellitus.
- Katichakrasana (Waist rotating pose) helps to remove it.
- Mandukasana: Beneficial for digestive disorders.
- Mayurasana (Peacock pose): This yoga asana is helpful in solving the problem of indigestion.
- Naukasana (Boat poses): Improves and activates the digestive system and intestine.
- Paschimottansana (Head to knee pose): Practicing yoga like this removes the severe condition.
- Pavan Muktasana: Improves gastrointestinal problems by stimulating abdominal region thereby correct flatulence. It also reduces abdominal fats.
- Pawan Sukhasana
- Sarvangasana (Shoulder stand): Improves digestion and relieves from the problem.
- Shalabhasana (Locust pose): Strengthens the abdominal muscles, beneficial for digestion.
- Supta Vajrasana (Sleeping pelvic pose): Aids in digestion and provides relief.

- Suryanamaskar
- Trikonasana (Triangular stretch pose) helps to pass stool easily and good for bowel movement.
- Vajrasana (Diamond pose): Improves the functioning of whole digestive system.

Piles, also known as haemorrhoids, are caused when the veins around the anal canal become swollen and inflamed. Even though this condition is not life threatening, it can become quite troublesome because of the pain it causes. The symptoms of piles are not always manifested in the same way for everyone. The most common symptom, however, is bright red blood present in the stool or on the toilet paper. Other symptoms include swelling or a hard lump present in the area of the anus, which is caused by blood clots. Although bleeding piles may be common it is not necessary for there to be bleeding in all cases of piles. Piles are normally the result of chronic constipation. Chronic constipation causes you to exert pressure on the rectum and the anus in an attempt to evacuate your bowels. This downward pressure results in constant pressure on the veins, their swelling and distension and subsequent rupture and other malfunctions. Hence you should get to the root of the problem and, first and foremost, deal with constipation or any other effort would be futile. If you have bloodied stools you ought to take it up even more seriously since ruptured veins could lead to further complications. Meanwhile this is the prescribed program of Yoga for constipation and piles. It includes a routine of Yogasana (physical postures), Pranayama (breathing exercises), Kriya (cleansing techniques) and Yoga diet for constipation and piles. Asanas (Yoga poses) subject to your age and physical fitness you should practise all the Yoga postures.

Irrespective of the nature or severity of the condition, treatment for piles should never be delayed. Any treatment for piles should begin by bringing relief to the symptoms the patient suffers from. It will be helpful to have a bath many times a day with warm water for around 10 minutes. Applying a haemorrhoid cream or a suppository prescribed by the doctor will also help in the treatment of piles. Drinking chamomile tea is also considered to be effective for people suffering from piles. Also, wearing cotton underwear will provide comfort. If the pain continues to be present, you could apply an ice pack that will soothe the area and also prevent swelling. Symptomatic treatment for piles however only relieves the symptoms and for a lasting cure the treatment for piles should address the underlying cause. To get rid of piles for good, doctors recommend an increased intake of fibre. Consuming plenty of fluids is also necessary, and you should drink 6 to 8 glasses of water, at the least, every day. By doing this, you will ensure that your stools are softer, thereby reducing the pressure put on the haemorrhoids. For the treatment of piles, natural methods like home remedies can also be effective. One home remedy is involves soaking 3 to 4 figs in hot water through the night; make sure to clean them properly. You should consume them as soon as you get up in the morning, together with the water you soaked them in. This should be done again in the evening, and you should continue this treatment for 3 to 4 weeks. This helps to eliminate the faeces easily, and it will clean the alimentary canal. The treatment of piles symptoms should be administered on time; otherwise, it will only get worse with considerable amount of pain. Along with treatment for piles, you should follow a proper diet to ensure effective results. Otherwise, the symptoms may only be relieved temporarily only to recur later. You should eat foods that are high in fibre such as vegetables, wholegrain and fruit. By eating the right foods and living a healthy lifestyle with enough exercise, you should be able to permanently get rid of piles.

Piles can be cured through various yoga asanas. Piles and yoga simply means that yoga helps a great deal to treat piles. Before we go onto exactly how piles and yoga works, it is important to know just what Piles are. Piles are enlarged blood vessels which are present near the anal region. This disease can affect people of all ages. The veins present in the rectal area get inflamed and this results in a great deal of pain. There are two types of Piles – external and internal. Internal piles are those which are found inside the body, close to the anal canal.

Yoga for Piles treatment can be done in the convenience of one's own home. Yoga can work wonders for the treatment of piles. Pile is a very common ailment these days. Haemorrhoids are balloon kind of swelling in the veins near the anus. It can be internal or external. External piles are not harmful but they cause pain at the time of excretion. Internal piles are a great cause of trouble as they cannot be dealt with immediately. Yoga helps greatly for the treatment of dry internal piles in the body.

Piles can be either caused due to heredity or at times due to sexual troubles or over indulgence. Lack of physical activity too can be a cause of piles. Constipation and mal functioning of liver can cause piles which may trouble the individual for a long period of time. When piles are caused due to improper circulation of blood in the veins of the body then the distant veins have blockage of blood causing piles.

The pouched blood causes the muscles to swell and causes inflammation in the nearby tissues. Various asanas can be used for the treatment of piles and a few which have guaranteed results like sarvangasana (shoulder stand), tadasana (mountain pose), Surya namaskar (sun salutation) and a few quite challenging poses like shirshasana (head stand).

Constipation can lead to piles and it can cause indigestion which may lead to several ailments of the stomach and intestine. It is also a known cause for the piles. Yoga helps in the removal of the toxins in the body which can give a free and active feeling to the body and once the toxins are out from the body, it helps to restore the normal balance of the body and provide freedom from the pain caused due to piles. Piles may cause back pain in several individuals because of its critical position in the body.

Yoga exercises can help greatly in the treatment of piles and the back pain. The stretch and strain provided as a part of yoga helps to regulate the body and provide freedom from the acute pain caused in the body. A few recommended asanas of yoga like sarvangasana (posture involving all body parts) helps to activate the glands of the body which can also help to heal the piles. Uttanasana (standing forward bend pose) and chakrasana (wheel pose) are highly recommended postures for the treatment of piles in the human body.

Yoga breathing exercises help stimulate bowel action. If you suffer from high blood pressure do not attempt Bhastrika and Kapalabhati Pranayama. Agnisar Pranayama (Abdominal Lifts) is an excellent exercise for getting relief from chronic constipation and indigestion. It also strengthens flabby abdominal muscles. Effective Pranayama for constipation cure are Alom- Vilom, Agnisar, Bhastrika and Kapalabhati.

Reduce constipation by yoga poses

Those having constipation should avoid taking the tablets on a daily basis to empty the stomach. Dear friends this habit is very dangerous for your intestine. The intestine will become weaker and will find unable to empty the stomach naturally. In the treatment for constipation yoga and Pranayama gives outstanding and very effective results.

Benefits of Yoga poses

- Cures constipation and indigestion
- Strengthens the stomach and abdominal muscles.

- Daily practicing yoga helps to become more active throughout the day.
- Helps to improve metabolism.
- It releases gases from the stomach
- Impoves overall good for digestive system.

Yoga Poses for Constipation and Indigestion

Important: Drink more warm water and chew food properly. Avoid eating when you are in stress. Drink more water one and half an hour after of your meal. Drink one glass of water one hour before having meal. These points are very helpful to cure constipation and indigestion. Let's see some effective yoga poses to cure constipation and indigestion one by one.

1. Kapalabhati Pranayama: Kapalabhati Pranayama is a well known breathing exercise to improve your digestive system. Regular practice of Kapalabhati will cure your stomach disorder, acidity and reduce your belly fat. Kapal in Sanskrit means the skull and bhati is Diya or a lamp. Doing Kapalabhati gives you shining and glow on your face. How? Performing this asana initiates the removal of carbon dioxide from the body; as a result it leads to blood purification. This makes your skin healthy and beautiful. You can sit in either Sukhasana (similar to sitting in a simple cross-legged position) or Padmasana (or Lotus pose is a cross-legged yoga posture which helps deepen meditation by calming the mind).

Kapalabhati	Ardh Matsyendrasana	Vrikshasana

Kapalabhati Technique: 1. First and foremost, sit in a comfortable position with your spine erect. Place your hands on the knees, palms open to the sky. Then take a deep breath in. 2. As you exhale, pull your stomach. Pull your navel backwards towards your spine. Now repeat the steps quickly and as many times as you can do comfortably. 3. You can keep your right hand on the stomach to feel your abdominal muscles contract. 4. When you relax your navel and abdomen, the breath flows into your lungs automatically. Take 20 such breaths to complete one round of Kapalabhati Pranayama. Performing Kapalabhati everyday can help you achieve that. Benefits: 1. It provides a flat and toned tummy. 2. Kapalabhati also rejuvenates the tired cells of your body, thus helping in reducing wrinkles and other signs of ageing. 3. Improves your digestive tract, absorption and assimilation of nutrients in your body. 4. Move over skin packs, performing Kapalabhati can give you a glowing and a healthy face. Caution: People with high blood pressure, heart problems should not perform this asana. Women who have recently given birth and girls during their Mensuration cycle should avoid this asana.

2.   Anulom Vilom Pranayama: This is one of the most effective Pranayama (breathing exercises) to purify your mind and body. Anulom Vilom offers benefits in curing most of the internal bodily conditions and is very useful in releasing stress and anxiety. Bonus points - Anulom Vilom Pranayama can be performed by people of all ages. Anulom Vilom Techniques: 1. to perform Anulom Vilom, sit in Sukhasana (similar to sitting in a simple cross-legged position) or Padmasana (or Lotus pose is a cross-legged yoga posture which helps deepen meditation by calming the mind). 2. Now place your left hand in chin mudra and right in Vishnu mudra. Vishnu mudra is when index finger and middle finger touch the base of the thumb. The ring finger, little finger and the thumb remain up. You should first close your eyes and relax all your muscles for a while. Then, inhale from your left nostril while keeping your right nostril closed with the thumb of your right hand for the count of 4. 3. Retain the breath for a 16 counts and exhale from your right nostril with your ring fingers and little finger closing your left nostril to the count of 8. Then, once again take in the breath from your right nostril. Finally, exhale from your left nostril while closing your right nostril with your thumb. This will complete one round of the Pranayama. You could perform this exercise for around 15 minutes while taking a minute rest after every 5 minutes. Benefits: 1. Anulom Vilom benefits us by balancing the body's three dosha - Vata (Wind), Pitta (A bilious humour, or that secreted between the stomach and bowels and flowing through the liver and permeating spleen, heart, eyes, and skin) and Kapha (body fluid principle which relates to mucus, lubrication, and the carrier of nutrient.) Any imbalance in the three dosha will lead to illnesses. 2. Anulom Vilom also benefits you by bringing relief to conditions like sinus, respiratory problems, and asthma. Removing of artery blockages and maintenance of cholesterol levels are some other benefits of this asana. It is also effective in dealing with conditions like constipation, flatulence, diabetes, and obesity.

"As Anulom Vilom has no side effects it is considered to be very effective for weight loss," says Fitness trainer Kiran Sawhney." Caution: Women should avoid performing Anulom Vilom during pregnancy and periods. Individuals who suffer from heart troubles should not perform this exercise with too much force and should practice it under the guidance of a qualified instructor. You to reap from the Anulom Vilom benefits, it is important that you practice it daily. It is also essential for you to combine it with a yogic diet that is purely vegetarian and do Kapalabhati daily.

3.   **Half a Spinal Twist or Ardh Matsyendrasana:** Spinal Twist Technique: 1. Sit with your spine erect and legs straight ahead of you. Now fold the left knee like sitting in cross-legged position. 2. Fold the other knee. Keep the right foot close to the knee of left foot. Take the knee over and above the left knee. 3. Then take the right hand behind your back. Now lift the left hand up. Stretch it. Take it across the right knee and towards the right ankle. 4. Twist the waist and the spine. Look across your right shoulder behind you. If you can go deeper then, join both the hands from under your right knee. Benefits: 1. it improves the flexibility of the spine and makes it supple. 2. It improves the breathing capacity. 3. The chest and hip joints also become more elastic. Caution: Avoid doing this asana if you are pregnant or have periods as the asana requires strong twist in the abdomen. People with Heart, abdominal or brain surgeries should not practice this asana. If you have peptic ulcer or hernia, you should first consult your doctor before doing this asana. If you have severe spinal problems then this asana should be avoided.

4.   **Vrikshasana (Tree pose):** Vrikshasana Technique: 1. Start by standing tall and straight with arms by the side of your body. 2. Now bend your right knee and place your right foot high up on the left thigh. The sole of the foot should be placed flat and firmly near the root of the thigh. Note: Ensure your left leg is straight. 3. Once you have found your balance start taking a deep breath in. Then raise your arms over your head from the side, and bring your palms together in 'Namaste' position (hands-folded position). 4. You should be looking straight, see some distant object in front of you. 5. Make sure that your spine is straight. Keep taking in long, deep breaths. With each exhalation, relax the body more and more. Now with slow exhalation, gently bring down your hands from the sides. You may gently release the right leg too. Stand tall and straight as you did at the beginning of the posture. Repeat this pose with the left leg off the

ground on the right thigh. Benefits: 1. Performing tree pose can strengthen your thighs, calves, ankles, and spine. 2. It stretches the groins and inner thighs, chest and shoulders, thus improving your sense of balance. 4. Tree pose is very beneficial for relieving sciatica which is a pain affecting the back, hip, and outer side of the leg. It also reduces flat feet. Caution: Do not practice Tree Pose if you are experiencing headaches, insomnia, low blood pressure, or if you are feeling dizzy. If you have high blood pressure then you should not raise your arms over ahead while doing this asana.

5.3 Acupressure to prevent Constipation

Mainly constipation occurs because of two reasons. Firstly constipation occurs due to dehydration, when our colon absorbs more amount of water from stool and hence the muscles of the colon act so poorly that the stool finds difficult to move ahead and loses more water. Secondly it occurs due to poor diet, particularly eating one high in processed foods like dairy products, animal protein; caffeinated drinks, such as, sodas, coffee, energy drinks; fatty Meats, such as, steak, veal, brisket, pork; fast & fried foods, such as, pizza, burgers, tacos, fried chicken; dairy products, such as, butter, ice-cream; carbonated drinks high in Sugar, such as, sodas, cold drinks, energy drinks; refined sugars, such as, chocolate, cake, pie, candy-bars, alcohol, beer, wine, mixed drinks; and enriched white flour, such as, white bread, doughnuts, some varieties of tortillas having no fibre. Followings are Iso causes of constipation relted to Acupressure:

1. Nutritional Stress: Disease and nutrition are intimately linked. Our food supply has become saturated with processed foods that are largely foreign to the human body. Chiefly derived from wheat and corn, these abnormal foods are the driving force behind obesity, cardiovascular disease, diabetes, digestive problems, cancer, and most all other diseases.

2. Emotional Stress: A baseline of chronic stress is much more prevalent than most people realize. Chronic emotional stress robs the body of vital energy, suppresses immune function, and disrupts hormonal systems. The cumulative result can be devastating; elevated blood pressure, increased blood clotting, compromised digestive function, elevated blood sugar, chronic sleep disturbances, weight gain and especially suppressed immune function. Uncontrolled stress sets the stage for all diseases.

3. Toxins: There are up to 200,000 man-made chemicals in the environment that were not present a hundred years ago. Most are petroleum derived. Everyone is exposed and trace amounts can be found in every living creature on earth. The role that toxins play in disease and cancer is hard to absolutely define, but it is certainly a factor. Because toxins can only enter the body by three different pathways (ingestion, breathing, and through the skin), limiting this risk factor is fairly simple.

4. Physical Stress: Three types of physical stress can affect your body—trauma (wear & tear), temperature, and pressure. Even everyday physical stress (minor trauma, being too cold or too hot, pressure changes) can aggravate established disease processes. For some people, extreme physical stress (severe trauma, severe hypothermia, severe hyperthermia, altitude sickness) can be the primary trigger for allowing disease processes to occur.

5. Free Radicals (Inflammation): Inside each of the trillions of cells that make up your body, free radicals are being continually generated as a by-product of energy production. Free radicals can damage all parts of the cell, including DNA. It is the most significant factor in aging and contributes to all disease. Other sources of free radicals in the body include abnormal fats from processed foods and toxins. In addition, white blood cells actually generate free radicals to destroy foreign substances in the body; this is the root of inflammation in the body.

6. Radiation: Like all living creatures, you are exposed to a certain level of background radiation from gamma rays, x-ray and UV radiation from the earth, sun and space or electronic items. Though these forms of radiation are a force of disease and aging, exposure from natural sources has been relatively constant since humans began walking the earth. Of greater concern are the increased levels of radiation from artificial and unnatural sources (such as electronics).

7. Microbes: The role that microbes play in acute disease is well understood. Diseases like strep throat, influenza, malaria, small pox, polio, and the plague cause acute illness in most people who are exposed. Collectively, these aggressive types of microbes (which include viruses, bacteria, fungi, & protozoa) can be referred to as high virulence microbes. In chronic disease, however, a different sort of microbe plays a prominent role. You (and everyone around) are almost continually exposed to these types of microbes (also composed of viruses, bacteria, fungi, & protozoa, but different than above). They actually have a low potential to cause disease and most of the time, they pass by hardly noticed. However, if immune function

is compromised by other factors, chronic low grade infection can occur.

8. Disease: The term disease broadly refers to any condition that impairs the normal functioning of the body. For this reason, diseases are associated with dysfunction of the body's normal homeostatic process. Commonly, the term disease is used to refer specifically to infectious diseases, which are clinically evident diseases that result from the presence of pathogenic microbial agents, including viruses, bacteria, fungi, protozoa, multicellular organisms, and aberrant proteins known as prions.

9. Disorder: In medicine, a disorder is a functional abnormality or disturbance. Medical disorders can be categorized into mental disorders, physical disorders, genetic disorders, emotional and behavioural disorders, and functional disorders. The term disorder is often considered more value-neutral and less stigmatizing than the terms disease or illness, and therefore is a preferred terminology in some circumstances. In mental health, the term mental disorder is used as a way of acknowledging the complex interaction of biological, social, and psychological factors in psychiatric conditions. However, the term disorder is also used in many other areas of medicine, primarily to identify physical disorders that are not caused by infectious organisms, such as metabolic disorders.

10. Mental illness: Mental illness is a broad, generic label for a category of illnesses that may include affective or emotional instability, behavioural deregulation, cognitive dysfunction or impairment. Specific illnesses known as mental illnesses include major depression, generalized anxiety disorders, schizophrenia, and attention deficit hyperactivity disorder, to name a few. Mental illness can be of biological (e.g., anatomical, chemical, or genetic) or psychological (e.g., trauma or conflict) origin. It can impair the affected person's ability to work or study and can harm interpersonal relationships. The term insanity is used technically as a legal term.

11. Organic disease: An organic disease is one caused by a physical or physiological change to some tissue or organ of the body. The term sometimes excludes infections. It is commonly used in contrast with mental disorders. It includes emotional and behavioural disorders if they are due to changes to the physical structures or functioning of the body, such as after a stroke or a traumatic brain injury, but not if

Important Acupressure Points for Constipation

Constipation is a common disturbance of the digestive tract. A lot of patients complain about having constipation. It's very difficult to pass the stools sometimes or feel something inside my bowel. In this condition, the bowels do not move regularly, or are not completely emptied when they move. The disease in which chronic constipation is an important predisposing factor is appendicitis, rheumatism, arthritis, high blood pressure, cataract and cancer. Constipation is one of the most common of all digestive disorders and it can affect people of all age groups, from toddlers to the aged. Long term chronic constipation when neglected can lead to conditions like faecal impaction, piles or haemorrhoids, anal fissures and faecal incontinence. Acupressure Points for Constipation are helpful to get faster relief in constipation problem. Acupressure can relive Constipation in a natural way. By stimulating Acupressure Points frequently, you can relieve constipation. Constipation, for some people, is an occasional problem caused by some foods, in others it reveals itself as a chronic health issue where they need to take regular medication or laxatives to keep things moving. Constipation can occur in people of all ages, from new-born babies to elderly. Medications and laxatives, in general, is a way of treating constipation which provides temporarily relief with many side-effects. Other than medications and laxatives, acupressure is an effective natural way of treating constipation which provides lasting relief without any side-effects. Acupressure Technique works on twelve different meridians in Human Body to regulate Energy pathways. Acupressure has some specific pressure points for constipation. Applying proper pressure on Acu-Points will cure the constipation problem sooner. You must know the applying technique and edge of pressure on various body parts regarding Acu-Points to prevent constipation. Acu-Points are very useful to relive constipation and maintaining better health. They also help in relieving the associated symptoms of constipation such as abdominal pain, bloating and gas. Stimulating these acupressure points along with a healthy fibre rich diet and optimum intake of fluids can go a long way in relieving constipation without depending on laxatives and medicines. Precautions: It is strongly recommended that pregnant women shall not do it. Please do not apply any of the Acupressure Points for constipation on a pregnant woman. Applying pressure on Acu-points to any pregnant woman may lead to worse situations like premature baby birth and other labour pains/problems.

Acupressure Points for Constipation are situated at various parts of body. Here we will discuss about Acu-Points for relieving constipation and how to get rid of it. The method for applying pressure and the load of pressure are important keys of healing constipation with Acupressure Points.

So if you have constipation problem, do massage some acupressure points. Press deeply till it 'hurts' i.e. mild pain. Massage each point for 1 minute and do it 2-3 times a day. Stimulating these acupressure points with your fingers can help relax the abdomen and promote regular bowel movement without any pain or discomfort. They also help in relieving the associated symptoms of constipation such as abdominal pain, bloating and gas. There are the acupressure points for relieving Constipation. Working on these points can help you get better quicker. You do not have to use all of these points. Using just one or two of them whenever you have a free hand can be effective.

There are different types of constipation in Chinese Medicine. It could be due to excess of heat and Qi (air) or deficient in Qi, Yang Qi, and blood.

Regardless types of constipation, there are some acu-pressure points you could use to massage yourself. It is an easy way to prevent and improve the condition, as there is no side effect and you can do it yourself. Acupressure uses a system of 365 pressure points along the 12 energetic meridians used in Traditional Chinese Medicine, which is also called TCM. Proponents of TCM believe that stimulating these points, by using fingertip pressure or acupuncture needles, can restore balanced health. Several points are traditionally stimulated to relieve constipation. You can balance the flow of energy by pressing on body points. Focus on the liver and conception vessel channels to assist constipated clients.

However, it is advisable to take care of your fibrous diet with sufficient intake of liquid (water) and do some exercise to avoid constipation and other digestion related problems. But Acupressure has been succeeded to relieve constipation faster. Acupressure Points for Constipation relieves the illness by stimulating the pressure points which are directly or indirectly associated with Stomach and Digestion System. Stimulating these acupressure points along with a healthy fibre rich diet and optimum intake of fluids can go a long way in relieving constipation without depending on laxatives and medicines. Acupressure Points are very helpful to give relief, heal and cure Constipation problem. You just need to practice the pressure points on a regular basis to get the benefits sooner. Stimulating these specific points can help in relieving indigestion and treating problems like constipation, diarrhoea, abdominal pain, gas and bloating. Stimulate the intestines reflex. Roll the ball around in the lower area of the palms or heels of the hands. Do this for a minute once or twice a week to help with digestion. Our modern eating habits and increasing dependence on packed and ready to eat meals has lead not only to increased risk of heart diseases, obesity and diabetes, it has also disrupted our digestive system causing problems like indigestion, gas, constipation, Irritable Bowel Syndrome (IBS), heart burn, sour stomach, diarrhoea, etc and most of us suffer from at least one of these problems although we don't really speak up or do something to relieve it. The best way to treat all these issues is changing the eating pattern for good, but in the meantime Acupressure and reflexology can be used effectively to relieve the painful side effects of an upset digestive system. So, now that you know the important acupressure points for relieving digestive problems of heartburn, acid reflux, and GERD, use them yourself and stimulate them in your loved ones for natural and lasting relief from these problems. Acupressure Points for Constipation are described as under.

Tips of Auc-pressure points to relief constipation

Your hand is a good measuring tool. A couple of tips to remember for acupressure:

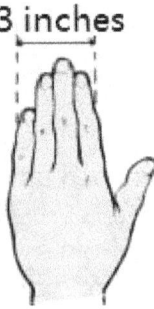

3 inches

Always measure any 'finger widths' with the fingers of the person being acupressure. That keeps the ratios the same. Don't push on the spot if you have long fingernails. You can use the eraser on the end of a pencil.
Use firm pressure, but not super hard.

Back off if this causes pain. If this happens, retry it very gently, slowly and steadily increasing the pressure. Also, focus on the breath if this happens, as it can help to release stress and pain.

Sometimes this works in as little as 5 or 10 seconds. If it doesn't, feel free to continue applying pressure for 1 to 3 minutes. Don't hold it for more than 5 minutes, though.

I would also like to add that, in our house, we don't have problems with chronic constipation and this method has consistently worked within a minute or two. For cases of chronic constipation, it might require more frequent (and maybe shorter) sessions of acupressure.

Practice following Auc-pressure points to relief constipation

1). Three Point Mile/"Leg three miles" or "Below Kneecap Point" (ST 36): The acupoints known as Stomach 36 (ST-36) is also called Zu San Li, which means "leg three miles". The name refers to the ability of this point to greatly strengthen energy, so that a person can walk another three miles, even when exhausted. Location: This point is located on the outer edge of the leg, three fingers width below the knee. Acupressure "Below Kneecap Point" is situated in lower of Kneecap, 3 to 4 centimetres below the kneecap. The exact spot for Point is below the kneecap and one centimetre outer side of shinbone as displayed in picture. Slightly bend your leg and place three fingers just below the kneecap. Begin with the index finger at the base of the kneecap. The point is where the little finger rests, on the outside aspect of the hard shinbone. Feel around for the tender spot. This acupoints can boost the immune system, and it can also strengthen overall energy. It is often used to strengthen weak digestion and improve digestive disorders, ranging from constipation to diarrhoea, gas, bloating, vomiting, and nausea. It gives you an immune system boost, addresses digestive problems from nausea and vomiting to gas and bloating, reduces swelling in the legs, reduces coughing and wheezing, and aids in sleep. To find exactly the point, measure three thumb widths below the bottom of your knee along the bone. Once you've measured down, let your finger slide to the outside of the bone. You might feel that achiness or a dip at the location of the point. If you're having trouble finding it, you can rub down along the side of the bone toward your feet from your knee to your shin--you'll hit this point and others on the Stomach meridian. The exact spot for Acupressure "Below Kneecap Point" is below the kneecap and one centimetre outer side of shinbone. Find "Below Kneecap Point" as displayed in picture and apply soft pressure on this Point on daily basis. Applying pressure on this Point will help you to cure stomach disorders, improves digestion ability and regulates the intestine. Below Kneecap Point is the last pressure point among Acupressure Points for Constipation. Stimulating this point helps in relieving ulcer, enteritis, nausea, gas, Gastric pain, vomiting, dysphasia, abdominal distention, borborygmus, diarrhoea, indigestion, dysentery, constipation, abdominal pain and bloating.

2). Sea of Energy (CV 6): Conception Vessel 6 is an important acupressure point for treating constipation. It is also named the "Sea of Qi" and this point is located exactly three finger widths below the belly button, directly below the belly button. This point should be stimulated using the fingertips gradually. The pressing should be no more than 1 inch deep. You will peel something firm with your fingers as you press. Maintain this firm pressure for 30 seconds as your breath normally keeping your eyes closed. This point helps in relieving pain in the abdomen, constipation, colitis and gas and is used to tone the abdominal muscles, as well relieve constipation and gas. The Sea of Energy moniker refers to the location of many organs in this area. This point should be stimulated using the fingertips gradually. The pressing should be no more than 1 inch deep. You will peel something firm with your fingers as you press. Maintain this firm pressure for 30 seconds as your breath normally keeping your eyes closed. It is also useful for treating hernia, irregular menstruation, and impotence in men, digestive disorders and fatigue. Benefits: Relieves pain in the abdominal muscles, constipation, colitis, and gas. It's important to drink plenty of warm water after the massage, to help clear away toxic substances in our body. Caution: If you have a serious illness, or life-threatening illness such as heart disease, or cancer, please consult with your physician before practicing Acupressure. If you're dealing with constipation, there's no need to reach straight for the laxatives. A blogger has shared a secret trick to get your bowels moving once again – involving no medication or fancy teas.

3). Centre of Power (CV 12) or Solar Plexus Point: CV12 or Conception Vessel 12 or REN 12 or Ren 12 or Zhong Wan or "Middle Cavity," or "Solar Plexus Point" is a channel where all the yin fluids of the body collect or where the energy of the stomach gathers and collects. In Chinese medicine, the stomach is called the "sea of water and grain". One of its principle functions is to transform water and grain into usable nutrients.

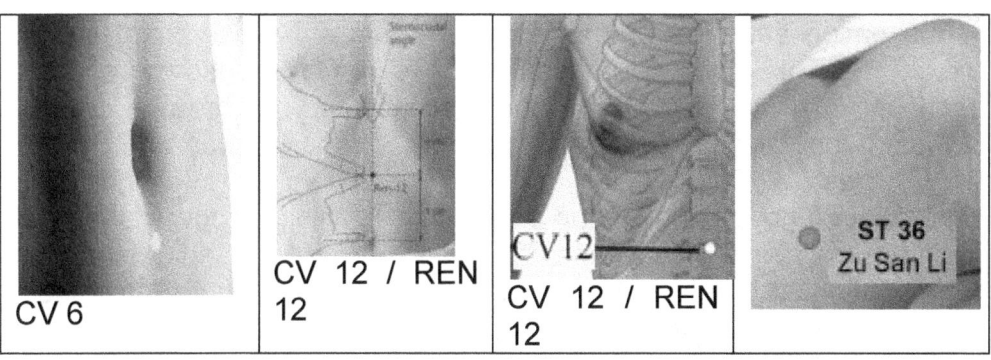

CV 6	CV 12 / REN 12	CV 12 / REN 12	ST 36 Zu San Li

Location: Find your belly button and locate the point where your ribs come together, where there will be a soft depression. If you draw a line from the point where your ribs meet to your belly button, Ren 12-Point is in the centre of this line or this point is located half way between the breast bone and the belly button, at the mid-line of the body. Stimulating this point helps in relieving heartburn, indigestion and abdominal pain and constipation. One of its principle functions is to transform water and grain into usable nutrients. In the chakra system, this relates to the solar plexus. This acupoints is used for setting of the "Solar plexus" and to improve lack of appetite and indigestion. This acupoints relieves stomach upset that is related to emotions. It can also alleviate fullness from overeating, gas, bloating, and acid regurgitation. It is yet another vital acupressure point that is a solution for all types of digestive problems and provides quick constipation relief. It is known as the "Centre of Power". This point should be stimulated with great care and should not be pressed for more than 2 minutes at a stretch. It should be pressed on an almost empty stomach. It is best to avoid this point if you are suffering from heart disease, cancer or hypertension. It relieves constipation along with abdominal spasms, stomach pain, indigestion, heartburn and emotional stress. It is also an effective pressure point for dysentery, jaundice, insomnia and vomiting.

4). Crooked Pond/Elbow Point (LI 11-Large Intestine 11): LI 11 or Large Intestine 11 is a functional acupressure point that provides quick cure for constipation. This point is also called the "Crooked pond" and it is situated at the outer end of the elbow crease. Acupressure Elbow Point is situated on the external side of elbow. Firstly fold your hand from elbow. Then put your finger on external end of elbow and move towards internal side. As you find the Elbow Point as displayed in picture, apply gentle pressure with your thumb on Elbow point in daily routine. Applying pressure on Acupressure Elbow Point will help you to improve digestion functions, remove

Constipation and also helpful for fever. Elbow Crease Point is first pressure point among Acupressure Points for Constipation. Press this point firmly using your fingers for 1 minute as your breathe deeply. Switch hands and stimulate the point on the other arm as well. This is large intestine 11, a point that can help balance intestinal tone whether you have constipation or diarrhoea. This is a powerful trigger point for the colon. This is an effective point to relieve indigestion and constipation. It also aids to reduce high fever, skin diseases, diarrhoea and heat stroke. It is also a local point for elbow pain and tennis elbow. Large Intestine 11 is a functional acupressure point that provides quick cure for constipation.

Crooked Pond Elbow Point	Grandfather-Grandson (Spleen- 4)	Inner Gate (Pericardium 6)	Union Valley

5). Grandfather-Grandson/Gang sun (Spleen-4) Point: Location of Spleen 4: In the arch of the foot, in a depression at the base of the first metatarsal bone. Find Spleen 3 in a depression at the ball of the toe, and then slide your finger up the shaft of the metatarsal until you are at the base of the bone. This point is located on the side of inner side of the foot, four finger width away from the big toe. In Gong sun – Grandfather Grandson Point, we find that it acts upon the abdomen in multiple ways. It is a powerful point of the Spleen channel and the luo-connecting point of that meridian. And it is the master point of the Chong Mai (Penetrating Vessel) which influences the whole of the abdomen and all its organs. Stimulating this point harmonizes energy flow in the stomach and relieves indigestion, constipation, stomach ache and nausea. SP 4 exerts a pronounced influence over the emotions. Because of Spleen's connection to the Heart, SP 4 can settle the spirit when there is restlessness, agitation, insomnia, mania and depression. The point also addresses an imbalance of sympathy, where a person suffers self-pity and feels unsupported by others and by the world at large, or relies too heavily on others to meet their needs. It therefore exerts a strong regulating effect on Blood and Qi. As the master point of the sea of blood, SP 4 regulates blood circulation, stops bleeding and addresses all menstrual irregularities.

It has an influence on the uterus and treats gynaecological disorders, constipation, such as endometriosis, fibroids and cysts. As the master point of the sea of the meridians, it ensures good circulation of Qi throughout the 12 meridians. It addresses counter-flow Qi, for example where Stomach Qi is rising rather than descending and causing chest or gastric pain. Apply firm pressure directed towards the ankle. It is believed that the Extraordinary Vessels develop at conception and form the basis of the energy network of the body, well before the development of the 12 organ meridians. Treating the Vessels therefore treats the depth and foundation of who we are as humans. Spend some time with Gong sun and become master of your own inner seas.

6). Great Rushing Point: This point is located in the webbing between the big and the second toes. Stimulating this point helps in improving gall-bladder health and relieving nausea, vomiting and abdominal pain.

Great Rushing	Heaven's pivot ST-25	Hand Valley (LI 4)	Inner Gate Point (P-6)
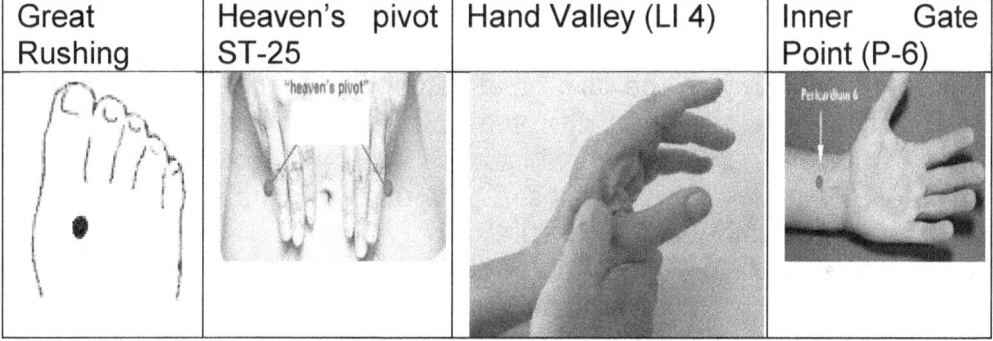			

7). "Hand Valley" Point (LI 4-Large Intestine 4) or "joining of the valley" Point: Hand Valley Point is second pressure point among Acupressure Points for Constipation. Acupressure Hand Valley Point is situated in the valley between Index Finger and Thumb. Find the Hand Valley Point same as displayed in the picture. It is close to the thumb and the index finger, the highest point on the back of your both hands Slide your fingertip from "He Gu Xue" toward your wrist, feeling for a bony bump at about the halfway point. Location: At the highest spot of the muscle on the back of the hand that protrudes when the thumb and index finger are brought close together. This is point LI 4 on the large intestine meridian, traditionally used to stimulate intestinal contractions. In TCM, constipation is considered a blocked passage; "joining the valley" refers to creating a passage, which creates a state of balance in your overall health. Caution: This point is forbidden for pregnant women, because its stimulation can cause premature contractions in the uterus. Benefits: Relieves constipation, headaches, toothaches, shoulder pain, arthritis, and labour pain. Joining Valley point (LI 4 - Large Intestine 4) is by far the most famous acupressure point that is a solution for various health issues and is an important point for constipation acupressure. It is called the Joining Valley point and it is located on the fleshy muscle between the index finger and the thumb. Spread your thumb and in index finger apart and stimulate this point by squeezing the fleshy webbing with your fingertips for 1 minute while you take long, deep breaths. Now, switch sides and press the point on the other hand for 1 minute. It helps to relieve constipation, chronic pains, eye problems, toothache, and allergies and boosts the immune system. This point is forbidden for pregnant women because stimulating this point can lead to premature contractions of the uterus. Applying pressure on Acupressure Hand Valley Point will help you to reduce Headache, Toothache. It relives Constipation and Shoulder tension.

8). Heaven's pivot (ST 25)/Tian Shu Point: Location: The Heaven's Pivot points are located three finger widths on the left and right side of the navel. It is 2 inches lateral to both sides of your navel. To locate: Place three fingers parallel and alongside the centre of the bellybutton. The point is at the edge of the last finger, three fingers away from the centre of the bellybutton. Method: you need to relax and take in a few deep breaths. Then, use your index, middle, and ring finger to lightly apply pressure on the Heaven's Pivot Points, but only till it feels a little tight. Keep the pressure from light to moderate for about thirty seconds, and then release. You may also massage with light, circular motions. Repeat it another two times. It has been observed that stimulating these points may lead to a bowel movement within a few minutes. However, remember that you must immediately halt the massage if you happen to experience any pain. Pregnant women are strictly advised against using this technique to relieve constipation, as it may trigger premature labour. Stimulate this point for 30 - 40 seconds on each hand. Repeat this 3 - 4 times a day. Regular stimulation of these points is known to help in alleviating constipation in the long run. However, ensure that you exercise caution while practicing acupressure. Even though this acupoints is located on the stomach meridian, it is where all the energy of the large intestine gathers and concentrates. The name for Stomach 25 (ST-25) is Tian Shu, which means "heaven's pivot". This acupoints is where the upper and lower gastrointestinal tract meet and relate to each other. Stomach 25 is especially useful in alleviating constipation, diarrhoea, and any other kind of intestinal disorder. Stimulating ST-25 also moves abdominal blood.

9). Inner Gate Point/Nei Guan (Pericardium 6): PC6 or Pericardium 6 is an effective acupressure point that is located on the medial aspect of the hand, four finger widths below the wrist, in the hollow between the tendons. To find the point, from the centre of the underside of your wrist measure two thumb widths down your arm. You might be able to find two tendons running along your arm there-- the point is in the middle of the two tendons. This point is also called the Inner Gate point and it should be stimulated by pressing the point with your fingertips. Apply pressure on the point for 1 minute and then switch side and apply pressure on the other arm. In addition, it is also used to treat upset stomach, motion sickness, constipation, headache, nausea, carpal tunnel syndrome, asthma, and angina and chest tightness. Pericardium 6 is great for motion sickness, morning sickness, or any kind of nausea. It's also amazing at taking down chest tightness from anxiety or full on anxiety attacks.   This one can be really sensitive for some folks so starting out with gentle pressure is a good idea. Same thing here--follow the thin line down toward the skin from the red handle to see where the point is.

Grandfather-Grandson (Spleen-4)	ST-36	Three Yin Crossing (Spleen 6)	Union Valley (LI 4)

10). Inner Court/Nei Ting/ST Water Point (ST 44): Nei Ting, or Stomach 44 (ST44), is the second to last point on the Stomach meridian in acupuncture. It is two finger widths directly below the belly button. It is a special point on the Stomach meridian, called the Ying Spring point. The Ying Spring points on all the meridians clear heat from that particular meridian and energy system. So we use ST44 to treat heat-type disorders of the stomach, including ulcers, acid reflux, abdominal pain, and GERD. To activate your body's self-healing power, first locate of the acupressure points that you need to work on for your specific needs. Apply firm pressure is the most fundamental technique. Use thumbs, fingers, palms, the side of the hand, or knuckles to apply steady, stationary pressure to the point for 1-2 minutes. A general guideline to follow is that the pressure should be firm enough so that it hurts a little. The more developed the muscles are, the more pressure you should apply. If you feel extreme sensitivity or pain, gradually decrease the pressure until you find a balance between pain and pleasure. Do not continue to press a point that is excruciatingly painful. It's important to drink plenty of warm water after the massage, helps to clear away toxic substances in our body. Caution: please consult with your physician before practicing Acupressure. ST44 also clears Damp-Heat from the intestines. Damp-Heat refers to a build-up of toxic heat and excess fluid accumulation and treats things like diarrhoea, dysentery, constipation, or acute abdominal cramping.

ST44 can clear "excess" type heat from our system, heat that comes from an acute stomach bug, or from a build-up of stress, or a sinus infection. But it can also be paired with other points to clear "deficient" type heat and heat that comes from a weakness in our own body. In this way, we can effectively use ST44 to treat more chronic digestive issues, chronic sinus pain, and even some kinds of chronic viral infections. Benefits: It cools heat in the Stomach and Intestines and moves the stools easily, Benefits: It relieves water retention, chronic diarrhoea, constipation, and gas. It relieves toothache, frontal headache, nasal congestion, and dental anaesthesia, and laryngitis, pain during menstrual periods, nose bleed, abdominal pain, food retention, and fever.

11) Three Yin Crossing: This point is located three finger widths above the inner ankle bone. Place your four fingers at the top of the inside ankle bone as shown in the picture above to find the point. The point is right there along the side of the shin bone. Look at the last picture for good idea of where it is. Stimulating this point helps in overall healing of diseases related to the lower abdomen. It relieves colitis, abdominal distention, constipation, flatulence, reproductive disorders, including menstrual cycle irregularity, pre-menstrual discomfort, and menstruation pain. There's a wonderful point on the leg which is commonly used in acupressure and is very versatile. It can treat many conditions associated with all three organs. If you have digestive, gynaecological or emotional conditions, just find the point and massage it. It may be tender, but do this for two minutes. The tenderness should subside and so should the symptoms.

12). Union Valley/He Gu Xue (LI 4): Location: This point is located in the webbing between the index finger and the thumb. Stimulating this point improves over all intestinal function and helps relieve diarrhoea, constipation and abdominal pain. It is found on the webbing between your thumb and pointer finger, the He Gu Xue point stimulates contractions in the digestive system, and is helpful for relieving insomnia and shoulder tension. An acupressurist might hold this point firmly for up to two minutes in a session. Pregnant women should avoid stimulating this point, as it can induce labour contractions. Acupressure Point LI 4 is called Union Valley, (Hegu/ He Gu in Chinese) and is referred as a channel of energy associated with the large intestine. I personally apply acupressure on this point two times daily to get relief from pain or aches and easy bowel movement and to prevent constipation. It also helps in many other ailments. For any kind of discomfort and pain, acupressure therapy is suggested along with Li 4 point because it helps in getting relief from pain or aches. Benefits: One of the keys to maintaining wellness is regular bowel movements. Diet, stress and other factors can often interfere with the body's natural elimination. According to the theory of Acupressure, this important source point helps re-establish the energy balance of the meridian. Application of thumb pressure on LI 4 has been shown to help alleviate constipation and has also been beneficial for some in helping to relieve headaches.

(13) Stretching to open all the Digestive Channels: It is important to stretch the entire body before beginning the acupressure session in order to unblock the blocked meridians and help the "qi" flow throughout the body that will make the session more effective. Raise your arms above your head while breathing in and stretch backwards as much as you can without hurting yourself. Count till 3 and come back to the original position while exhaling slowly. Inhale and bend forward in the rag doll position while exhaling. Count till 3 and come back to the starting position while inhaling. Bring your arms above your head and lean your body to the right side while exhaling. Come back to the starting position while inhaling. Now lean your body to the left side while exhaling. Come back to the starting position while inhaling. Repeat this whole stretching workout 3 times to open all digestive channels. All these pressure points helps in opening up the digestive channel and it will benefit any digestive condition in an effective way. So the next time you feel bloated and full, don't just reach out for an antacid, try out these easy and simple reflexology procedures and get long term relief from digestive problems.

(14) Appetite, Hiccups and Nausea: Point Di Er Li Dui: Location: This is another of the pressure points on feet that is located in the toe area. It can be found on the upper side of your second toe, just below your toenail. Uses: Appetite, hiccups and nausea

Burping and Heartburn: Point Di San Li Dui: Location: This point is found right below the toenail of your middle toe. Uses: Excessive burping and heartburn.

(15) Digestive System Calmness: LI 4 acupressure point: Location: It is located on the top side of the hand, between your thumb and your index finger. To locate it, squeeze the thumb against the base of the index finger. The point you are looking for is located on the highest point of the bulge of the muscle. Press this point for about 30 seconds to induce calmness and for a health-inducing digestive detoxify. However, you should NOT try this technique if you are pregnant. It is really difficult to determine the root cause of Digestive Problems, but it is often treated according to the symptoms, but here are a few most common causes for digestive disorder.

Ileocecal Valve Functions and its Opening:

Constipation symptoms can sometimes be caused by an ileocecal valve that isn't working properly. The ileocecal valve, which is located between the small and large intestine, serves two purposes. First, it acts as a block that prevents the toxic contents of the large intestine from backing up into the small intestine. Second, it keeps the food products in the small intestine from passing into the large intestine before the digestive processes have been completed. The Ileocecal Valve sticks shut sometimes and the faeces stay in the small intestine, unable to move any further. This back-up causes constipation. When the ileocecal valve isn't working right, it can cause these symptoms and many more. Just look at the list of things that it can cause:

- Shoulder pain
- Light-headedness
- Nausea
- Ringing in the ears
- Bursitis-like pain in the shoulders and hip joints
- Low back pain for no reason
- Recurrent sinus infections
- Dizziness
- Chest pain
- Heart fluttering
- Headaches
- Fever

Causes of Ileocecal Valve Problems:

There are several reasons why the valve doesn't always work right. There are a few common reasons why the ileocecal valve doesn't always work right, resulting in constipation symptoms. Sometimes spicy or roughage-type foods will irritate the valve and cause it to get stuck. Stress and emotional trauma can also cause the valve to malfunction. Those who have had their appendix removed seem to have more problems with the valve than others.

Sometimes spicy or roughage-type foods will irritate the valve and cause it to stick shut or open.

Another factor that greatly influences the valve is stress or emotional trauma. Almost everyone is exposed to these factors, but some of us are more sensitive than others.

I personally find that those who have had their appendix removed seem to have more problems. Some researchers believe that the appendix, which is located right next to this valve, acts like "an overflow bag for toxins" and holds these until the body can work them out slowly and not interrupt the workings of the ileocecal valve.

Closing an Ileocecal Valve that is Stuck Open: When the valve is open (diarrhoea, loose stools, and symptoms like those mentioned earlier), there are some temporary things that can be done first. The valve is located about halfway between the belly button and the "hip bone." Many times you can get relief in one of two ways. First, you can sometimes hold the valve shut for several minutes. These are done by placing your hand over the valve and while pushing in, pull up toward the left shoulder. The second way is to place a cold pack made of cold water or ice over the valve for about 15 to 20 minutes. This process can be repeated if necessary.

Maintaining the Health of Your Ileocecal Valve: Except for the two things to do for diarrhoea and an open ileocecal valve (which I also find works quite well for travellers in Mexico who are suffering from the famous so-called "tourist" or Montezuma's revenge); there are several things that need to be done for both the open and the closed valves.

Opening up an ileocecal valve

Luckily, there are a couple of simple things you can do to open up an ileocecal valve that is stuck closed and causing constipation symptoms. Do as follows:

- First, the toxic food products that are either backing up or that are blocked up in the intestines need to be detoxified, and the best method to do this is to use either garlic or chlorophyll. I find that chlorophyll works the best and is easy to obtain at any health food store. Initially, either two capsules or tablets or 1/2 teaspoon of chlorophyll liquid should be taken every two hours for about six to eight hours, and the same amount with each meal for the next three or four days.

- Next, the diet should be modified in such a way that spicy foods be eliminated for a week or so.
- Modify your roughage-type food intake. If the problem is diarrhoea, it is helpful to eliminate all roughage-type food for a short period of time. If it is a closed valve and constipation is a problem, then increase the roughage.
- Eliminate alcohol, cocoa, chocolate and caffeine products from the diet.
- For a closed valve (constipation), add calcium and vitamin D to the diet.
- For an open valve (diarrhoea), add lactic acid yeast wafers to the diet, which can be obtained at any health food store. This product alone can sometimes stop even the most stubborn cases of chronic diarrhoea.
- Most importantly, however, you can relieve problems almost instantly by rubbing out the following "reflex" points for both the open and the closed ileocecal valve. The areas illustrated should be massaged with firm pressure for about 10 to 20 seconds each (it is not beneficial to rub the points any longer than that. In fact, it may negate the effect). Most of the points will be extremely sore if the problem is long standing. If a cooperating friend or a vibrator is available, they can be used to work out the points. Massage your ileocecal "reflex" points. By rubbing out the points illustrated below, you can unstick the valve to relieve constipation. The areas illustrated should be massaged with firm pressure for about 10 to 20 seconds each. Note: It is not beneficial to rub the points any longer than that. In fact, it may negate the effect.)
- Detoxify the toxic food products that are backing up in the intestines, causing the constipation symptoms. The best method to do this is to use chlorophyll, which is easy to obtain at any health food store. Initially, either two capsules or tablets or a ½ teaspoon of chlorophyll liquid should be taken every two hours for about six to eight hours, and the same amount with each meal for the next three or four days.

- Modify your diet to relieve constipation. Eliminate spicy foods, alcohol, cocoa, chocolate, and caffeinated products for a week or so. Also, take additional calcium and vitamin D.

5.4. Unani for constipation:

- Grind 25 gm Halaila siyah (Black variety) and 25 gm of Almond separately and add honey. The mixture may be taken twice a day. It is a useful remedy for it as well as piles.
- 6 gm of Asapaghol along with milk may be taken daily at bed time to get relief.
- Take equal quantity of sana, sonth, sonf and sendha namak. Grind it properly, may be taken at bed time to cure the condition. The mix is an effective unani treatment for it.
- 10 gm of Itrifal Zamani should be taken with lukewarm water before going to bed.
- 2 tablespoon of Itrifal Mulayyan is a valuable unani medicine that is recommended with warm water at bed time.
- 6 ml of Rogan Badam with milk at bed time is useful.
- About 30 ml of Sharbat Arzani + water is a good.
- Gulqand and Majoon Anjeer are also beneficial.

5.5 Ayurveda remedy for constipation:

- Soak the mix of Amaltas fruit + Tamarind, keep it overnight, before drinking mashed and filter it. This is the good Ayurvedic remedy for it.
- 10-20 ml real home made fruit juice twice a day is useful.
- Increased the use of coconut oil, especially in diet as it is the effective Ayurvedic treatment.
- 5 ml ghee along with warm milk may be taken at bed time without sugar as a good natural remedy.
- Spinach juice helps to relieve it.
- Isabgol (Plantago ovate) and vitis vinifera boiled with milk take the mix at bed time with 5 ml ghee. It is Ayurvedic remedy for sluggish bowel movements.
- Triphala powder is an excellent cleanser and natural colon cleanser.
- Warm lemon juice helps in clearing motion.
- Aloe vera juice cleanses the intestine.
- Isabguha or psyllium husk is quite effective treatment.

- Rhuharb cures chronic constipation and use as constipation remedy.
- Bael fruit juice, an ayurvedic food, is helpful in removing waste from the body.
- As an herbal medicine for acute constipation, it is better to take the ripe fruit of Belleric Myroblan.
- Cassia is a good remedy in the treatment of it.
- Castor oil is beneficial for the disease.
- Chicory, a natural laxative, used as Ayurvedic medicine.
- Haritak, an Ayurvedic herb, helpful for treating it.
- Spices like cumin seeds, coriander, and turmeric powder easily digested the foods. All these are good Ayurvedic product.

5.6 Homeopathy medicine for constipation, Piles and Anal Fissures:

- Homeopathy has proper and effective solution for constipation, irritable bowel syndrome, haemorrhoids, anal fissures, piles, etc. It also eases hard stool. Homeopathic medicine helps to work the body efficiently by treating the condition from its root. Here, few of the important homeopathic remedies are being mentioned.

Advantage of Homeopathy treatment naturally:

There are added advantages of Homeopathy. First and foremost, homeopathic treatment is completely natural. There are no chemical or synthetic preparations that are used in homeopathic medicines. All homeopathic medicines are made from natural sources like plants and minerals. Even during the preparation, these natural medicines are not put through any chemical processes. Therefore, one can always remain assured that whatever homeopathic medicines you take are purely natural and will be safe. There is no chance of any side effect or any adverse reaction either. The fact remains that Homeopathy is the safest system of medicine. There are no side effects. You can rest assured that you will not be suffering from a dozen other problems while taking medicines for one problem. Also, it is much more economical than the allopathic system of medicine or the surgical option which can cost a bomb. Moreover, taking Homeopathic treatment is as effortless as breathing. The homeopathic medicines are easy to take. You can carry them in your pocket anywhere and take them at the appointed time. At the same time, there is no problem of taste with the homeopathic medicines also. In fact, the taste is one of the reasons that children crave for the medicines more and more.

5.6.1 Best Homeopathic medicines for Constipation

Source: (1. Dr. Vikas Sharma MD-Homeopathy (Gold Medallist); and 2. Dr Shah's, MD-Homeopathy of "Life Force Homoeopathy")

The above Doctors of Homeopath MD, have had the experience of treating millions of cases of anal fissures and piles with homeopathy medicines in their clinic as well as on line in the last 2 decades. The fact remains that homeopathy is very effective at curing anal fissures. Dr. Vikas Sharma (MD-Homeopathy) says that the biggest reason to choose homeopathic medicine for piles is the permanency and safety of the treatment. Once treated with homeopathy, piles tend to not to recur (under conditions where lifestyle modifications are sustained for long). Homeopathic medicines are very safe and side effects with homeopathy while treating piles are unheard of.

I, as an author, have just noted down this information from their website on line and put here for the purposes and benefits of millions and millions of people in the world suffering from Anal Fissure and Piles. When it comes to alternative or complementary treatments for piles or haemorrhoids, Homeopathy offers the best treatment for piles. The doctors say it is best not only because the cure rate is exceptionally good but also because Homeopathic treatment for piles offers several more advantages. It is very economical when compared to any other alternative or complementary treatment for piles. At the same time, the homeopathic medicines do not have any side effects. This is one of the biggest advantages of Homeopathy over any other system of medicine. While you are under treatment of any other system of medicine, you run the risk of getting one or the other side effect while Homeopathic treatment for piles is absolutely safe. That is why Doctors say that Homeopathy is the best when it comes to alternative or complementary treatment for piles or Haemorrhoids. In Homeopathy, there are very effective medicines that can cure Piles or Haemorrhoids very easily. Long standing constipation may lead to piles, anal fissures and rectal prolapsed. Abdominal hernia (inguinal hernia/umbilical hernia) may also arise from long standing constipation. Piles are swollen, dilated veins in rectal canal or anus. Anal fissure refers to a tear in the tissue lining of

210

the anus. Rectal prolapsed refers to protrusion of a part or the entire rectum from the anus. Abdominal hernia is the protrusion of an organ through the abdominal wall or cavity which normally contains it.

Excessive gas and distended abdomen with constipation point toward irritable bowel syndrome. The irritable bowel syndrome is a functional bowel disorder without any pathological changes in bowels. In irritable bowel syndrome, constipation and/or diarrhoea can predominate or alternate. Other symptoms include bloated abdomen, gas, cramps in abdomen and mucus in stool.

Best Homeopathic medicine for constipation with particular Symptoms

Homeopathy offers a wide range of medicines for constipation. Among these, the medicines, the Doctors rate top grade are Nux Vomica, Alumina and Bryonia Alba. Nux Vomica is most helpful in case of unsatisfactory stool. The urge to pass stool is frequent, yet scanty stool is passed each time. Alumina is indicated when a person skips days without stool. The urge to pass stool is absent for days together. The stool passes only when there is large accumulation in the intestines. Homeopathic medicine Bryonia Alba is used to treat constipation where the stool is hard and dry. Homeopathic medicines that can help treat hard stool in constipation are Bryonia Alba and Opium. Bryonia Alba works well where a person passes hard, dry stool in large lump. Opium is the best Homeopathic medicine for constipation where the person passes hard, dry stool in the shape of a ball.

Homeopathic medicine Nitric Acid shows the most wonderful results where hard stool tears the anal lining and leads to blood with stool.

Homeopathic medicine Alumina works wonders in cases where a person goes days without passing stool. The intestine movements are very sluggish. Alumina helps in such cases by improving the bowel movements.

Homeopathic medicines that work best for constipation with hard, dry, round ball-like stool include Opium and Chelidonium Majus.

Homeopathy uses Lycopodium Clavatum to treat constipation where it is attended with excessive flatulence and bloated abdomen.

Getting fresh in the morning is a normal thing for most people. For some others, it is a big task. The stool may be dry, hard or even normal. There may be constant urge to pass stool. At the same time, when one tries to pass stool, he is unable to do so in a satisfactory manner. The urge for stool remains even after passing stool.

This is the incidence of constipation, which is to be shared by the modern day lifestyle. The situation in the modern world is such that one is mentally overworked and physically underworked. The work culture everywhere is demanding. One has to constantly run against time. The race to complete targets never ends. It is a corollary of this culture that one has little time or inclination to go out for a walk or a game of one's favourite sport. To add to it, there is the added allure of fast food. This fast food is rich in calories but low in fibre content. Raw fruits and vegetables are not a part of the modern menu. Tea, coffee, smoking and liquor add further fuel to the fire. One drinks little water but glasses of colas are gulped down day in and day out. All the above mentioned things are the cause of the scourge of constipation.

Homeopathy intends to cure the root cause of constipation. It is therefore natural that these medicines are going to take some time to get things going. Ultimately, it is effective at restoring this peristaltic movement to the normal self. Here are the best 5 homeopathic medicines for constipation as per my experience.

Nux Vomica: One of the best homeopathic medicines for constipation due to sedentary lifestyle. Nux Vomica is the most commonly indicated medicine these days. In fact, it fits the bill most effectively. The modern day lifestyle being the culprit, Nux Vomica is one of the best homeopathic medicines for constipation. It is very effective when a lot of laxatives have been taken regularly. The patient is habituated to stimulants like tea, coffee or alcohol. There is frequent, ineffectual urge for stool. One is able to pass only a small quantity at a time. At times, diarrhoea and constipation alternate. There is a constant feeling of unease in the rectum. The patient is usually chilly. He gets angered easily. He is an achiever and a go-getter.

Bryonia: One of the best homeopathic medicines for constipation with intense thirst. In cases, where there is constipation despite increased thirst and intake of lot of water, Bryonia is one of the best homeopathic medicines for constipation. There is dryness of all mucous membranes and that of the whole system. The mouth feels dry and so do the lips. It is due to this dryness that one has constipation. Even the stool is dry. At times, the stool looks as if burnt.

Graphites: One of the best homeopathic medicines for constipation with obesity. In cases where there is constipation along with obesity, Graphites is one of the best homeopathic medicines for constipation. There is hardly any urge to stool. There are large knotty stools that are united by mucous threads. Soreness of the anus may be seen.

There is a tendency to form fissures. Other skin affections may also be present ailing with the constipation.

Alumina: One of the best homeopathic medicines for constipation in children. In cases where there is constipation even in early childhood, Alumina is one of the best homeopathic medicines for constipation. It is all the more indicated in children who have been artificially fed. This may mean that they have had little breast milk and have been fed bottle milk or formula feed. There is intense dryness of the intestinal tract. The stool is also dry, hard and knotty. The stool may resemble that of sheep. Even a soft stool requires great straining and is passed with great difficulty.

Silicea: One of the best homeopathic medicines for constipation with receding stool. In cases where the stool is partly expelled and then recedes back, Silicea is one of the best homeopathic medicines for constipation. The patient is usually chilly. The faces remain a long time in the rectum but are not expelled. There is great straining but hardly effective. In females, the constipation is aggravated before and during menses.

Nitric Acid: Homeopathic medicine Nitric Acid shows the most wonderful results where hard stool tears the anal lining and leads to blood with stool.

Other Homeopathic medicines for Treatment of Constipation

Bryonia Alba: Excellent Homeopathic medicine for constipation with dry, hard, stool in lump form. For constipation with hard, dry stool that passes in lump form, Bryonia Alba is considered one of the best Homeopathic medicines for constipation. The stool is dry, as if burnt, and is passed with much difficulty. Abdominal distension is also noted in some cases. Headache from constipation may also be effectively treated with Homeopathic medicine Bryonia Alba.

Lycopodium Clavatum: Effective Homeopathic medicine for constipation with flatulence and bloated abdomen. Lycopodium Clavatum works wonders in cases where constipation is attended with flatulence and a bloated abdomen. Lycopodium Clavatum is also the most helpful Homeopathic medicine for constipation in elderly people. It is very useful in irritable bowel syndrome as well.

Antimonium Crudum and Podophyllum Peltatum: Valuable Homeopathic medicines for cases where constipation and diarrhoea alternate. Antimonium Crudum and Podophyllum Peltatum are two prominent Homeopathic medicines for constipation alternating with diarrhoea. Antimonium Crudum also effectively treats soreness of rectum, anal itching and mucus piles. It is extremely useful for alternating constipation and diarrhoea in elderly. Some unique features to look out for while prescribing Homeopathic medicine Podophyllum, apart from alternating constipation and diarrhoea, are gurgling in bowels, prolapsed of rectum with stool, clay coloured stool or greenish stool and highly offensive stool.

Aesculus Hippocastanum and Collinsonia Canadensis: Best Homeopathic medicines for constipation with piles. Aesculus Hippocastanum and Collinsonia Canadensis have shown the most remarkable recoveries in cases of constipation with piles. Homeopathic medicine Aesculus Hippocastanum is advised in case of dry, hard, knotty stool with painful piles. There is a sensation of small sticks stuck in the rectum. Pain may worsen while walking. Aesculus Hippocastanum is useful for piles that are bleeding or blind type. A severe lower back ache attends piles complaints, which it also treats. The characteristic features to look out for using Collinsonia Canadensis are protruding piles with hard stool. Itching or constriction at the anus may also be noticed. Collinsonia Canadensis is also well indicated for constipation during pregnancy.

Ratanhia and Nitric Acid: Highly recommended Homeopathic medicines for anal fissures with constipation. Ratanhia and Nitric Acid are well recognised Homeopathic medicines for anal fissures with constipation. Ratanhia is more useful in case of anal fissure with burning pain and constriction at the anus while passing stool. The stool is passed with great effort and strain. Burning may continue for hours after stool is passed. Cold water application may relieve the burning pains. Homeopathic medicine Nitric Acid is the choice where there is bleeding and pain while passing stool. The pain may be tearing, cutting or stitching in nature.

Natrum Mur: Top rated Homeopathic medicine for constipation when stool is passed on alternate days. In cases where stool is passed on alternative days, Homeopathic medicine Natrum Mur is what the doctor orders to regularise bowel movements. The attending features are constriction in the rectum, smarting, burning or tearing pain at the anus.

Opium and Chelidonium Majus: Top Homeopathic medicines for constipation with dry, hard stool in ball form. Homeopathic medicines Opium and Chelidonium Majus work well in cases of constipation where the stool is hard, dry and passed in ball-like form. In addition, Opium is also the Homeopathic medicine for constipation where the person has been taking laxatives to pass stool for a long time.

Homeopathy Medicine for Constipation in children and infants:

Homeopathic medicine for constipation is natural and safe for administering to children, even infants. Alumina and Calcarea Carb are mostly prescribed for constipation in children and infants. Alumina is prescribed where a child skips days without passing stool. The stool, though soft, requires straining. Calcarea Carb is a good choice where the first part of stool is hard, followed by soft stool.

Homeopathy Medicine for Constipation in elderly people:

The elderly people often suffer constipation. For elderly people with constipation, Lycopodium Clavatum, Alumina and Opium are ideally suited. Lycopodium is used where constipation is accompanied with gas in abdomen. Homeopathic medicine Alumina is advised where the aged person goes days without passing stool while Alumina works well where the stool is soft, but passes with much straining and difficulty. Opium is selected where the stool is hard, dry and passed in ball-like form.

5.6.2 Best Homeopathic medicines for Piles (Haemorrhoids)

The term haemorrhoids or piles refer to a condition in which the veins around the anus or lower rectum are swollen and inflamed. Haemorrhoids are very common in both men and women. About half of the population has haemorrhoids by age 50. Piles or Haemorrhoids (called Bawasir in Hindi language) is a disease affecting the anal region. In Piles, the veins in the rectal area swell due to stagnation of blood. The swollen veins cause pain, itching and discomfort while passing stool, sitting, standing or walking. The pain may last for a long time after passing stool. In some patients, there may be bleeding while passing stool. This is known as bleeding piles. The piles may be internal or external depending upon the location of the veins. When the problem is severe, the piles may protrude from the rectum and may have to be pushed back manually.

Haemorrhoids may result from straining to move stool. Other contributing factors include pregnancy, ageing, chronic constipation or diarrhoea. Haemorrhoids are either inside the anus (internal) or under the skin around the anus (external). Although many people have haemorrhoids, not all experience symptoms. The most common symptom of internal haemorrhoids is bright red blood covering the stool, or in the toilet bowl. However, an internal haemorrhoid may protrude through the anus outside the body, becoming irritating and painful. Some simple lifestyle modifications can help one, prevent and even cure piles. A softer stool and regular bowel movements are its primary goals. A softer stool makes emptying the bowels easier and lessens the pressure on haemorrhoids caused by straining. Warm Baths- bathing the perennial area in warm water can ease out the acute pain in a significant manner. This possibly relaxes the anal sphincter and gives relief from the pain. Increasing fluid intake can help in reducing the hardness of the stools. Drinking 12 to 15 glasses of water will help in softening and passing bulky stools. High-fibre diet like good sources of fibre fruits, vegetables, and whole grains can be very helpful. Regular exercise including walking can be very useful in regulating your digestive system.

Out of all the diseases, the most feared are the ones are that remind one of surgeon's knife. Piles are just one out of those diseases. But with Homeopathic medicines for piles one can be saved from the surgeon's knife; moreover they are entirely safe, gentle and the cure of piles is mostly permanent. This means that homeopathy can help in the complete recovery of piles. Homeopathic Remedies for haemorrhoids aim at correcting the internal disturbances of venous system by making the vein valves more strong which helps in a complete recovery. The sooner the patient approaches a homeopathic physician for piles treatment, higher are the chances of a complete recovery and avoidance of surgery. Homeopathy should be the preferred and the first mode of treatment in piles owing to the use of safe, natural nature of medicines before.

Symptoms of Haemorrhoids (Piles):

The following common symptoms that are seen in the majority of piles or haemorrhoids patients happen to be: There is pain while passing stool. The character of the pain may vary from one patient to the other. While some experience excruciating pain, others have only mild discomfort. Some patients describe the pain as if some splinter or a glass is pricking in the anal canal while others may feel burning pain. Often patients keep on feeling this pain for hours after passing stool. This pain can make sitting or standing difficult. Symptoms of haemorrhoids may include painful swelling or a hard lump around the anus. In addition, excessive straining, rubbing, or cleaning around the anus may cause irritation with bleeding and/or itching, which may produce a vicious cycle of symptoms. When one has been diagnosed with piles, the next obvious thing that comes into one's mind is its treatment. The only treatment for piles or haemorrhoids that is offered by Allopath is the surgical option. There is no other treatment in allopath. Most of the patients are afraid or wary of getting a surgery done. There are some disadvantages of this surgical option. Surgery is cumbersome and expensive. At the same time, the very purpose of surgery is lost when this problem recurs after some time of getting surgery done. At times, people are not aware of the possibility of piles being treated in any other way and end up getting surgery done. They do not look around or ask around for other possibilities i.e. alternative or complementary treatment for piles. It is only later when the problem recurs that they regret their decision of getting surgery done and start looking for some alternatives. At times some patients are lucky enough to be given the right guidance by a friend or family member or a relative to look for other alternatives to surgery. Some patients are themselves smart enough to look around before taking the surgeon's word as the gospel truth. There are still others who are not lucky enough and get a surgery done but look around only when the problem recurs. Having got themselves surgically treated once, they realize that they cannot keep on getting surgeries every now and then. So they start searching the internet or ask friends for some alternative or complementary treatment for piles.

Homeopathic Medicines for Piles:

Source: (1. Dr. Vikas Sharma MD-Homeopathy (Gold Medallist); and 2. Dr Shah's, MD-Homeopathy of "Life Force Homoeopathy")

The above Doctors of Homeopath MD, have had the experience of treating millions of cases of anal fissures and piles with homeopathy medicines in their clinic as well as on line in the last 2 decades. The fact remains that homeopathy is very effective at curing anal fissures. Dr. Vikas Sharma (MD-Homeopathy) says that the biggest reason to choose homeopathic medicine for piles is the permanency and safety of the treatment. Once treated with homeopathy, piles tend to not to recur (under conditions where lifestyle modifications are sustained for long). Homeopathic medicines are very safe and side effects with homeopathy while treating piles are unheard of.

I, as an author, have just noted down this information from their website on line and put here for the purposes and benefits of millions and millions of people in the world suffering from Anal Fissure and Piles. When it comes to alternative or complementary treatments for piles or haemorrhoids, Homeopathy offers the best treatment for piles. The doctors say it is best not only because the cure rate is exceptionally good but also because Homeopathic treatment for piles offers several more advantages. It is very economical when compared to any other alternative or complementary treatment for piles. At the same time, the homeopathic medicines do not have any side effects. This is one of the biggest advantages of Homeopathy over any other system of medicine. While you are under treatment of any other system of medicine, you run the risk of getting one or the other side effect while Homeopathic treatment for piles is absolutely safe. That is why Doctors say that Homeopathy is the best when it comes to alternative or complementary treatment for piles or Haemorrhoids. In Homeopathy, there are very effective medicines that can cure Piles or Haemorrhoids very easily. By opting for Homeopathy treatment for piles problem, one can avoid surgery, which is the only option that is offered by Allopath. In my experience in the last 2 decades of practice in Homeopathy, the Doctors (MD Homeopath) have found a few medicines to be very effective in Homeopathic treatment for piles. A lot of cases were really bad ones. Some had been suffering for decades and had tried lots of piles medicines including creams for applications, home remedies or Ayurvedic medicines. From the vast experience of treating such difficult and chronic piles cases, the Doctors (MD Homeopath) have compiled this list of the best Homeopathy medicines for Piles problem for you. At the cost of being repetitive, Doctors have emphasized that this list of homeopathic piles medicines is not an exhaustive one. They often have to use other medicines depending upon the symptoms of the patient. Nonetheless, these 5 piles medicines can be called the first 5 best homeopathic remedies for piles problem. The best Homeopathic medicines for Piles treatment are:

Aesculus: Aesculus is one of the top Homeopathic Medicines for piles with a backache. Aesculus is a homeopathic medicine for piles when it is accompanied with a backache. Severe, sharp, shooting lower backache in the lumbosacral region with haemorrhoids is sure shot sign for Aesculus to be used. Aesculus is mainly a remedy for blind piles. Lower backache accompanies piles. Constipation is also present with dry, hard stool. Piles appear purple, painful, burning with rawness, soreness, and itching. The stool is also constipated and is hard, dry and difficult to expel. Rectum feels full of small sticks. Piles are purple in colour and accompanied with hard, dry stool. This is one best Homeopathic remedy for Haemorrhoids or Piles problem with pain in the back. If the patient has pain in the back along with piles, Aesculus Hippocastanum is the best Homeopathic remedy for piles or haemorrhoids. There is pain in the back along with the piles and there is no explanation for this backache except that it is occurring along with the piles. There may be pain in the rectum as if it is full of small sticks. More often, the piles is blind in character, which means that there is no bleeding. In some patients, there is itching or irritation in the anal canal. Bleeding may or may not be present. In those cases, where bleeding occurs, it is mostly while passing stool. The blood is often fresh red blood.

Aloe Socotrina: A Top grade Homeopathic medicine for Protruding Piles. Homeopathic medicine Aloe Socotrina is a highly ranked homeopathic medicine for treating protruding piles. They are very tender, sore and painful. Burning at anus also accompanies. Intense itching may also appear. Relief from cold applications in piles symptoms is also a guiding feature to use Aloe. A history of long-standing diarrhoea may be present in persons needing Aloe in haemorrhoid complaint.

Aloe: Aloe is a homeopathic medicine of much help when piles appear blue like a bunch of grapes around anus with extreme tenderness, soreness and pain. Cold applications may soothe the pain.

Calcarea Fluor: Calcarea Fluor seems most applicable to persons who have internal or blind piles with backache. Calcarea Fluor may be used for painless, non bleeding piles with backache.

Causticum: Causticum is a homeopathic medicine of much help when piles are very large, painful, burning and hinder the passage of stool and walking worsens the pain.

Collinsonia: Collinsonia is the best choice when obstinate constipation is present with piles. Stool is dry, hard, and knotty.

Graphites: This is one of the Best Homeopathic medicines for Piles or Haemorrhoids with Constipation. If the patient has constipation along with piles, Graphites is the best homeopathic medicine for piles and has shown wonderful results in my practice. The stools are hard, knotty and united by mucous threads. Obesity is another strong indication for this medicine. Skin eruptions are another common symptom seen in such patient. When one finds such a patient who is obese, has skin eruptions or any history of skin eruptions and is constipated, Graphites is most likely to cure such a patient. In females, there is menstrual disturbance too. Most of the times, menses are scanty and delayed.

Hamamelis: In homeopathy, Hamamelis is a top grade remedy for venous congestions and bleeding tendencies and for bleeding piles. It is very effective in controlling haemorrhages. It can be used confidently with great results in bleeding piles. Piles that bleed profusely require Hamamelis without a second thought. Burning and soreness in the rectum may appear with bleeding. Few may also complain of a backache with bleeding piles. Pain or rawness at anus is also marked. Extreme weakness also accompanies bleeding piles. Hamamelis is the best homeopathic remedy for arresting acute bleeding from piles. Bleeding is profuse and is often accompanied by backache and utmost weakness. Such patients are usually quite worried and anxious. The best way to ease their anxiety is to stop the bleeding as soon as possible. In such cases, It is rarely required any other medicine to stop the bleeding. Any form of venous congestion and venous bleeding comes under the purview of this medicine and the rectal region is the most prominent. There is a feeling of soreness and bruised sort of sensation which is another important guiding symptom for the use of this medicine.

Muriatic acid: Muriatic acid is useful when piles prolapsed even while urinating. Piles are swollen blue and very painful to touch. Muriatic Acid works well when the piles are intensely swollen, sore and painful to slightest touch.

Nux Vomica: Nux Vomica can be used when constant ineffectual urging for stool is present with piles. The stool passed is always scanty and unsatisfactory. Nux Vomica is helpful when constipation appears with blind piles. There is constant, ineffectual urge to pass stool. Stool is scanty and always unsatisfactory. Nux Vomica is for Piles accompanied with constipation. Homeopathic medicine Nux Vomica is a top grade remedy for piles with constipation. A person needing Nux Vomica has piles with frequent- ineffectual urging for stool but passes little stool at a time. The urge for stool is renewed shortly after one has defecated. The stool is always unsatisfactory. Nux Vomica is highly beneficial for blind piles. Blind piles with pressure/sticking/burning/shooting pains calls for use of Nux Vomica. Subjects with sedentary habits developing piles with constipation fit the complete picture for Nux Vomica to be used. This is one of the best Homeopathic medicines for Piles or Haemorrhoids due to sedentary lifestyle. The modern day lifestyle has become more and more sedentary. One tends to work a lot but only on the mental plane while there is little physical activity. At the same time, one tends to take lot of rich food and also non veg. Use of stimulants like liquor or cigarettes is also quite high. This causes a lot of problems, piles being one of them. In such cases, Nux Vomica is the best Homeopathic medicine for piles. It not only cures the piles but also sets the gastrointestinal system in order again. Such a patient is usually an aggressive person who is a go-getter. He is a chilly patient who means he cannot tolerate cold air or cold weather.

Phosphorus: Phosphorus is top grade homeopathic remedies for haemorrhoids that bleed. Homeopathic medicine Phosphorus is indicated for piles which bleed frequently and blood is bright red colour.

Ratanhia: Ratanhia is a best choice when piles are accompanied with utmost burning and pain lasting for hours together after stool. This is usually referred to as painful piles. When it comes to curing painful piles, Ratanhia is the best homeopathic remedy for piles. Doctors place Ratanhia as the best homeopathic piles medicine when it comes to the use of Homeopathic medicine to cure painful piles. There is pain while passing stool and the pain persists for hours afterwards. The character of the pain is such as if there is broken glass inside the rectum. Sometimes there is pain as if a knife is thrust inside. Dry heat or burning may also be felt. This burning may be relieved by cold water. Homeopathic medicine Ratanhia offers a great help in piles which marked by burning and pain for many hours after stool. The character of Pain is 'as if broken glass pieces are placed in the rectum.' A knife like stabbing pain also indicates the use of Homeopathic medicine Ratanhia. Ratanhia is the best homeopathic medicine for piles with a fissure too.

Sedum acre: Sedum acre can work wonders for piles that cause pain which lasts for hours after passing stool.

Silicea: Silicea to be the best homeopathic medicines for piles that is accompanied with fistula.

5.6.3 Best Homeopathic Medicines for Anal Fissures

An anal fissure is a shallow ulceration or a small tear in the tissue or crack in the lining of the anus (the opening through which stool passes out of the body) that extends upwards into the anal canal or ulcer in the lining of the anal canal that extends into the anal canal. It is a common cause of red blood in the stool (faeces) and toilet paper. It may occur when passing large or hard stools, straining during childbirth, or experiencing bouts of diarrhoea. Fissures are a common condition of the anus and anal canal and are responsible for 6% to 15% of the visits to a colon and rectal (colorectal) surgeon. They affect men and women equally and both the young and the old. Fissures usually cause pain during bowel movements that often is severe. Anal fissure is the most common cause of rectal bleeding in infancy. An anal fissure can cause sharp pain and bleeding during and after bowel movements. It may also cause itching and burning in the anal area. An anal fissure is usually a minor condition that goes away within six weeks. Anal fissures occur in the specialized tissue that lines the anus and anal canal, called anoderm. At a line just inside the anus (referred to as the anal verge or intersphincteric groove) the skin (dermis) of the inner buttocks changes to anoderm. Unlike skin, anoderm has no hairs, sweat glands, or sebaceous (oil) glands and contains a larger number of sensory nerves that sense light touch and pain. (The abundance of nerves explains why anal fissures are so painful.) The hairless, gland-less, extremely sensitive anoderm continues for the entire length of the anal canal until it meets the demarcating line for the rectum, called the dentate line.

The crack in the skin exposes the muscle tissue underneath, causing severe pain and bleeding during and after bowel movements. An anal fissure can affect people of all ages, but it's most often seen in infants and young children. An anal fissure usually isn't a serious condition. In most cases, the tear heals on its own within four to six weeks. Certain treatments can promote healing and help relieve discomfort, including stool softeners and topical pain relievers. If an anal fissure doesn't improve with these treatments, surgery may be required or your doctor may need to look for other underlying disorders that can cause anal fissures. An anal fissure that fails to heal within six weeks is considered chronic and may need further treatment. Once you've experienced an anal fissure, you are prone to having another one. A tear extends to surrounding muscles. An anal fissure may extend into the ring of muscle that holds your anus closed (internal anal sphincter), making it more difficult for your anal fissure to heal. An unhealed fissure can trigger a cycle of discomfort that may require medications or surgery to reduce the pain and to repair or remove the fissure.

These are known as chronic anal fissures. These require treatment. Anal fissures mainly result from straining while passing hard or large stool. In some persons, chronic diarrhoea may also lead to anal fissures. Anal fissures may arise in women from trauma caused to the anal canal during childbirth. Anal fissures are very common in infants (children aged 1 month to 12 months). The main symptoms of anal fissure are pain during defecation and anal bleeding. The pain from anal fissures may last for hours after passing stool. The pain is often accompanied by marked burning in the anal area. Anal fissures can be quite painful. Passing the stool becomes a difficult and painful exercise and the result can be nothing short of traumatic for the patient. Itching around the anus and malodorous discharge from the anal fissure are other symptoms that present themselves. Anal

Fissure is a result of the trauma caused by the passage of hard, long stool (constipation) and repeated episodes of diarrhoea. Anal Fissure actually refers to a tear in the anus. Anus, of course, is the opening that marks the lower end of the gastro-intestinal system of the body or the opening through which stool are passed out of the body. Homeopathic remedies can be quite beneficial in the treatment of Anal Fissures. The typical symptoms of an anal fissure are extreme pain during defecation and red blood streaking the stool. Patients may try to avoid defecation because of the pain. The pain is usually felt while passing stool and may remain for a long time afterwards. The pain may be burning or stinging in character. There may be discharge of pus or some foul matter too. An anal fissure is just a cut or a crack in the mucous membrane lining the anal canal. It may occur due to hard stools. When one is constipated, one has to strain to pass stool. This can also cause a break or a crack in the mucous membrane. At times, diarrhoea can also cause anal fissures. In females, anal fissures occur commonly after a vaginal delivery. Homeopathic remedies for fissure promote the natural healing of anal fissure. Homoeopathic treatment mainly improves the entire process of digestion thus helps patient to get relief from constipation and straining from stools which is the main causative factor for fissure in anus. Homeopathic remedies commonly used for the treatment of anal fissures are capable of completely curing the problem. You can easily get yourself cured and that too without any surgery

Symptoms of Anal Fissure:

The symptoms of anal fissure are in many ways similar to piles. In some cases it may be difficult for the patient to understand whether he or she is suffering from anal fissure or piles. An experienced doctor or a surgeon is the best person to diagnose it properly. The common symptoms of anal fissure are as follows-Onset of acute anal fissure is characterized by tearing, cutting, or burning pain during or immediately after bowel movement. A few drops of blood may streak toilet paper or underclothes. Painful anal sphincter spasms result from ulceration of "sential pile" (swelling at the lower end of the fissure).

Best Homeopathic Medicines to treat Anal Fissures:

Source: (1. Dr. Vikas Sharma MD-Homeopathy (Gold Medalist); and 2. Dr Shah's, MD-Homeopathy of "Life Force Homoeopathy")
The above Doctors of Homeopath MD, have had the experience of treating millions of cases of anal fissures and piles with homeopathy

medicines in their clinic as well as on line in the last 2 decades. The fact remains that homeopathy is very effective at curing anal fissures. Dr. Vikas Sharma and Dr Shah's say that the reasons to choose homeopathic medicine are the permanency and safety of the treatment. Once treated with homeopathy, piles and fissures tend to not to recur (under conditions where lifestyle modifications are sustained for long). Homeopathic medicines are very safe and side effects with homeopathy while treating piles are unheard of. I, as an author, have just noted down this information from their website on line and put here for the purposes and benefits of millions and millions of people in the world suffering from Anal Fissure and Piles. The medicines that have most frequently been used and found effective are being given here with a brief description of symptom of diseases so that you can select as per your symptom the best one for you.

Homeopathy is natural mode of treatment that assures permanent cure for anal fissures. Homeopathic medicines help to manage the most troublesome symptoms of pain, bleeding and itching from anal fissures. They also aid in healing of the cuts and tears in anal canal thus effecting a permanent cure. Homeopathy is a great alternative treatment method for anal fissures that can be safely used among person of any age group. Doctors have treated many cases of anal fissures in their clinical practice with homeopathic medicines. The homeopathic medicines that they have found to be most effective in curing anal fissures are Nitric Acid, Ratanhia, Graphites, Paeonia and Thuja. Here is the list of best homeopathic medicines for anal fissures:

Dose of Homeopathy Medicines

Graphites-200; is the top third, prescribed daily at bed time for six weeks.

Natrum muriaticum-200; is prescribed daily at bed time for six weeks.

Nitricum acidum-200; is prescribed daily at bed time for six weeks.

Silicea-200; is prescribed daily at bed time for six weeks.

Bryonia-200; is prescribed daily at bed time for six weeks.

Nitric Acid-200; is the top one, prescribed daily at bed time for six weeks.

Nitric Acid and Phosphorus-200; is prescribed daily at bed time for six weeks.

Paeonia-200; is the top fourth, prescribed daily at bed time for six weeks.

Paeonia and Silicea-200; is prescribed daily at bed time for six weeks.

Phosphorus-200; is prescribed daily at bed time for six weeks.

Ratanhia-200; is the top second, prescribed daily at bed time for six weeks.

Sulphur-200; is prescribed daily at bed time for six weeks.

Thuja-200; is the top fifth, prescribed daily at bed time for six weeks.

Aesculus and Ratanhia: Aesculus and Ratanhia are Homeopathic medicines as a remedy for pain after stool. Homeopathic medicine Aesculus can be of great help if you are experiencing severe pain in the anus following stool passage. The stool or poop passed is mainly hard and large followed by severe pains. Homeopathic medicine Ratanhia is the best remedy when both pain and burning in anus follow the passage of stool. This burning and pain continue for several hours after passing stool. But it is Ratanhia, which has zero side effects, which can be really beneficial as a remedy for the pain.

Aesculus hip: anus, dry, itching; rawness and soreness is marked; burning sensation; itching and fullness; pain like a knife sawing backward; pain in anus about an hour after stool; burning in anus with chills up and down back.

Bryonia: Bryonia relieves from dry stools, dryness in the rectum and acute pain in the stomach and is a well-known homeopathic treatment.

Bryonia, Alumina and Natrum Mur: Homeopathic medicine Bryonia can be used in all cases where the stool is very hard, dry and large, leading to Anal Fissures. Bryonia will help in softening the stool and thereby preventing the tears in the anus that occur due to hard stool. Homeopathic medicine Alumina is mainly given when constipation is of the worst kind. The stool remains in the rectum for very long. The stool is hard and knotty and passes with difficulty, causing cracks and bleeding from the anus. Homeopathic medicine Natrum Mur provides help when the stool is hard and dry. Stool breaks frequently while passing due to constriction of anus. Bleeding and pain of burning, smarting and stitching nature follow the passage of stool.

Graphites: Graphites is one of the best Homeopathic medicines for anal fissure with large, difficult, constipated burning stool. When there is burning pain and the stool may be hard, large, and knotty and joined by mucous threads. Amongst all the homeopathic medicines for anal fissures, Graphites is seen to give excellent results. The stool tears the anus while defecating. Smarting pain in the anus is well marked. Intense soreness of anal area is also prominent. Graphites help in relieving constipation and anal pain. Anal fissures which have recently occurred; caused by large faecal masses; irritability; frequent desire for passing stool is not often associated with anal fissures; soreness and smarting in the anus; aggravation of complaints from sitting and night; severe constipation with smarting of parts and fissure of the anus; and the anus is very sore associated with knotty stool covered with mucus. When complaints of anal fissure are seen in obese individuals who also complain of having a very long standing constipation and intolerance for cold, graphite is often the remedy of choice. This homoeopathic remedy for fissure is chosen when the stools are knotty and covered with mucus.

Hydrastis: anal fissure with burning and smarting pain in the anus and rectum after each stool; this pains lasts for hours after stool, hot sensation in bowels, pain in abdomen and giddiness is also associated with; nodulated, dry, hard stool.

Ignatia: prolapsed of rectum with fissures and haemorrhoids; pains shooting upward after stool, even after a loose stool; pain in the rectum at the same hour each day, aggravation from walking or standing.

Lachesis: anal fissure with sensation as if little hammers pecking away in fissured parts; tormenting urging, but not to stool; itching at anus, worse after stool.

Natrum muriaticum: Natrum Muriaticum is an interesting example of homeopathic medicine prepared from a common food substance, the common salt, sodium chloride. As a rule, the common salt undergoes a special procedure called potentiating, whereby its inner healing power is activated to make it available for healing.

Nitric Acid and Phosphorus: Nitric Acid and Phosphorus is a Natural remedy for fissures with bleeding in anus. Homeopathic medicine Nitric Acid can be used to control bright red blood passing from the anus along with stool. The bleeding is accompanied by a tearing and stitching pain in the anus. Phosphorus is yet another Homeopathic medicine that can be used as a treatment for bleeding from the anus when the stool is long and hard with much offensiveness.

Nitric Acid and Sulphur: Nitric Acid and Sulphur is a Natural Homeopathic medicine for anal fissures with painful stools. The pain in anus while passing stool is best controlled with the use of Homeopathic medicine Nitric Acid. Nitric Acid can be used for various kinds of pain in the anus like stitching, tearing, stinging or cutting pains that occur while passing stool. The stool is constipated. In cases of Anal Fissure with burning pains in anus during passage of stool; Homeopathic medicine Sulphur is the best choice. Sulphur will effectively help in reducing the burning pains while passing stool.

Nitric Acid: One of the best Homeopathic remedies for anal fissures with bleeding after stool. This homoeopathic remedy for anal fissure selected by your doctor when there is severe pain in anus, felt for many hours after passing the stools. This remedy is chosen for people when they describe a sensation of splinter or stick in the anus, sharp, sphincter like cutting pains in the rectum during stool; there is sensation of burning after stool; sensation of constriction in the anus. When there is bleeding after passing stool, Nitric Acid is one of the best Homeopathic remedies for anal fissures. There is splinter like pain in the anal or rectal region. It feels as if some splinter has lodged in the area. Another feeling is as if the rectum is torn. There is offensive discharge from the fissure. This offensiveness of discharges may even extend to the urine, stool and even perspiration. The patient is quite prone to take colds. Diarrhoea is also quite frequently present. The stool is quite soft. Despite the stool being soft, one has to strain to pass the stool. Nitric Acid is one of the top grade homeopathic medicines for anal fissure. The classic symptoms guiding its use are violent anal pains, bleeding with passing stool and constipation; pains that are cutting or tearing in nature; Bleeding with stool that is of bright red colour; Stool is passes with much straining and it tears the anus (even if it is soft).

Paeonia and Silicea: Homeopathic remedies for anal fissures with offensive anal discharge. Homeopathic medicine Paeonia can be used when offensive fluid is discharged from the longstanding Anal Fissures. The anus seems ulcerated and torn with intolerable pain during and after stool passage. Homeopathic medicine Silicea is the best choice when the discharge contains the pus of offensive odour. The stool is passed with difficulty and straining. The stool comes out partially and then recedes again.

Paeonia: One of the Best Homeopathic Medicines for Anal Fissure with itching and offensive discharge. The pains may continue for some hours after passing stool too. The guiding symptom for its use is that the patient complains of a constant sensation of wetness and moisture in the anal area. Paeonia is a Homeopathic remedy for Anal Fissures violent pains in the anus during and after passing stool. There is intolerable itching and constant oozing of moisture. There is a severe pain in anus felt during and after passage of stools for many hours. The itching in the anus is lasting for several hours after stool.

Phosphorus: One of the best Homeopathic remedies for anal fissures with painlessness. When there is little pain despite the presence of anal fissure, Phosphorus is one of the best Homeopathic medicines for anal fissures. The patient is usually tall, thin and narrow chest. There is increased thirst and that too for cold water. The patient is unable to tolerate warm water and as soon as the water turns warm in the stomach, it is vomited. This medicine is known to irritate, inflame and cause degeneration of the mucous membranes all over the body. The stool is long, narrow and hard, like that of a dog. The stool may be white and hard too. The patient is very sensitive to light, sound and all sorts of external impressions.

Ratanhia: In doctor's opinion and experience, Ratanhia is one of the Homeopathic medicines for Anal Fissure that almost always shows satisfactory results in cases of this type. It is the Best Homeopathic Medicines for Anal Fissure with long lasting pain in anus after stool. Ratanhia is used very frequently for anal fissures. The Most prominent symptom for it is- intense pain in anus that last for many hours after stool; Burning in anus and rectum also appear along with pain; The anus burns like fire; Cold water application may give little relief in burning; Along with burning pains, constricted sensation in anus may also indicate the use of Ratanhia. Homeopathic medicine Ratanhia is also indicated in cases of fissures when pains are splinter like and knife like cutting in nature. Passing of stool is very painful. When there is pain while passing stool and the pain lasts for hours afterwards, Ratanhia is one of the best Homeopathic medicines for anal fissures. The prominent symptom is intense pain in the anus that lasts for several hours after passing stool. Burning in the anus and rectum also appear along with the pain in such cases. The anus feels like it is on fire. The prominent symptom is intense pain in the anus that lasts for several hours after passing stool. Burning in the anus and rectum also appear along with the pain in such cases. The anus feels like it is on fire.

Sedum Acre: Sedum Acre is a Homeopathic treatment for anal fissures with post-stool pains. It may be a lesser known Homeopathic medicine, but Sedum Acre can be very beneficial in providing relief and reducing the anal pains of constricting character following stool.

Silicea: Silicea is a Homeopathic treatment for anal fissures caused due to constipation; stool is very hard, has to remove mechanically; sphincter any seem tightly to resist the effort till suddenly stool passes. Here the irritable sphincter comes to mind and the slipping back of the partially expelled stool. It also has great pain, coming on half an hour after stool and lasting several hours. Platina has fissure of the anus, with crawling and itching every evening. Silicea is a homoeopathic remedy for fissure, when the patient complains of having a very peculiar type of constipation where stools are partly expelled out from anus, and partly stools will recede back into anus. Silicea is a strongly indicated remedy for fissure in anus in female patients who complain of getting constipation always before and during menses and straining for stools ultimately results into fissure in anal region. Silicea is given to smooth bowel movement.

Lycopodium: Lycopodium, being a good homeopathy treatment cures excessive gas.

Alumina: Alumina is good for children who faces hard stool.

Causticum: Causticum may be helpful in difficulty of passing stool.

Sepia: Sepia is beneficial in case of rectum sensation and hard stool.

Sulphur: Sulphur is a top Homeopathic medicine for Anal Fissure pains. Sulphur is the best Homeopathic medicine when the stool is hard and dry, causing tears and immense pain in the anus while passage. The patient is fearful of even going to the toilet as he thinks of the pain that will accompany the passage of stool. Sulphur is of great help in reducing the pain and softening the stool. The pain is almost always accompanied by burning. Itching in anus due to fissures is best controlled with the use of Sulphur. Sulphur is the best natural medicine for dealing with itching in anus. Sulphur has a very powerful ability to control itching in anus. Itching in anus may also be accompanied by a burning sensation. Sulphur helps when the anus itches and burns; but is relieved by cool compresses; the area around the anus is extremely red, usually from painless diarrhoea; the person wants to have a bowel movement immediately after waking up early in the morning. This homoeopathy remedy is extremely effective to relieve the itching in anus and dry hard stools resulting into the fissure of anus and is often selected as constitutional medicine for anal fissure. Redness in anal region with severe burning smarting pain is another strong indication for selection of Sulphur as a remedy to relieve the anal fissure.

Thuja: Thuja is one of the best Homeopathic medicines for Anal Fissure that is highly tender. Doctors have found Thuja as one of the most helpful medicine for intensely tender anal fissure. The pain gets worsened from slight touch and sitting. Constipation and rectal pains are also well marked. The stool passes with much effort with violent rectal pains. Swelling stitching and burning pain is also present with above mentioned symptoms. The prominent symptoms to look out for before prescribing Thuja are extremely tender anal fissure with pain that gets worse with the slightest touch and with sitting. Constipation and rectal pains are also well marked. Stool is passed with much effort and with violent rectal pains. Swelling, stitching and burning pain is also noted along with the symptoms mentioned above. Thuja, like all the medicines above, is natural and set off the body's own restorative processes to heal the condition.

5.7 Naturopathy Management for constipation:

It is a common disturbance of the digestive system where the bowel didn't move properly. This is a common problem of elderly people of age 60 plus where use of laxative is frequent. Appendicitis, rheumatism, arthritis, high blood pressure, cataract and cancer are the diseases where chronic constipation is a predisposing factor. Prevention of constipation is not a tough task; simply, you have to follow some simple methods, eat high fibre diet, drink enough fluids, adopt a healthy lifestyle and develop regular bowel habits. All these can prevent the onset of constipation symptoms, bloating and ulcer. Poor diet, poor bowel movement and poor hydration are some of the causes that delay prevention of constipation, especially in pregnant women. Lack of exercise, frequent intake of beverages too intensifies constipation.

Constipation preventing Foods, Liquid and Styles

The observance of regular hours for meal, elimination and sleep, balanced diet, and sufficient exercise are essential in the treatment of it.

- The most important factor in curing the condition is natural and simple fibrous diet.
- Regular drinking of water is essential as it cleans the system.
- All fruits except jack fruits are beneficial in the treatment.
- Pear is regarded as one of the best laxative fruits.
- Guava due to roughage helps in the normal evacuation of the bowel.
- Grapes contain cellulose, sugar and organic acid that make them a laxative food.
- Drinking lukewarm water with lime juice twice a day is a highly effective remedy.
- Copper vessel water is too beneficial.
- Linseed is extremely useful in difficult cases.
- The bowel may be cleansed daily by sitting in warm water tub.
- A warm friction bath is also useful.
- Exercise is beneficial to ease it.
- Taking warm milk with half lemon juice before going to bed
- Bale fruit is excellent for constipation.

- 3 tsp of castor oil in milk may help in chronic situation.
- Drinking 3-4 glasses of Luke warm water early morning and before bed helps in bowel movement and normal stool.
- Add more fibrous fruits and leafy green vegetables in your diet.
- Taking 2 tsp of molasses is good to treat it.
- Sleep at least 6-8 hours.
- Proper cooked vegetables should consume.
- Eat only whenever you are feeling hungry.
- Use spices like cumin, turmeric and coriander, all helps to digest your food.
- Avoid non-vegetarian, deep-fried, junk food etc.
- Cabbage juice is beneficial in treating it.
- Heat some dry grapes in milk, drink it after straining, a natural remedy.
- Spiegel seeds in warm milk are good for it.
- Water and Epsom salt in the ratio of 2: 1 helps to ease it.
- More fibrous nature of orange easily digests the food and helps in bowel movement.
- Fruits like papaya and figs act like as cleanser for the bowel.
- Fennel seeds are beneficial in its treatment.
- Food should be properly chewed and each morsel for at least 15 times.
- Wholesome diet, fruits, boiled vegetables and soup is a good remedy.
- Vegetables like radish, turnip, peas, carrot, tomato, bitter gourd, beetroot, sprouts, coriander, cabbage, mints are useful to relieve from constipation.
- Eat fresh fruits like avocado, guava, mango, orange, jamun, papaya, grapes, etc.
- Increases the quantity of salads in your diet.
- Increase the intake of watermelon, mangoes, cucumber.
- Drink more quantity of water.
- Eat whole grain cereals, bran, honey and lentils.
- Milk products like butter, ghee and cream.
- Dry fruits like fig, apricot and dates
- Restrict your non-veg., fried, oily and junk foods are considered as constipated diet.
- Bread, cakes, pasta, maida, pizzas, burgers, cookies are responsible for constipation and comes under as unhealthy diet. Avoid it.

- Buttermilk, Cheese and Yoghurt are good for it.
- Avoid spices, fats, excessive salt.
- Avoid White flour, biscuits, preserves, white sugar, boiled egg etc.
- Hurried meals and meals at odd time should be avoided to skip from gastro intestinal, reflux.
- Give more thrust on high fibre diet is a good tool for prevention of constipation.
- Defecate at the appropriate time to avoid stomach pain.
- High sugary and fatty food should be avoided as these steal B vitamins from the body without which the intestine function irregularly.
- Take adequate quantity of water and juices.
- Do regular exercises.
- Avoid more uses of laxatives.
- Avoid caffeine, soda and alcohol.
- Avoid back bowel movement.
- Avoid three white things Maida, Sugar and Salt.
- Avoid white rice, white bread and white flour.
- More quantity of vitamin and Magnesium Supplements should be taken.
- Avoid taking too many varieties at one meal.
- Relax after meal.
- Don't spend more than 10 minutes in toilet.
- Chew your food properly so to facilitate easy digestion and avoid abdominal pain.
- Eat only whenever you feel hungry.
- Take adequate sleep.
- Don't ignore bowel movement
- Don't peel the fruits

5.8 High-Fibre diet to prevent constipation, Piles and Anal Fissures:

Constipation is usually easier to prevent than to treat. Following the relief of constipation, maintenance with adequate exercise, fluid intake, and high-fibre diet is recommended. Children benefit from scheduled toilet breaks, once early in the morning and 30 minutes after meals. Treatment of constipation may include dietary fibre. Eat foods that contain plenty of fibre. We need enough fibre in our diets, but most of us fall short of it. The recommended daily intake of fibres are 50 for adults and younger; 25 grams for women and 38 grams for men.

High Fibber: High Fibber helps to regulate bowel functions, reduce cholesterol and triglycerides, and strengthens the colon walls. In addition, it helps in weight loss, management of blood sugar levels, and may prevent insulin resistance and associated diseases. Dietary fibre intake may prevent insulin resistance and disease. In addition, a recent study found that women who eat a high fibre diet (38-77 grams per day) had a greater than 20% reduction in risk for developing ovarian cancer.

After the discussion of the high fibre foods, let's take a look at just what fibre is. First, it is important to note that fibre only occurs in fruits, vegetables, and grains. It is part of the cellular wall of these foods. Diets high in fibre may reduce the risk of obesity, heart disease, and diabetes. Along with fibre and adequate fluid intakes, fibre is responsible for quickly moving foods through the digestive tract, helping it function optimally. Fibre works by drawing fluids from the body to add bulk to the stool. When increasing dietary fibre in your diet it is essential to start slowly, and increase gradually. Recommended Daily Fibre is 25 grams for Women and 35-40 grams for Men. The vast majority of the people get less than half of the daily recommended fibre. Without fibre, our digestive tract suffers, we develop high cholesterol that may lead to heart disease, and inflammation may increase in the body. High fibre diets help to lower the risk of some cancers, diverticulitis, heart disease, irritable bowel syndrome, kidney stones, and obesity. Some studies show that women with PMS or those that are menopausal can experience some relief from symptoms with high-fibre diets. For individuals with digestive tract conditions, dietary fibre may help to relieve symptoms. High fibre helps to shift the balance of bacteria, increasing healthy bacteria, while decreasing the unhealthy bacteria that can be the root of some digestive problems.

The Difference between Soluble Fibre & Insoluble Fibre: Insoluble fibre's job is to provide bulk in the intestines, while helping to balance the pH levels in the intestines. It promotes regular bowel movements, and helps to prevent constipation. Insoluble fibre doesn't dissolve in water, and doesn't ferment with bacteria in the colon. It is believed to help prevent diverticulitis and haemorrhoids, while sweeping out carcinogens and toxins from the system. Nuts, seeds, potatoes, fruit with skin, and green vegetables are excellent sources, as mentioned above. The job of soluble fibre is much the same; however it creates a gel in the system binding with fatty acids. Studies show that it prolongs stomach emptying to allow for better absorption of nutrients. Soluble fibre helps to lower cholesterol and helps to regulate blood sugar levels for individuals with diabetes. It is present in beans, legumes, oats, barley, berries, and some vegetables. It does ferment in the stomach, which can lead to bloating and gas. Increase these foods gradually, and drink plenty of water. Both soluble fibre and insoluble fibre has recently been show to be important in helping to control and manage hypertension.

Harms of getting fibre foods Supplements: The supermarket and drug store shelves are packed with fibre supplements, so the natural question is why not just taking those supplements instead. I hope in this article we have sold you on the benefits of eating high fibre foods mentioned above, because of their health benefits.

As another consideration, fibre supplements typically only contain a small fraction of necessary fibre. The sources of the fibre are often suspected. Beware of any supplements that contain methylcellulose (synthetic cellulose), calcium polycarbophil, or wheat dextrin as they provide no food value and nutrients, and are synthetic.

In addition, according to a study from the Maryland Medical Centre, people taking some medications including for diabetes, cholesterol-lowering drugs, seizure medications, and some antidepressants are advised not to take fibre supplements as it may interfere with the absorption of these medications and some minerals. These ultimate high fibre foods in this book are the best way to get the fibre you need; incorporate fibre slowly, and drink plenty of water and non-caffeinated beverages to help the fibre do its job and prevent constipation and making the bowel movement healthy. Fibre (roughage) is the part of plant food that is not digested. It stays in your gut and is passed in the stools (faeces). Fibre adds bulk and some softness to the stools. There are many foods you can eat to help relieve constipation and foods to avoid that can make constipation worse. Fibrous foods help relieve your constipation. When planning a healthy diet, it helps to include plenty of high-fibre choices food to help you stay regular. Aim to eat whole grain meal, bread (Roti) made of wheat flour, and at least, five portions of a variety of fruit and vegetables each day. One portion is one large fruit such as an apple, pear, banana, orange, or a large slice of melon or pineapple; or two smaller fruits such as plums, Satsuma, or one cup of small fruits such as grapes, strawberries, raspberries, cherries, etc; or one tablespoon of dried fruit; or a normal portion of any vegetable about two tablespoons; or one bowl of salad, wholegrain breakfast cereals. A simple thing like changing your regular breakfast cereal can make a big difference to the amount of fibre you eat each day. Although the effects of a high-fibre diet may be seen in a few days, it may take as long as four weeks. You may find that if you eat more fibre (or take fibre supplements - see below), you may have some bloating and wind at first. This is often temporary. As your gut becomes used to extra fibre, the bloating or wind tends to settle over a few weeks. Therefore, if you are not used to a high-fibre diet, it is best to increase the amount of fibre gradually and then you must have lots to drink when you eat a high-fibre diet or fibre supplements. Drink at least two litres (about 8-10 cups) per day. This is to prevent a blockage of the gut, which is a rare complication of eating a lot of fibre without adequate fluid. You will pass much of the fluid as urine but some is passed out in the gut and softens the stools. Most sorts of drink will do but alcoholic drinks can lead to a lack of fluid in the body (dehydration) and may not be so good. As a start, try just drinking a glass of water 3-4 times a day in addition to what you normally drink. Sorbitol is a naturally occurring sugar. It is not digested very well and draws water into the gut, which has an effect of softening the stools. In effect, it acts like a natural osmotic laxative (osmotic laxatives are explained later). So, you may wish to include some foods that contain sorbitol in your diet. Fruits and their juices that have high sorbitol content include apples, apricots, gooseberries, grapes and raisins, peaches, pears, plums, prunes, raspberries and strawberries. The concentration of sorbitol is about 5-10 times higher in dried fruit. Dried or semi-dried fruits make good snacks and are easily packed for transport in a packed lunch. Eat a well- balanced diet with plenty of fibre. Good sources of fibre are fruits, vegetables, legumes, and whole-grain bread and cereal (especially bran). Eat the best High-Fibre Foods, such as:

- Wheat,
- Oats
- Flax seed
- Split Peas, which contain Fibre 16.3 grams per cup, cooked.
- Lentils, which contain Fibre 15.6 grams per cup, cooked.
- Black Beans, which contain Fibre 15 grams per cup, cooked.
- Lima Beans, which contain Fibre 13.2 grams per cup, cooked.
- Artichokes, which contain Fibre 10.3 grams per medium vegetable, cooked.
- Peas.
- Broccoli.

- Brussels sprouts.

The benefits of an efficient bowel of a high-fibre diet are that it reduces the risk of stroke, hypertension, and heart disease. Unfortunately, fibre consumption is currently at an all-time low, with less than three percent of the recommended intake.

Fibre is something the body needs but never actually digests; in fact, it remains more or less the same from plate to toilet. It comes in two varieties, soluble and insoluble, and most plant-based foods contain a mixture of the two. Soluble fibre turns to gel in the stomach and slows digestion, which helps lower cholesterol and blood glucose. Insoluble fibre, on the other hand, remains unchanged all the way to the colon, making waste heavier and softer so it can shimmy through the intestines more easily. Regardless of these differences, neither type of fibre is ever absorbed into the body.

Skipping out on a daily dose of fibre often leads to constipation, which can make going to the bathroom painful and uncomfortable and hence the term "backed up." Eating too little fibre can make it tough to control blood sugar and appetite because fibre regulates the speed of digestion and contributes to satiety (aka feeling full). There can be too much of a good thing, though. Overdoing it with fibre can move food through the intestines too quickly, which means fewer minerals get absorbed from food. It can also result in uncomfy gas, bloating, and cramping, especially when fibre intake is dramatically increased overnight.

The Institute of Medicine recommends that men under 50 eat about 38 grams of fibre each day and women consume 25 grams. Adults over 50 require less fibre (30 grams for dudes and 21 grams for ladies) due to decreased food consumption. To put that into perspective, a young man is supposed to eat the same amount of fibre found in 15 slices of whole-wheat bread or two to three (Roti) every day.

1. Raw Seeds (hemp seeds, flax seeds, pumpkin seeds, sunflower seeds and sesame seeds): Consuming raw seeds have many of the same health benefits as raw nuts do. They will not only give you lots of energy, but they are also very high in fibre, Vitamin E, protein, zinc and other essential nutrients. Try to stay away from roasted or irradiated seeds if possible, as raw seeds contain higher amounts of nutrients. The best raw seeds to consume during a cleansing program include – hemp seeds, flax seeds, pumpkin seeds, sunflower seeds and sesame seeds.

High Fibres Food Grains:

Most of us get both types of soluble and insoluble fibres from foods grains. "Functional" fibre is extracted from its natural sources, and then added to supplements or fortified foods and drinks to boost their fibre content. Most nutritionists say to get fibre from whole foods because they're healthy in other ways, too. But if you don't get enough from your diet, fibre supplements can help fill in the gap. And evidence shows that most of us aren't getting enough. The average person only gets about half of the fibre needed daily. Aim to eat a wide variety of different types of fibre. This chart shows the most common types of dietary and functional types and explains where they come from and how they can keep you healthy. Maintaining a balanced diet is a key to living a healthy life. If you find yourself excessively consuming any foods that cause constipation, primarily dehydrating fluids and low fibre foods that are high in fat (fried foods, refined sugars, dairy products, coffee, coke, alcohol, etc), you are depriving your digestive system of vital nutrients including vitamins and minerals necessary to regulate your intestinal tract, not to mention relieve the symptoms of constipation.

When consuming large amounts of fibre, be sure to increase your intake of fluids. Live fibre foods are already high in water content. When doing a colon cleanse, it is important you follow a healthy, low-fat diet. If you eat unhealthy foods, you're not going to get the full potential of the cleansing program. It is important to stay away from all junk foods, fast food and microwave meals. Be sure to drink lots of purified water throughout the day, and not coffee or sodas. The amount of fibre in these foods can vary slightly between the raw and cooked versions.

1). Wheat:

Wheat is probably the most common cereal available all over the world and is in even higher demand in recent years due to its abundant health benefits. Over the years, it has shown itself to be one of the most successful and sustainable cereals crops in the world. It originated in south western Asia, but today it is grown in countless countries. Commonly, wheat cultivation is done at higher latitudes and is primarily used for baking bread products. Foods like bread, pasta, crackers, bagels, cakes, and muffins are just a few common examples of wheat sources. Wheat is believed to be one of the most wholesome food items, and it ensures a diet rich in nutrients. Research has already proven that wheat is extremely beneficial for healthy living. It considerably lowers the hazards of heart diseases, owing to its comparatively low fat content. It also regulates blood glucose levels in diabetic patients.

Wheat is able to provide you with an immense energy source due in all parts of the grain kernel, including the bran, germ, and endosperm. The nutrient value of wheat is retained even after processing it into flour. However, if you wish to get the maximum benefit out of wheat products, it's advisable to choose those products that are made from whole-wheat flour rather than the refined varieties.

Wheat Diet Varieties: The health benefits of wheat greatly depend on the form in which you consume it. While whole wheat is extremely nutritious, the benefits of wheat are reduced if you eat bleached white flour which is obtained by processing after only 60% extraction from the grain. In the United States, most wheat products undergo 60% extraction; you see this in noodles, breads, and pasta, as well as in baked goods like rolls, biscuits, and cookies. In these foods 40% of the original wheat grain was removed, and you get only the remaining 60%. Usually the 40% that is removed – the outer brown layer – contains the highly nutritious bran and the germ of the wheat grain. In the process of making 60% abstraction flour, more than half of the vitamin B1, vitamin B2, vitamin B3, vitamin E, calcium, phosphorus, folic acid, copper, zinc, iron, and fibre are lost. If you buy 100% whole wheat products, you are assured of all the nutrients of the bran and the germ, as well as the endosperm.

In recent years, the nutritional value of whole wheat is being recognized by consumers. Low-carob diets and an increase in the whole wheat cereal market are prevalent around the world, especially in the Mediterranean. Just like in whole wheat, wheat germ is a rich source of nutrients. Wheat germ has an abundance of vitamins and minerals, but it is particularly rich in vitamin E. Wheat germ is known to be a main source of the vitamin B complex in dietary structures throughout the world, and includes vitamins like thiamine, folic acid, vitamin B6 and minerals like manganese, magnesium, and zinc. The wheat germ oil improves strength and increases life span.

Cooking of Wheat: Wheat is consumed in the form of Cracked Wheat (Dalia), Sandwiches and bread (Roti). Wheat flakes at breakfast are undoubtedly a delicious and appetizing choice for your morning meal, and you can also use sprouted wheat berries in vegetables and various kinds of grain salads. Opt for whole wheat pita breads for your pizza crust, and if you are a pasta lover, make sure that it is whole wheat pasta. You can find it in all different forms like spaghetti, spirals and penne. In India, wheat is consumed in the form of breads called roti or chapatti.

Nutritional Value of Wheat: Wheat is rich in catalytic elements, mineral salts, calcium, magnesium, potassium, sulphur, chlorine, arsenic, silicon, manganese, zinc, iodide, copper, vitamin B, and vitamin E. This wealth of nutrients is why it is often used as a cultural base or foundation of nourishment. Issues like anaemia, mineral deficiencies, gallstones, breast cancer, chronic inflammation, obesity, asthenia, tuberculosis, pregnancy problems and breastfeeding problems are quickly improved by consuming whole wheat. It is also recommended to treat sterility. Since germinated wheat comprises 2 or 3 times more vitamin B than the common kind; the seeds are used for useful for treating gastrointestinal conditions, skin diseases, respiratory illnesses, and cardiovascular ailments. It is also known to help balance cholesterol levels and protect the heart. Health Benefits of Wheat: Controls Obesity (especially in women): Wheat has a natural ability to control weight in everyone, but this ability is more pronounced among women. Improves body metabolism: Saturated and Tran's fats increase the chances of cardiovascular diseases, while omega-3 fats decrease cardiovascular disease risk. Whole grains like wheat are immensely effective on patients with metabolic disorders. Common types of metabolic syndromes include visceral obesity, also known as the "pear shaped" body, high triglycerides, low levels of protective HDL cholesterol, and high blood pressure. It protects against all of these conditions. Research has shown that foods made from refined grains not only tend to increase weight but they also increase the hazards of insulin resistance. Doctors recommend eating whole wheat bread and other fibre-rich foods. The majority of fibre works to help the digestive process in the body and improve the overall metabolism. Having a whole wheat diet is probably the most effective, quick, and enjoyable way to reduce metabolic syndrome, but also to stay slim and healthy throughout your life.

a). Prevents Type 2 Diabetes: Wheat is rich in magnesium, which is a mineral that acts as a co-factor for more than 300 enzymes. These enzymes are involved in the body's functional use of insulin and glucose secretion. The FDA permits foods that contain whole grain by at least 51% weight and are also low in saturated fat and cholesterol, which means a lower risk of coronary ailments and certain types of cancer. Moreover, regular consumption of whole grain wheat promotes healthy blood sugar control. People who suffer from diabetes are able to keep their sugar levels under control by replacing rice with wheat in their diet.

b). Prevents Gallstones: It has been proved that breads and cereals made from whole wheat help women to avoid gallstones. Since whole wheat is rich in insoluble fibre, it assures a quick and smooth intestinal transit time and lowers the secretion of bile acids. Excessive bile acids are a major cause of gallstone formation. Moreover, a high intake of wheat increases insulin sensitivity and thereby lowers triglycerides or fat in the blood. Besides wheat, you also get insoluble fibre from the edible skins of fruits and certain vegetables like cucumbers, tomatoes and squash,
berries, apples, and pears. Beans also provide both insoluble and soluble fibre.

c). Assured Healthy Lifestyle: Wheat is the most popular and easily available bulk laxative. Three cups of wheat consumption per day is enough for an individual to live a long, healthy and disease-free life. When you maintain a fibre-rich diet comprised of wheat breads and cereals that are high in bran, you can be confident that problems such as pain, flatulence, nausea, constipation, and distension will be alleviated in no time. Diverticulitis often occurs due to inflammation and lower intestinal pains. This can also lead to chronic constipation and unnecessary straining, which can result in a sac or a pouch in the wall of the colon. Such cases can be easily dealt with naturally by keeping up with a fibre-rich diet and including whole grain wheat on a regular basis.

d). Promoting Women's Gastrointestinal Health: Benefits of wheat bran are bountiful, and promoting overall women's health is yet another important role of this cereal variety. Wheat acts as an anti-carcinogenic agent, particularly in women. Wheat bran enhances the metabolic rate of estrogens, which often leads to breast cancer if left at an excessive level. In one survey of pre-menopausal women in the age group of twenty to fifty, they ate three to four high-fibre muffins per day made from wheat, and they showed reduced blood estrogens levels by 17% in only 2 months. The other group of women eating corn bran did not show this result. Wheat contains contain lignans, which are phytonutrients acting as hormone-like substances. The lignans often occupy the hormone receptors of our body, thereby alleviating certain risk factors for breast cancer. This effectively checks the high circulating levels of estrogens. Wheat increases the metabolic rate of estrogens production and protects women against this key factor of cancer. Wheat bran considerably reduces bile acid secretion and bacterial enzymes in the stool, thereby cutting down chances of colon cancer. If you include bread, pasta, and bran cereals in your daily diet, these ailments will be avoided.

e). Protective against Breast Cancer: Research at the UK Women's Cohort Study found that a fibre-rich diet is extremely important for women to keep breast cancer at bay. Foods from whole grains like wheat and fruits provide significant safeguards for pre-menopausal women against breast cancer. Studies say that around 30 grams of wheat consumed daily is enough for women to reduce the risks of breast cancer. Reports say that pre-menopausal women who have consumed wheat had a 41% reduced risk of breast cancer in comparison to others who ate other forms of fibre.

f). Prevents Childhood Asthma: The American Lung Association says that around 20 million Americans experience some form of asthma. Studies have stated that whole grains and fish in the diet can lower the chances of childhood asthma to a great extent. The International Study on Allergy and Asthma in Childhood proved through numerous studies that a wheat-based diet has the capacity to lower chances of developing asthma by almost 50%. During the survey, the wheat diet was increased considerably and the mothers were given special diets high in fish and whole grains; this showed an almost 66% reduction in the possibility of becoming asthmatic.

Bronchial hyper-responsiveness is the key factor that encourages asthma. This condition is characterized by the narrowing of the airways and increased sensitivity. In many surveys, it has been seen that children who eat wheat and fish in high amounts do not suffer from such ailments. The magnesium and vitamin E provided by wheat also contributes in reducing the problem of asthma. However, in some cases, wheat consumption may be harmful for asthma patients, since wheat also happens to be a food allergen closely linked with asthma. Consult a doctor who can give you a complete examination and diagnosis of possible allergies you may have.

g). Protects against Coronary Diseases: Plant lignans, a type of phytonutrient, is abundant in whole wheat. These lignans are converted by responsive flora in the human intestines into mammalian lignans. One of these lignans is called enterolactone, which protects against breast and other hormone-dependent cancers, as well as heart disease. Wheat is not the only source of lignans; nuts, seeds and berries are also rich sources of plant lignans, as well as various other vegetables, fruits, and beverages like coffee, tea and wine. A Danish journal published in a recent article that women eating the most whole grains were found to have considerably higher blood levels of this defensive lignan.

h). Improves Cardiovascular System in Postmenopausal Women: Whole wheat is supposed to be a primary element in the diet of a post-menopausal woman so as to avoid any kind of cardiovascular problems. Daily intake of this whole grain cereal is the best way to avoid such ailments. Doctors prescribe a high wheat intake diet for women who are dealing with conditions like high blood pressure, high cholesterol, or other signs of cardiovascular syndromes. A survey has concluded that this kind of diet slows down the progression of atherosclerosis, which is the building of plaque in the arteries and blood vessels, as well as reducing the frequency of heart attacks and strokes.

i). Prevents Heart Attack: In the United States, heart failure is the prime cause of hospitalization and death of elderly people. The medicinal drugs have been successful in certain cases, but natural remedies work much faster and with less of an impact on the rest of the body's systems. Hospitals use ACE inhibitors and beta-blockers, but the long-term effects are not yet clear. Whole grain products and dietary fibre have been shown to considerably reduce blood pressure levels, thereby checking the possibility of a heart attack. Of course, confounding factors like age, alcohol consumption, smoking, exercise and proper nutrition are equally important. Ample vitamins, vegetables and fruits are extremely important in such cases as well. The start of your day can be both healthy and tasty with a daily bowl of whole grain cereal. There are various other forms in which you can serve wheat like bread, puddings and a variety of baked goods.

The health benefits of wheat are no longer unknown, and people all over the world have experienced them by including wheat in their daily diet. This "health food" reputation is due to the important B vitamins, such as thiamine, foliate, and vitamin B6, and the minerals magnesium, zinc, and manganese content. Wheat can be easily integrated into cakes, burritos, brownies, waffles, bread, muffins, patties and pancakes or simply sprinkled over your favourite cereal or yogurt.

Caution: There are some limitations to wheat consumption as well. If you are susceptible to allergic reactions, whole wheat consumption can enhance your allergies, such as hives, itching, skin rash, and eczema. Thus, it is advised to check with your physician to be sure that you are not allergic. Whole wheat contains oxalates, which are the naturally-occurring substances in animals, plants, and human beings. However, too much oxalate in bodily fluids can lead to crystallization, thereby causing health problems like gallstones, kidney stones, and gout.

Cracked Wheat (Dalia):

A bowl of Cracked Wheat (Dalia), high fibre content, is a hot Cereal, simply the finest hard red whole wheat that has been cut into a few pieces. Nothing fancy, just whole grains as nature intended. The nutty flavour and chewy texture make this one of our most popular hot cereals. Whole grain wheat delivers a healthy dose of protein, dietary fibre and is a great source of calcium and iron, all of which work together to keep your body strong and healthy. Whole wheat is also a good source of foliate, which helps with cell production and is especially critical for pregnant women and infants. Cracked Wheat is, indeed, very popular as a cereal, but you can also add cracked wheat to your favourite bread recipe for a crunchy texture, or use as a meat extender to add fibre and nutrition. It can be cooked and used in place of bulgur in salads, soups and sides. Bulgur is simply cracked wheat that has been parboiled to save on cooking time. Both are wonderful additions to your fibrous diet.

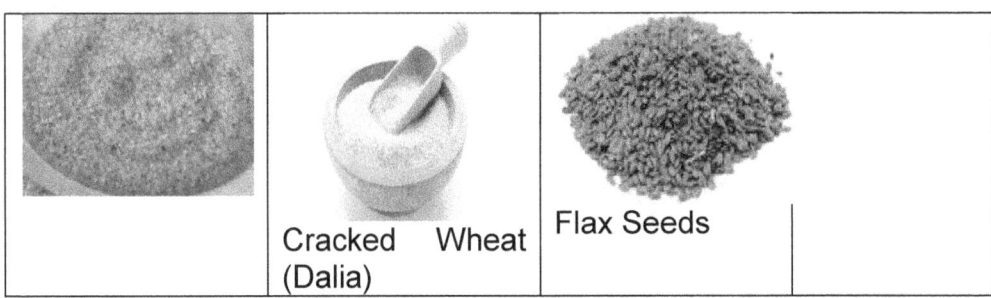

Cracked Wheat (Dalia)

Flax Seeds

Benefits: 1. Preventing constipation: A bowl of Dalia contains 2.5 gm of fibre that not only helps in the digestion but also prevents constipation. It works by absorbing water from the digestive water and adding bulk to stools. It also improves the consistency of stools, which helps relieve constipation. 2 Aid in weight loss: The high fibre content in Dalia gives you a feeling of fullness and thus, prevents you from binging. Eating a bowl of milk Dalia in the morning provides you 218 calories, which is less than other Indian breakfast options. It makes you feel full and also provides you with the energy required for the rest of the day. Dalia is low in fats that not only aids in weight management but also prevents obesity. So replacing wheat Roti (Bread) or rice with Dalia is not a bad idea to prevent your constipation and boost your weight loss too. 3. Good for diabetics: If you are a diabetic, Dalia is a must include food in your diet. It has a low glycemic index and contains complex carbohydrates, which ensure a slow and steady release of glucose into blood thereby preventing your blood sugar levels from spiking. With high fibre content and fewer calories, eating a bowl of Dalia when you are hungry helps you to manage blood sugar. A bowl of Dalia salad at night or Dalia upma in the evening keeps hunger pangs, even night cravings, at bay. 4 Nutritious weaning foods: Your baby's transition from breast milk to semi-solid food requires careful planning. A weaning food should be filling as well as easy on the stomach and Dalia fits the bill perfectly. A small bowl of Dalia kheer (made with milk and sugar or and jiggery added) can fill a 7-month old's stomach and also aid indigestion. 5 Helps in build muscles: Dalia is a rich source of proteins. If gaining muscle weight or building muscles top your list, ensure to include Dalia in your diet plan. It also contains various essential vitamins and menials that can replenish the lost nutrients from the body if had after a workout. Eat a bowl of Dalia porridge or Dalia upma with lentils to up your protein intake.

As Dalia is simple to make, easy-to-digest and low in fat, even pregnant women and older people can eat it. However, make sure you don't eat more than two bowls of cooked Dalia (which accounts to 50 gm of uncooked) in a day.

Popularly known as broken wheat, Dalia is a healthy alternative to whole wheat as it contains the outer bran, which makes it an excellent source of dietary fibre. Fibre helps you stay healthy. A powerful breakfast option, unlike other cereals, Dalia doesn't take a long time to cook. You can prepare many healthy recipes like Dalia vegetable upma, Dalia kheer or khichdi with this cereal.

Cracked Wheat (Dalia) Nutrition value: Cracked wheat, a product made by crushing whole raw wheat berries into smaller pieces is known as Dalia and is used to add texture to baked goods. Do not confuse cracked wheat with bulgur. Both are made in the same way, the wheat bulgur or kernels are cracked wheat steamed and toasted prior to crushing. Calories and Fat: A 1/4-cup portion of cracked wheat serves as a good source of iron. A popular brand offers 8 percent of the daily recommended intake of this mineral. The iron in your diet contributes toward the oxygen levels in your body because it helps make red blood cells, which delivery oxygen. Iron you don't need immediately stores in your muscles, liver, bone marrow and spleen; despite your body's capability to stockpile iron when you need it, many people still suffer from an iron deficiency -- the World Health Organization reports that nearly 80 percent of the world's population doesn't consume enough iron, and 30 percent of them have anaemia. This medical condition is marked by headaches, dizziness, fatigue and breathing problems. Protein: The protein you consume plays a critical role in the health of your immune system, fighting infections and keeping you healthy. It also serves as a secondary energy supply and helps you body make hormones and enzymes. Protein is best known for helping you build muscle. A 1/4-cup serving of cracked wheat contributes 5 g of protein to your meal plan, or 8.9 to 10.8 percent of the amount recommended for daily consumption by the Institute of Medicine. Carbohydrates: Carbohydrates serve as your body's main source of energy. This macronutrient breaks down into glucose and enters your bloodstream as fuel. Cracked wheat contains 29 g of Carbohydrates, nearly one-quarter of the amount you should ingest every day; the Institute of Medicine suggests ingesting 130 g of daily carbohydrates. Fibre: In addition to keeping your body moving throughout the day, some carbohydrates take the form of fibre, a type of Carbohydrates your body does not digest. Each serving of cracked wheat has 5 g. Fibre promotes the health of your digestive system and influences your bowel health; prevent constipation, helping to decrease your risk of developing haemorrhoids and diverticulitis. Eating a carbohydrate and fibre-rich diet aids in maintaining a steady blood sugar level, preventing spikes that can damage your health.

Wheat Burghol/Bulgur:

Bulgur is a cereal food made from the groats of several different wheat species, most often from durum wheat. Bulgur is a kind of dried cracked wheat. It is most common in European, Middle Eastern, and Indian cuisine.

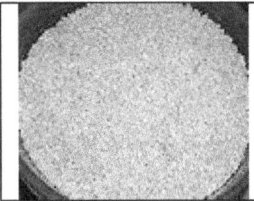 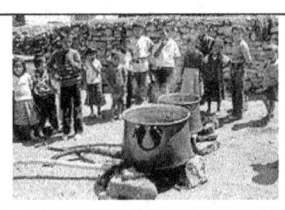

Fig: Parboiling of bulgur in central Turkey

Bulgur is usually sold parboiled and dried, with only a very small amount of the bran partially removed. Bulgur is recognized as a whole grain by the U.S.D.A. and the Whole Grains Council. Bulgur is sometimes confused with cracked wheat, which is crushed wheat grain that has not been parboiled. Whole-grain, high-fibre bulgur and cracked wheat can be found in natural food stores, Middle Eastern specialty grocers, and some traditional grocery stores. Bulgur is a common ingredient in Armenian, Assyrian, Kurdish, Syrian, Israeli, Jordanian, Palestinian, Lebanese, T urkish, Middle Eastern, and Mediterranean dishes. It has a light, nutty flavour. In Turkey, a distinction is made between fine-ground bulgur, called koftelik bulgur, and a coarser grind, called pilavlık bulgur. In the United States, bulgur is produced from white wheat in four distinct grinds or sizes (#1 Fine, #2 Medium, #3 Coarse and #4 Extra Coarse). The highest quality bulgur has particle sizes that are uniform thus allowing a more consistent cooking time and result.

It is also known as "Dalia" in North India. Dalia is popular all over the wheat-consuming regions of North India. It can be consumed as sweet Dalia or regular Dalia.

Bulgur can be used in pilafs, soups, bakery goods, or as stuffing. In breads, it adds a whole grain component. It is a main ingredient in tabbouleh salad and kibbeh. Its high nutritional value makes it a good substitute for rice or couscous. In Indian cuisine, bulgur or daliya is used as a cereal with milk and sugar. In the United States is often used as a side dish, much like pasta or rice. In meals, bulgur is often mistaken for rice because it can be prepared in a similar manner, although it has a texture more like couscous than rice. A popular South American carnival food, bulgur is often prepared with flower pollen and tapioca syrup and fried in patties.

Nutrition facts: Compared to unenriched white rice, bulgur has more fibre and protein, a lower glycemic index, and higher levels of most vitamins and minerals. As below:

Bulgur (dry) Nutritional value per 100 g (3.5 oz)	
Energy	342 kcal (1,430 kJ)
Carbohydrates	75.87 g
Sugars	0.41 g
Dietary fibre	18.3 g
Fat	1.33 g
Protein	12.29 g
Vitamins:	
Vitamin A	9 IU
Thiamine (B1)	(20%) 0.232 mg
Riboflavin (B2)	(10%) 0.115 mg
Niacin (B3)	(34%)

	5.114 mg
Vitamin B6	(26%) 0.342 mg
Foliate (B9)	(7%) 27 µg
Vitamin C	(0%) 0.0 mg
Vitamin E	(0%) 0.06 mg
Minerals:	
Calcium	(4%) 35 mg
Iron	(19%) 2.46 mg
Magnesium	(46%) 164 mg
Phosphorus	(43%) 300 mg
Potassium	(9%) 410 mg
Sodium	(1%) 17 mg
Zinc	(20%) 1.93 mg

2). Oat Grains (Raw):

Oats are a whole-grain cereal, known scientifically as Avenal Satva. They are a very good source of fibre, especially beta-glucan, and are high in vitamins, minerals and antioxidants. Whole oats are the only source of a unique group of antioxidants called avenanthramides, believed to have protective effects against heart disease.

The oat is a species of cereal grain grown for its seed. Oats are generally considered healthy due to their rich content of several essential nutrients. In a 100 gram serving, oats provide 389 calories and are an excellent source (20% or more of the Daily Value, DV) of protein (34% DV), dietary fibre (44% DV), several B vitamins and numerous dietary minerals, especially manganese (233 % DV). Oats are 66% carbohydrates, including 11% dietary fibre and 4% beta-glucans, 7% fat and 17% protein. The established property of their cholesterol-lowering effects has led to acceptance of oats as a health food.

Oat	Chocolate Oat Fondant	Oat Crunches	Chickpeas

My grandmother started her day with a steaming bowl of freshly cooked oats doused in milk. It is a healthy diet; one can really have it every single day. Nutritionist says that "Oats are rich in soluble and insoluble fibres which help in preventing constipation and lowering cholesterol levels. These soluble fibres help increase intestinal transit time and reduce glucose absorption. Oats also contain beta glucan which is a lipid lowering agent. A very healthy breakfast option - you can spruce your oats with fruits and crunchy nuts." Oats is the one super food that can easily fit itself to suit your needs. Protein-packed, full of fibre and low on fat, oats are designed to boost your energy levels and help you lead a healthy lifestyle. They are not only good for the stomach but are interestingly super filling, satisfying and versatile. Oats contain a wide range of nutrients like fibre, vitamin E, essential fatty acids, etc. which make them top the healthy food charts.

Cooking with Oats: Followings are recipes to make your morning diet and healthy. Cooking with oats like never before:

1. Chocolate Oatmeal Bars Recipe:

Crust and Topping: Ingredients:

1⅓ cups oatmeal

1 cup all-purpose flour

1⅓ cups light brown sugar

½ tsp baking powder

10½ tbsp butter

Filling: Ingredients:

½ cup all-purpose flour

½ cup light brown sugar

2 cups semisweet chocolate chips

4 tbsp butter

3 large eggs

Instructions: Preheat the oven to 325 degrees and line an 8x8-inch baking pan with aluminium foil and add some oil. Combine flour, oats, 1⅓ cups light brown sugar and baking powder in a medium bowl, add

10½ tablespoons melted butter and stir to combine. Press half of mixture firmly into the pan and bake about 8 minutes, cool it. To make the filling, melt the butter and chocolate chips together and stir until it's smooth. Whisk together flour and sugar in a bowl. Whisk eggs into cooled chocolate mixture, and then stir in the flour mixture. Pour chocolate filling over cooled crust and top with remaining oatmeal mixture. Bake 35 to 40 minutes. Note: Cool completely before serving.

2. Banana Oats Smoothie:

Ingredients:

¼ cup rolled oats

½ cup yogurt

1 banana, cut into thirds

½ cup milk

2 tbsp honey (optional)

½ tsp ground cinnamon

Instructions: In a blender, combine all the ingredients and blend until smooth. Top it off with a pinch of cinnamon and serve immediately.

3. Chocolate Oat Fondant: Here is a classic French dessert with a healthy addition of oats. The sinfully flavourful chocolate soaks in the aromatic goodness of oats, and in the end it's what you call - having the best of both worlds.

Ingredients:

Melted butter for brushing the ramekins

Cocoa powder for dusting

200 gms good-quality dark chocolate, chopped into small pieces (70 %)

150 gms butter, cut in small bits

3/4 cup Demerara sugar (ground)

4 whole eggs

4 yolks

3/4 cup flour

3/4 cup oats (ground)

1 tsp baking soda

1 Tbsp of cocoa

1/2 cup milk to loosen batter (optional)

For the strawberry compote:

1 cup freshly cut strawberries

1 tsp lemon juice

1 Tbsp brown sugar

1/2 tsp balsamic vinegar

Instructions: Brush butter on the insides of your ramekins, and dust with cocoa powder. Put them in the freezer to set. Take a pan of simmering water, and place another bowl that fits snugly over it, without touching the water. Slowly melt the chocolate and butter together. Remove the bowl from the heat and allow it to cool for 5 minutes. In a separate bowl whisk the eggs and yolks together with the sugar until the whisk leaves a trail. Now add the flour, oats and baking soda into the eggs and beat it well. Pour the melted chocolate into this batter bit by bit, beating well in between each addition. Add a little milk to loosen the batter. Take the ramekins out of the fridge and pour this batter in equal quantities into the ramekins. Put these back in the freezer, and take them out just before you're ready to bake them. Bake in a preheated oven at 190 degrees till the fondant rises and flowers out of the ramekin.

4. Strawberry compote: In a pan add butter, strawberries and sugar. Add the lemon juice and vinegar. Let the strawberries leave a little juice. Your compote is ready.

5. Oat Crunches:

150 g butter
2 tbsp golden syrup
¾ cup brown sugar
½ cup coconut
2 cups rolled oats
½ cup flour

Instructions: Melt butter, syrup and brown sugar in a saucepan and keep stirring. Mix in coconut, oats and flour until combined. Roll table spoonful of oats into balls. Spread on a greased oven tray and flatten with a spoon. Bake it at 180C degrees for 10 minutes or until it is lightly browned. Cool on a rack and voila.

6. Chocolate Banana Oatmeal:

Ingredients:

1 cup water
1 tsp brown sugar
1/2 cup old-fashioned rolled oats
1/2 banana, sliced
1 tbsp chocolate-hazelnut spread
Pinch of salt

Instructions: Bring water and a pinch of salt to a boil in a small saucepan. Stir in oats; reduce heat to medium and cook, stirring occasionally, until most of the liquid is absorbed, about 5 minutes. Remove from heat, cover and let stand 2 to 3 minutes. Top it off with banana and a yummy chocolate spread.

What better way to gain the strength and energy to carry you through a hectic morning schedule than with a steaming bowl of freshly cooked oatmeal. Oats are harvested in the fall but are available throughout the year and can add extra nutrition to a variety of healthy dishes.

Oats, known scientifically as Avena Satva, are a hardy cereal grain able to withstand poor soil conditions in which other crops are unable to thrive. Oats gain part of their distinctive flavour from the roasting process that they undergo after being harvested and cleaned. Although oats are then hulled, this process does not strip away their bran and germ allowing them to retain a concentrated source of their fibre and nutrients.

Oats, unprocessed, dry 0.25 cup (39.00 grams) – Calories = 152 GI, low. Manganese 96%; molybdenum 64%; phosphorus 29%; copper 27%; biotin 26%; vitamin B125%; magnesium 17%; fibre 17%; chromium 15%; zinc 14% and protein13%.

This chart graphically details the %DV that a serving of Oats provides for each of the nutrients of which it is a good, very good, or excellent source according to our Food Rating System. Oats enhance Immune Response to Infection.

Buy small quantities of oats at one time since this grain has a slightly higher fat content than other grains and will go rancid more quickly. Oats are generally available in pre-packaged containers as well as bulk bins. Just as with any other food that you may purchase in the bulk section, make sure that the bins containing the oats are covered, free from debris and that the store has a good product turnover so as to ensure its maximal freshness. Smell the oats to make sure that they are fresh. Whether purchasing oats in bulk or in a packaged container, make sure there is no evidence of moisture. If you purchase prepared oatmeal products such as oatmeal, look at the ingredients to ensure that the product does not contain any salt, sugar or other additives. Nutritional Profile: Oats are an excellent source of manganese and molybdenum. They are also a very good source of phosphorus as well as a good source of copper, biotin, vitamin B1, magnesium, dietary fibre, chromium, zinc and protein. Oats and oatmeal shall be regularly included in the diet for those with constipation problems. Oats contain both soluble and insoluble fibre - 8 grams in one cup of uncooked oatmeal. In addition to containing the most soluble fibre of any food (55 percent), oats contain 45 percent insoluble fibre. Insoluble fibre, the portion of the plant that can't be broken down by your digestive system, which absorbs water and swells, making the stool bulky, soft, and easy to pass and relieves constipation. This is the reason why we always need to increase our water intake when we increase the fibre in your diet.

When you buy oats, don't get instant oatmeal, which has already been partially cooked and often contains sugar, salt, or other unnecessary ingredients. Use whole grain oats, which take a little longer time to cook, fifteen minutes will be well worth the wait. You shouldn't buy oats in large quantities. The beneficial fats in oats can go rancid with time. Fresh oats should smell fresh. Generally, if they are in an airtight container in a cool, dry, dark area, you can expect them to last about two months.

Due to their beneficial health effects, such as lowering blood sugar and cholesterol levels, oats have gained considerable interest as a health food. Oats are most commonly rolled or crushed, and can be consumed as oatmeal (porridge), in baked goods, bread, muesli and granola. Whole grain oats are called oat groats. The oat groats are most commonly rolled or crushed into flat flakes and lightly toasted to produce oatmeal.

Quick or instant oatmeal is made up of more thinly rolled or cut oats that absorb water much more easily and therefore cook faster. The oat bran (the fibre-rich outer layer of the grain) is often consumed separately as a cereal, with muesli or in breads. To produce infant oatmeal, oats are often further processed into powder that becomes a thick porridge when mixed with water.

Nutrition Value: Oats have a well-balanced nutritional composition, and one serving (30 grams) of oats contains 117 calories. By weight, raw oats are 66% carbohydrates, 17% protein, 7% fat and 11% fibre. The table below contains detailed information on the nutrients in oats:

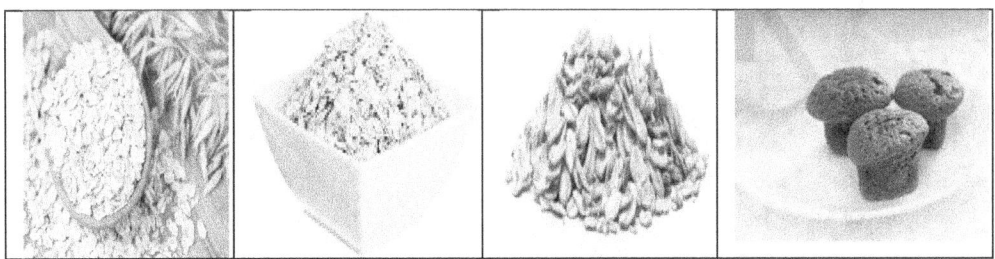

Fig: Rolled oats

Table: Oats - Nutrition Facts (Amounts per 1 cup - 94g):

Amounts Per Selected Serving % DV

Calorie Information:
Total Calories 231 (967 kJ) 12%
From Carbohydrate 146 (611 kJ)
From Fat 55.3 (232 kJ)
From Protein 29.6 (124 kJ)
From Alcohol 0.0 (0.0 kJ)

Carbohydrates:
Total Carbohydrate 62.3g 21%
Dietary Fibre 14.5g 58%
Starch ~
Sugars 1.4g
Fats & Fatty Acids:
Total Fat 6.6g 10%
Saturated Fat 1.2g 6%
Monounsaturated Fat 2.2g
Polyunsaturated Fat 2.6g
Total Omega-3 fatty acids 114mg
Total Omega-6 fatty acids 2487mg

Protein & Amino Acids:
Protein 16.3g 33%

Vitamins:
Vitamin A 0.0IU 0%
Vitamin C0.0mg 0%
Vitamin D ~ ~
Vitamin E 0.9mg 5%
Vitamin K 3.0mcg 4%
Thiamine 1.1mg 73%
Riboflavin 0.2mg 12%
Niacin 0.9mg 4%
Vitamin B 6 0.2mg 8%
Foliate 48.9mcg 12%
Vitamin B12 0.0 mcg 0%
Pantothenic Acid 1.4mg14%
Choline 30.3mg
Betaine 18.4mg

Minerals:
Calcium 54.5mg 5%
Iron 5.1mg 28%
Magnesium 221mg 55%
Phosphorus 690mg 69%
Potassium 532mg 15%
Sodium 3.8mg 0%

Zinc 2.9mg   19%
Alcohol 0.0g Water 6.2g Ash 2.7g Caffeine 0.0mg Theo bromine 0.0mg

The carbs in oats are mostly made up of starches and fibre. Oats are a good source of a unique type of fibre called beta-glucan, which is associated with a range of health benefits.

Protein: Oats are a good source of quality protein, ranging from 11-17% by dry weight, which is higher than most other grains.

Fat: Whole oats contain more fat than most other grains, ranging from 5-9%. It consists mostly of unsaturated fatty acid.

Vitamins and Minerals: Oats are high in many vitamins and minerals.

Vitamins and minerals

Manganese: Typically found in high amounts in whole grains, this trace mineral is important for development, growth and metabolism.

Phosphorus: An important mineral for bone health and tissue maintenance.

Copper: An antioxidant mineral that is often lacking in the Western diet. It is considered important for heart health.

Vitamin B1: Also known as thiamine, this vitamin is found in many foods, including grains, beans, nuts and meat.

Iron: As a component of haemoglobin, a protein responsible for transporting oxygen in the blood, iron is absolutely essential in the human diet.

Selenium: An antioxidant, important for various processes in the body. Low selenium status has been associated with increased risk of premature death, and impaired immune and mental function.

Magnesium: Often lacking in the diet, this mineral is important for numerous processes in the body.

Zinc: A mineral that participates in many chemical reactions in the body and is important for overall health.

Oats contain high amounts of many vitamins and minerals, such as manganese, phosphorus, and copper, B-vitamins, iron, selenium, magnesium and zinc.

Whole oats are rich in antioxidants that may provide various health benefits.

Ferulic Acid: The most common polyphenol antioxidant in oats and other cereal grains.

Phytic Acid: Most abundant in the bran, phytic acid is an antioxidant that can impair the absorption of minerals, such as iron and zinc.

Oats are the only dietary source of powerful antioxidants called avenathramides. They also contain ferulic acid and phytic acid.

Health Benefits of Oats: Studies have repeatedly confirmed that whole grain Oats; oatmeal or oat bran can:

It lowers cholesterol levels reducing the risk of heart disease. Two suggested mechanisms for these cholesterol-lowering effects have been proposed. First, beta-glucan may slow the absorption of fats and cholesterol by increasing the viscosity of the digestive cotents. Normally, bile acids are recycled (re-absorbed) in the digestive system, but beta-glucan inhibits this recycling process, leading to reduced levels of cholesterol in the body. Authorities have approved the health claim that foods containing at least 3 grams of beta-glucan per day may lower the risk of heart disease. Oats contain high amounts of beta-glucans, which are very effective at reducing blood cholesterol levels.

Second, beta-glucan binds with cholesterol-rich bile acids in the intestine, produced by the liver to aid digestion. Beta-glucan then carries them down the digestive tract and eventually out of the body.

Oats have also been claimed to lower blood pressure and reduce the risk of obesity and type 2-diabetes.

Listed below are the main health benefits of oats and oat bran.

Reduce Heart disease, which is the leading cause of death worldwide.

Blood cholesterol is a major risk factor for heart disease, especially oxidized LDL-cholesterol.

Numerous studies have shown the effectiveness of oats or oat bran in lowering blood cholesterol levels, which is mainly attributed to their beta-glucan content.

Other Benefits of Oats in detail:

1. Prevents cardiovascular disease: "The antioxidants present in oats are beneficial for heart disease and the dietary fibres help lower the bad cholesterol (LDL) without affecting the good cholesterol (HDL)". Oats also contain plant lignans, especially enterolactone, which protect against heart disease. Thus, oats help reduce your cholesterol levels and keep your heart healthy. He adds, "It is a key food item that has proven to be good for the heart".

2. Prevents constipation: Oats are a rich source of fibre, both soluble and insoluble, which helps in regulating bowel movements and hence prevents constipation.

3. Controls blood sugar levels: Since oats help stabilise blood sugar and reduce risk of type-2 diabetes, diabetics should consume oats regularly. The high fibre and complex carbohydrates slow down the conversion of this whole food to simple sugars, and beta-glucan delays the fall in blood sugar levels before meals and slows the rise after a meal.

4. Reduces cancer risk: Lignan, the same compound which helps prevent cardiovascular disease also "helps reduce chances of hormone-related cancers like breast, prostate and ovarian cancer", according to the American Cancer Society. Therefore, eating oats is good for both men and women.

5. Reduces hypertension: If you suffer from high blood pressure, a daily dose of oats will help combat this problem and in turn, lower risk of hypertension.

6. Rich source of magnesium: Oats are also a rich source of magnesium, which is the key to enzyme function and energy production, and helps prevent heart attacks and strokes by relaxing blood vessels, aiding the heart muscle, and regulating blood pressure. The high levels of magnesium nourish the body's proper use of glucose and insulin secretion.

7. Supports weight loss: Oats is a low calorie food which slows digestion and makes you feel full longer. Thus, reducing your cravings and helping you shed a few pounds. Cholecystokinin, a hunger-fighting hormone, is increased with the oatmeal compound beta-glucan.

8. Enhances immune response to disease: The unique fibre in oatmeal called beta-gluten has been shown to help neutrophils travel to the site of an infection more quickly and it also enhances their ability to eliminate the bacteria they find there.

9. Protects skin: Oats have been used as a soothing agent to relieve itch and irritation while also providing an array of benefits for the skin. According to The American Academy of Dermatology, "Oatmeal is able to normalise the skin's pH. It also helps moisturise and soften the skin."

9. Modest amounts of beta-glucans from oats have been shown to moderate both glucose and insulin responses after carbohydrate-rich meals. In patients with type 2 diabetes and severe insulin resistance, a 4-week dietary intervention with oatmeal resulted in a 40% reduction in the insulin dosage needed for stabilizing blood sugar

levels. Studies suggest that beta-glucans may favourably alter insulin sensitivity, delaying or preventing the onset of type 2 diabetes, but a recent review study concludes that the evidence is inconsistent.

Boiled whole oats cause low glucose and insulin responses, but the responses increase significantly if the oats are ground to flour before cooking. Oats may reduce blood sugar and insulin responses following carbohydrate-rich meals. This makes them particularly beneficial for diabetics.

10. Oats and Increased Satiety: Satiety plays an important role in energy balance. It stops eating and prevents us from eating again until hunger returns. Altered satiety signalling has been associated with obesity and type 2 diabetes. In a study ranking the satiety effect of 38 common foods, porridge (cooked oatmeal) ranked 3rd overall, and 1st among breakfast foods.

Water-soluble fibres, such as beta-glucans, may increase satiety by delaying stomach emptying, increasing stomach distension and promoting the release of satiety hormones. Human trials have shown that oatmeal, rich in beta-glucans, may increase satiety and reduce appetite when compared to a ready-to-eat breakfast cereal and other types of dietary fibre. In addition to being highly satiating, oats, eaten as porridge, are low in calories and contain plenty of fibre and other healthy nutrients, making them an excellent addition to an effective weight loss diet.

Bottom line: Porridge (cooked oatmeal) is low in calories, is very filling and may decrease appetite, compared to other breakfast foods.

Oats is Gluten-Free Diets: A gluten-free diet is the only solution for individuals who suffer from celiac disease, as well as for many individuals with gluten sensitivity. Oats do not contain gluten, but they contain a similar type of protein, called avenin. Clinical studies have shown that moderate or even large amounts of pure oats can be tolerated by most celiac disease patients. Oats have been shown to enhance the nutritional value of gluten-free diets, increasing both mineral and fibre intakes, and individuals usually prefer to include oats in their gluten-free diets. The biggest problem with oats in a gluten-free diet is contamination with wheat, because oats are often processed in the same facilities as other grains.

Therefore, it is important for celiac patients to only eat oats that have been certified as "pure" or "gluten-free."Oats are naturally gluten-free, but they are often contaminated with wheat. Individuals sensitive to gluten should only consume oats that are certified as "pure" or "gluten-free".

Other Health Benefits of Oats: Oats are being extensively studied in many other areas, such as in cancer research, which is still in its early stages. There are a few other benefits that deserve mentioning.

Feeding oats to young infants, before they reach an age of 6 months, has been associated with decreased risk of developing childhood asthma.

A few studies indicate that oats may boost the immune system, enhancing the body's ability to fight bacteria, viruses, fungi and parasites.

In elderly people, consuming oat bran fibre may improve well-being and decrease the need for laxatives.

Bottom line: Oats have been associated with all sorts of benefits, including decreased risk of childhood asthma, enhanced immune system and decreased need for laxatives in the elderly.

Adverse Effects

Oats are usually well tolerated, with no adverse effects in healthy individuals.

Avenin-sensitive individuals may experience adverse symptoms, similar to those of gluten intolerance, and should exclude oats from their diet.

Oats may be contaminated with other grains, such as wheat, making them unsuitable for people with celiac disease (gluten intolerance) or wheat allergy.

It is important for individuals allergic or intolerant to wheat, or other grain types, to buy only oats that are certified as pure from contamination.

Bottom line: Oats are usually well tolerated, but they may be contaminated with gluten. Individuals who are sensitive to gluten should only consume "pure" and non-contaminated oats.

Summary: Oats are among the world's healthiest grains. They are a good source of many vitamins, minerals and unique plant compounds. Oats also contain large amounts of unique soluble fibres called beta-glucans, which provide numerous health benefits. These include lower cholesterol, reduced blood sugar and insulin responses, relieved constipation and improved immune function. In addition to all this, oats are also very filling, and may reduce appetite and help you eat fewer calories.

3). Beans and Legumes:

Rinse 1 pound of beans thoroughly. Beans do not have to be pre-soaked with this technique. Place in slow cooker and cover with 7 cups of water, and ¼ teaspoon baking soda. Cook on high for 3.5 –

4.5 hours or on low for 8 – 10 hours, until they reach desired doneness. This process creates a creamy bean, without being mushy. Note: It is imperative that you increase your water consumption, when you eat beans. Water helps to flush the toxins from your body, but also helps to reduce gas and bloating associated with eating beans.

4). Lima Beans:

Total Dietary Fibre is 13.2 grams of fibre per cup (cooked). Notable Nutrients are Copper, Manganese, Foliate, Phosphorous, Protein, B2, and B6. In addition to the outstanding fibre per serving, lima beans offers nearly 25% of the daily recommended iron for women. The manganese helps with energy production, and the antioxidants help to fight free radicals. Lima beans are part of my Healing Foods Diet plan. Fibre is 13.2 grams per cup, cooked Lima beans might sound unappetizing, but when cooked in bacon fat, paired with leeks, pureed into a soup, and topped with sour cream, they're pretty darn delicious.

5). Black Beans:

Total Dietary Fibre is 15 grams of fibre per cup. Notable Nutrients are Protein, Thiamine, Magnesium, Manganese, Phosphorus, and Foliate. Black beans are nutrient dense, and provide great protein and fibre to your diet. The high content of flavonoids and antioxidants help to fight free radicals, reducing your risk of some cancers and inflammatory diseases. Take healthy black bean brownie recipe; it is a great way to increase fibre, while enjoying a treat.

6). Chia Seeds:

Total Dietary Fibre is 5.5 grams per tablespoon. Notable Nutrients are Protein, Calcium, Phosphorus, Manganese, Omega-3 fatty acids, Omega-6 fatty acids. Chia seeds are a true super food that is easily incorporated into your diet. High in fibre, and essential nutrients, they help to increase energy, support digestive health, and have many more health benefits. Like beans and legumes, some people may experience gas and bloating; increase water intake to help minimize these symptoms. For some individuals, soaking chia seeds may help to prevent these symptoms, and may aid in absorption of nutrients. (Recommended photo: chia seeds in spoon). When they meet with water, they form a goopy gel that is great for thickening smoothies, making healthy puddings, or replacing eggs in cakes and cookies.

7). Chickpeas (Kabuli Chana):

Chickpeas, also called garbanzo beans, are one of the oldest consumed crops in the world and remain one of the most popular today across nearly every continent. Chickpeas have been a part of certain traditional diets for over 7,500 years. Chickpeas are a type of legume that offers a range of health benefits. Chickpeas help to increase satiety, boost digestion, and keep blood sugar levels stable, increase protection against disease and more. Chickpeas nutrition is a potent package of protein, vitamins and minerals, and so they are often included in many healing diets.

Chickpeas Nutrition Facts:

Chickpeas nutrition truly proves that they really are an amazing super food. Just one cup serving of chickpeas contains (in daily recommended values):

268 calories
12.5 grams of dietary fibre
14.5 grams of protein
4.2 grams of fat
84% manganese
71% foliate
29% copper
28% phosphorus
26% iron
17% zinc

Chickpea Health Benefits:

Chickpeas, or garbanzo beans, are a great source of plant-based protein and fibre, iron, zinc, phosphorus, B vitamins and more. With so many vitamins and nutrients, chickpeas benefit the body in a number of different ways. Here are the top six health benefits of chickpeas:

Chickpeas helps control Blood Sugar levels: Chickpeas, like all legumes, are a form of complex carbohydrate that the body is able to slowly digest and use for energy. This is essential, as all carbohydrates are not created equal; some quickly raise blood sugar levels and lead to "spikes and dips" in energy (these are called simple or fast carbohydrates); while others do the opposite and give us sustained fuel (these are called complex carbohydrates). Chickpeas nutrition includes starch, which is a slow burning carbohydrate that the body does not react to by suddenly spiking glucose in the blood. Unlike simple sugars- found in processed products like refined flour, white bread and pasta, soda, candy, and most other packaged foods-the starches found in chickpeas take an extended period of time to break down once consumed. Starches contain natural sugars called glucose, which the body uses easily for many essential functions; however glucose can be troublesome for people who are pre-diabetic or who have diabetes. The process of digesting and utilizing the glucose found in all beans and starches is drawn-out, which is extremely important for diabetics who have trouble reaching a stable blood sugar level after contain sugars due to a resistance to insulin.

Increases Satiety and Helps with Weight Loss: Chickpeas are high in both protein and fibre, which helps to make you feel full and to curb food cravings and unhealthy snacking. Studies have shown that consuming fibre is correlated with having a lower body weight. Frequently consuming foods like fat burning garbanzo beans is an excellent way to aid in healthy and sustainable weight loss. The feeling of satiety makes you less likely to snack on empty calorie, processed junk foods between meals which can stall your weight loss. Chickpeas are even more filling if you pair them with other nutritious whole foods, like vegetables or organic goat cheese. Because they are so low in calories but high in essential fibre and protein, they are a perfect food for those that need to lose some weight but who are watching calorie intake.

Chickpeas improve digestion: Chickpeas are one of the 20 Ultimate High Fibre Foods, with roughly 6-7 grams per half cup serving. Unfortunately the modern western diet that many Americans consume leaves them deficient in dietary fibre; in fact it's believed that less than 5 percent of Americans get the daily recommended amount of dietary fibre that they need to consume through food each day. Fibre facilitates in healthy digestion by quickly moving foods through the digestive tract, helping to decrease symptoms of IBS and constipation. Fibre works by drawing fluids from the body and binding them to the bulk of forming stool, which contains toxins and waste that must be removed from the body.

Chickpeas Fibre helps to balance pH levels and bacteria within the gut: Chickpeas fibre also helps to balance pH levels and bacteria within the gut, increasing healthy bacteria while also decreasing unhealthy bacteria. An imbalance in gut flora bacteria is often linked to many different digestive problems. The high amount of fibre in garbanzo beans is responsible for its filling effect and helps to improve digestion, but it does much more than this. Fibre aids in heart health, helps to control blood sugar levels, guards against cancer, heart disease, diverticulitis, kidney stones, PMS, obesity, and more.

Chickpeas help protect against Heart disease and Cancer: Chickpeas have been shown to help balance unhealthy cholesterol levels, to reduce hypertension, and to protect against heart disease in multiple ways. This may be partially due to the high amount of fibre found in chickpeas, which helps people to avoid overeating and gaining harmful excess weight, especially around the vital organs. Fibre works to create a gel-like substance in the digestive system that binds with fatty acids, helping to balance cholesterol levels. Both soluble fibre and insoluble fibre have been show to be important in helping to control and manage hypertension. Beans help to keep the arteries clear from plaque build-up, maintain healthy blood pressure levels, and decrease the chances of cardiac arrest and stroke. In fact studies show that having just one daily serving (about 3/4 cup cooked) of beans of any kind can help to decrease chances of a heart attack and to help balance "bad" LDL cholesterol. Consuming beans has also been shown in studies to have protective benefits against cancer, in particular colon cancer, due to their high fibre content. Garbanzo beans were demonstrated in studies to help stall cancerous cells from further forming. Because beans keep the digestive system, including the colon, free from harmful bacteria and toxic build-up, they create a healthier overall environment where pH levels are balanced, inflammation is reduced and therefore cancer cells cannot proliferate like they can in an unhealthy environment.

Chickpeas provide essential Vitamins and Minerals: Chickpeas nutrition boasts high levels of iron, zinc, foliate, phosphorus, and B vitamins, all of which are especially important for vegetarians and vegans who may be lacking in these essential nutrients due to avoiding animal products. Chickpeas are great source of foliate, also called Vitamin B6. Foliate is important for helping the body to effectively produce new cells as it plays a role in copying and synthesizing DNA. It also helps the body utilize other B Vitamins in addition to protein (in the form of amino acids). A deficiency in foliate can contribute to anaemia, poor immune function, and poor digestion; and for pregnant women, a deficiency can lead to neural tube defects such as spina bifida.

Chickpeas nutrition also includes zinc: Zinc is an essential trace mineral that plays a role in over 100 important enzymatic reactions in the body. Zinc facilitates in bodily functions including protecting against free radical damage (also called oxidative damage), helps speed up wound healing, plays a part in the copying of DNA, and helps with the formation of haemoglobin within the blood. A deficiency can include frequently getting sick with colds, leaky gut syndrome, and consistent digestive problems like diarrhoea, poor eye health, infertility, thinning hair, and even stunted growth in children. Legumes have an alkalizing effect on the body, which helps to balance pH levels by combating the high level of acidity that is common in most modern, western diets. When chickpeas are combined with a source of healthy fat, like olive oil for example which is the case with hummus, nutrient absorption is further increased. Additionally, chickpeas are a good source of 3 nutrients that help to reduce common symptoms associated with PMS: magnesium, manganese, and vitamin B6.

Chickpeas are great source of plant-based Protein: Protein is an essential macro-nutrient that plays an important role in nearly every function in the body, from our vital organs, muscles, tissues and even hormone levels. Consuming enough healthy protein helps you to naturally slow aging. Proteins that we acquire from our diet help to create haemoglobin and important antibodies, to control blood sugar levels, help with muscle building and maintenance, give us lasting energy, fight bacteria, make us feel full, and help to heal wounds and injuries too. Chickpeas nutrition not only contains important protein- about 15 grams per cup of cooked beans- but also has many other nutrients and fibre too. Those who are most at risk for not consuming enough protein are children, vegans and vegetarians. Not eating adequate amounts of protein on a regular basis can result in muscle weakness, fatigue, low energy, eye problems such as cataracts, heart problems, poor skin health, imbalanced hormone levels and more. Because chickpeas are a completely plant-based source of vital protein, they are an excellent choice for non-meat eaters who need to be sure to consume enough of this macronutrient. Chickpeas are often eaten with grains or vegetables, for example in stews or in hummus that is eaten with pita bread; these foods luckily work together to make up a "complete protein". This means they contain all of the building-blocks of protein, called essential amino acids that are necessary for the body to acquire from food in order to use for body function and energy.

Zucchini Falafel Recipe: This zucchini falafel recipe is not only delicious, but it's packed full of vitamin C and healthy fibre. It's easy to make and gluten free. Try this as a snack, side or meal.

Total Time: 20 minutes

Serves: 2

Ingredients:

1 can of Chickpeas, drained

1 cup Mary's Gone Crackers
1 Zucchini, chopped
1 sm. Red Onion
1 Egg
1 tsp. Sea Salt
1/4 cup coconut oil
1 cup Goat's Milk Yogurt or kefir
8 leaves of Lettuce
1 cup fresh Mint Leaves
Directions:
Blend Chickpeas, Mary's Gone Crackers, Zucchini, Onion, Egg and Sea Salt in blender or food processor.
Heat coconut Oil in pan over medium heat. Form into patties and cook until golden brown. 2-4 minutes on each side.
Top with yogurt and mint on bed of lettuce.
Hummus Recipe:
Total Time: 5 minutes
Serves: 8-12
Ingredients:
2 cans garbanzo beans
1/4 cup raw sesame seeds
1 tbsp olive oil
1/4 cup lemon juice
1 garlic clove, peeled
1 tsp cumin
Sea salt to taste
Directions:
1. Drain and rinse garbanzo beans, reserving 1/4 c. liquid. Place all ingredients in a blender and blend. Add more water or olive oil until desired consistency is reached.

Chickpeas Side Effects:

Some people experience digestive discomfort when eating beans, due to their high fibre and starch content. If this happens to you, try preparing beans from scratch (dried form) and soaking them overnight first. This helps to cut down on certain compounds that can cause digestive problems including gas and bloating.
If you aren't accustomed to eating high amounts of fibre, gradually introduce more into your diet instead of consuming a large amount of fibre-rich beans all at once. This will help ease digestion and avoid unwanted

8). Flaxseeds (linseeds)

The leaves, stems and seeds of the flax plant have been used throughout history in cooking and medicine. Flaxseeds are the tiny, sesame seed-size seeds from the plant. Although flaxseed can be eaten whole, grinding the seeds allows the body to fully benefit from flaxseed's many nutritional benefits. Flaxseed has been known as one of the best ways to relieve constipation for centuries. The whole seeds contain anywhere from six to 12 percent mucilage. Mucilage is a slimy, gum-like compound that provides a temporarily soothing and protective coating along the entire digestive tract. It provides both bulk and softness to the stool. These properties make it an excellent tool to relieve constipation, as well as stomach and intestinal inflammation.

Flaxseed is inexpensive and you should be able to find it at your local health food store. Keep in mind that if the seeds aren't crushed, ground, or broken, they will pass through your system intact and you'll lose the benefits. Except for decorating the outside of bread loaves or muffins, I would recommend grinding the seeds in a small food processor or a blender. Small, inexpensive coffee grinders also work well for this purpose. (If you intend to use a blender, adding a bit of water or liquid to the seeds will make the blending process much easier.) Grind the seeds just prior to using them. If you don't consume the ground powder rather quickly after grinding, you risk the chance of the precious oils oxidizing and going rancid.

Finally, any time you consume ground flaxseed, you need to make certain that you are drinking plenty of water. The fibre in flax soaks up water like a sponge. While this action is great for promoting soft stools and relieving constipation, it could actually cause constipation without adequate consumption of liquids.

Important Nutritional Benefits: Flaxseed offers a wealth of healthful nutrients:

- Protein
- Omega-3 fatty acids
- Fibres
- Vitamins, minerals, and phytoestrogens

Flaxseed is very promising in increasing the bowel movements by about one-third. A direct comparison of ground flaxseed and psyllium in patients suffering from constipation predominant irritable bowel syndrome (IBS-C) shows that flaxseed reduced the constipation, bloating and pain significantly as compared to the psyllium.

Flax Seed and Diarrhoea: Flaxseed increases the number of bowel movements, and so it should not be used if you suffer from diarrhoea predominant IBS (IBS-D).

Caution: Individuals who suffer from diverticulitis, a condition in which a person has small pockets in their intestine lining, need to be extremely cautious not to have seed fragments become trapped in those pockets and, thus, should only use finely ground flaxseed or flaxseed oil.

Whole flaxseed has a shelf life of up to one year. Ground flaxseed is best refrigerated and used within a few months. Flaxseed oil must be refrigerated to keep it from going rancid and should be used within a few weeks.

It is also important to bear in mind that flaxseed oil lacks fibre and some of the other major-nutritional benefits of flaxseed in its seed form. Whole flax seeds have a shiny, hard outer coating that can make it difficult for your body to break down. The starch and nutrients in whole flax seeds are less available when the seeds are eaten uncooked — in some cases, the seeds can pass whole through the body. In other instances, such as when flax is used as an egg substitute, soaking is needed to take advantage of the seeds' fibre content.

Benefits of Soaked Flax Seed: The gum or soluble fibre on the exterior of the seed is softened during even short periods of soaking. In addition to softening the seeds, the soaking process removes substances such as phytic acid and tannins that are hard on your digestive system. Soaking seeds can make some nutrients, such as protein, more available and the seeds easier to digest in general.

Flax Seeds Soaking Process: To soak, cover the flax seeds with at least 1 inch of water and cover the bowl with plastic wrap or a lid and let sit. Soak whole flax seeds for as little as 10 minutes or for as long as overnight. The cooler the water is, the more time the seeds need to be soaked. For water that is around room temperature, 70 degrees Fahrenheit, soak for a minimum of 2 hours and a maximum of 4 hours. In warm water, soak for at least 10 minutes, up to 30 minutes. Use the soaking liquid for cooking or baking to take full advantage of the nutritional and health benefits of flax.

Use of Soaked Flax Seeds: Soaked flax seeds can be used the same way as uncooked flax seeds. Sprinkle the soaked seeds over top of baked goods, into salads, soups or stews, or add them to smoothies for a quick, nutritious boost to a meal or dish. You can store soaked, drained, unused flax seeds in an air-tight container in the fridge for five days. If you are using flax seeds as an egg replacement, you must use soaked seeds, as the softened soluble fibre around the hull is needed to mimic egg's natural viscosity.

Sources of Flax Seed: Purchase whole flax seeds in health food stores, grocery stores and bulk food stores. If possible, choose flax seeds that have been packaged in an air-tight, opaque container. While whole flax seeds can stay fresh for up to one year, their high oil content means they can go rancid after a time. Look for shiny, unbroken seeds. You can use either golden yellow or dark brown flax seeds for soaking.

Flax Seed Benefits and Nutrition Facts: Flax seeds improve digestion, give you clear skin, lower cholesterol, reduce sugar cravings, balance hormones, fight cancer and promote weight loss. Flaxseeds, sometimes called linseeds, are small, brown, tan or golden-colour seeds that are the richest sources of plant-based omega-3 fatty acids, called alpha-linolenic acid (ALA) in the world and contain fibres. Another unique fact about flaxseeds is that they rank #1 source of lignans in human diets. Flaxseeds contain about 7 times as many lignans as the closest runner-up, sesame seeds. Flaxseed Nutrition Facts are stunning that catch our attention. A 1 ounce (3 tbsp) serving of flaxseeds contains:

- Omega-3 (ALA) 6,338mg;
- Fibre 8g; Protein 6g;
- Vitamin B1 31% RDA;
- Manganese 35% RDA;
- Magnesium 30% RDA;
- Phosphorus 19% RDA
- Selenium 10% RDA.

Also, flaxseeds contain a good amount of vitamin B6, Iron, potassium, copper and zinc. This flax seed nutrition profile makes it easy to see why it's one of the most nutrient dense foods on the planet. Benefits of Flax Seed include: 1. High in Fibre, but Low in Carbs; 2. contain high levels of mucilage gum content. Mucilage is a gel-forming fibre that is water soluble and gives incredible benefits to the intestinal tract. The mucilage can keep food in the stomach from emptying too quickly into the small intestine which can increase nutrient absorption. 3. Flax seeds contain extremely high, both soluble and insoluble fibre which can support colon detoxification, fat loss and reduce sugar cravings. We should aim to consume 30-40 g of high fibre foods daily. 4. Gives healthy Skin and Hairs. Add 2 tbsp of flax seeds to diet or 1 tbsp of flax seed oil to your daily routine, if you want healthier skin, hair and nails. The ALA fats in flax seeds benefits the skin and hair by providing essential fats as well as b-vitamins which can help reduce dryness and flakiness. It can also improve symptoms of acne, rosacea, and eczema. This also applies to eye health as flax can reduce dry eye syndrome. Flax seed oil is another great option since it has an even higher concentration of healthy fats. 5. Gives Weight Loss. Flaxseeds and Walnuts improve obesity and support weight loss. Since flax is full of healthy fats and fibre, it will help you feel satisfied longer so you will eat fewer calories overall which may lead to weight loss. ALA fats may also help reduce inflammation. This is important for weight loss in that an inflamed body will tend to hold on to excess weight. 6. It lowers Cholesterol. The soluble fibre content of flax seeds trap fat and cholesterol in the digestive system so that it unable to be absorbed. Soluble fibre also traps bile, which is made from cholesterol in the gallbladder. The bile is then excreted through the digestive system, forcing the body to make more, using up excess cholesterol in the blood and lowering cholesterol overall. 7. Flaxseeds are Gluten-Free. Using flax is a great way to naturally replace gluten-containing grains which are inflammatory where flax is anti-inflammatory. So, flax seeds are great for those who have Celiac disease or have a gluten-sensitivity. They may also be a good alternative to omega-3 fats in fish for people with a seafood allergy. 8. Flaxseeds are high in Antioxidants (Lignans). Amongst its other incredible nutrition facts, flax seeds are also packed with antioxidants. Lignans are unique fibre-related polyphenols that provide us with antioxidant benefits for anti-aging, hormone balance and cellular health. Polyphenols support the growth of probiotics in the gut and may also help eliminate yeast and candida in the body. Lignans are also known for their anti-viral and antibacterial properties; therefore consuming flax regularly may help reduce the number or severity of colds and flues. 9. It gives Digestive Health. Maybe the biggest flax seed benefits come from its ability to promote digestive health. The ALA in flax can help protect the lining of the digestive tract and maintain GI health. It has been shown to be beneficial for people suffering from Crohn's disease or other digestive ailments, as it can help reduce gut inflammation.

Flax is also very high in soluble and insoluble fibre which can also improve digestive health and is one of the highest magnesium foods in the world. Two tablespoons of flaxseeds contains about 5 g of fibre or 1/4 of the RDA. The fibre found in flaxseeds provides food for friendly bacteria in colon that can help cleanse waste from your system. 10. Flax Seeds control Cancer. Flax seed benefits have been proven time and time again and even including fighting breast, prostate, ovarian and colon cancer. It is discovered that consuming flax seeds may decrease the risk of breast cancer. The three lignans found in flaxseeds can be converted by intestinal bacteria into enterolactone and enterodiol which naturally balance hormones which may be the reason flax seeds reduce the risk of breast cancer and also reduce the risk of endometrial and ovarian cancer. 11. It is very high in Omega-3 Fatty Acids. We hear a lot about the health benefits of fish oil or omega-3 fats. Fish oil contains EPA and DHA, two omega-3 fats that are critical for optimal health. Although flaxseeds do not contain EPA or DHA, they do contain ALA, another type of omega-3 fat. So, approximately 20% of ALA can be converted into EPA, but only .5% of ALA is converted into DHA and accordingly, provides optimal health. 12. The lignans in the flax have benefits for menopausal women. It can be used as an alternative to hormone replacement therapy because lignans do have estrogenic properties. These properties may also help reduce the risk of osteoporosis. It can even help menstruating women by helping maintain cycle regularity. Use of Flax Seeds: There are many great ways to add these super seeds into your diet including adding them to homemade muffins, breads and cookies. One of the most common questions about baking with flax seeds is that does baking have any effect on omega-3 fatty acid. According to many studies, you can bake flax seeds at 300F for 3 hours and the omega-3's (ALA) in flax seeds remained stable. Flaxseeds are best consumed ground as our bodies cannot access the nutrients if they are eaten whole and they will pass through undigested. You can grind the flax in a coffee grinder, this is best done immediately before eating them so they do not spend much time exposed to air or you can buy them pre-ground and add in your diet (i) to a morning smoothie, (ii) Mix a tablespoon in with yogurt and raw honey, (iii) Bake ground flaxseeds into muffins, cookies and breads, or (iv) It can be mixed with water and used as an egg substitute. However the very best way to experience flax seed benefits is to consume them in their sprouted form. Soaking flax seeds and then sprouting them eliminates phytic acid and may greatly increase mineral absorption. Like other sources of fibre including chia seeds and hemp seeds, make sure to take them with plenty of water or other fluids. The flaxseed deserves to be top of the list of the world's most powerful medicinal foods. For just pennies a day it may protect against dozens of life-threatening health conditions. Flaxseeds prevents Cardiovascular disease and Cancer; Heal Arteries; Contain beneficial Plant Estrogens; Reduce Breast Cancer Mortality by 70%;

269

Protect Against Ovarian Cancer; Protect against Radiation Toxicity; Dilate Arteries; and Treat Carpal Tunnel Syndrome.

Table 1: Flaxseed Protein and Amino Acid Content

Protein & Amino Acids		
Amounts Per Selected Serving		%DV
Protein	30.7 g	61%
Tryptophan	499 mg	
Threonine	1287 mg	
Isoleucine	1505 mg	
Leucine	2075 mg	
Lysine	1448 mg	
Methionine	622 mg	
Cystine	571 mg	
Phenylalanine	1608 mg	
Tyrosine	828 mg	
Valine	1801 mg	
Arginine	3234 mg	
Histidine	793 mg	
Alanine	1554 mg	
Aspartic acid	3437 mg	
Glutamic acid	6785 mg	
Glycine	2096 mg	
Proline	1354 mg	
Serine	1630 mg	
Hydroxyproline	294 mg	

Eating Flaxseeds Ground or Whole: Flaxseeds are Nature's ingenious design for preserving the precious cargo inside human body and is highly therapeutic, though fragile polyunsaturated fatty acids, amino acids, and other fat soluble vitamins. You don't have to worry about refrigerating it. Once the seed is ground up and exposed to air, light, ambient fluctuations in temperature, and time, it begins to "go bad," i.e. oxidize and degrade. This is why many make a daily practice of grinding up their own seeds in a coffee grinder to ensure maximum freshness. As far as whole flaxseed, make sure that you chew it well, if you primary objective is to obtain the beneficial nutrients, lignans, and fibre from them. Also, consider that flaxseed produces a very soothing mucilaginous gel when exposed and/or soaked in water. You can pre-soak a tablespoon in a glass of water overnight to produce a very good concoction for constipation by drinking it in the morning. Because flaxseed will naturally soak up water, remember not to consume too much dry, whole flaxseed without adequate hydration, as it could be a bit binding – the exact opposite effect. Never heat flaxseed oil as oils is rich in monounsaturated and polyunsaturated fatty acids and is prone to enhanced oxidation (rancidity) when heated.

Table 2: Flaxseed Vitamin Content

Vitamins		
Amounts Per Selected Serving		%DV
Vitamin A	0.0 IU	0%
Retinol	0.0 mcg	
Retinol Activity Equivalent	0.0 mcg	
Alpha Carotene	0.0 mcg	
Beta Carotene	0.0 mcg	
Beta Cryptoxanthin	0.0 mcg	
Lycopene	0.0 mcg	
Lutein+Zeaxanthin	1094 mcg	
Vitamin C	1.0 mg	2%
Vitamin D	~	~
Vitamin E (Alpha Tocopherol)	0.5 mg	3%
Beta Tocopherol	0.0 mg	
Gamma Tocopherol	33.5 mg	
Delta Tocopherol	0.6 mg	
Vitamin K	7.2 mcg	9%
Thiamin	2.8 mg	184%
Riboflavin	0.3 mg	16%
Niacin	5.2 mg	26%
Vitamin B6	0.8 mg	40%
Folate	146 mcg	37%
Food Folate	146 mcg	
Folic Acid	0.0 mcg	
Dietary Folate Equivalents	146 mcg	
Vitamin B12	0.0 mcg	0%
Pantothenic Acid	1.7 mg	17%
Choline	132 mg	
Betaine	5.2 mg	

Oral Dietary Fibre is 3 grams of fibre per tablespoon of whole flax seeds. Notable Nutrients are Protein, Thiamine, Manganese, Phosphorus, Magnesium, Copper, Omega-3 fatty acids. Tons of nutrients, packed in a little seed, flax seeds reduce cholesterol and help to ease the symptoms of menopause. Grind in a small coffee grinder, and add to smoothies, salads, and soups.

Table 3: Flaxseed Mineral Content

Minerals

Amounts Per Selected Serving		%DV
Calcium	428 mg	43%
Iron	9.6 mg	53%
Magnesium	658 mg	165%
Phosphorus	1079 mg	108%
Potassium	1366 mg	39%
Sodium	50.4 mg	2%
Zinc	7.3 mg	49%
Copper	2.0 mg	102%
Manganese	4.2 mg	208%
Selenium	42.7 mcg	61%
Fluoride	~	

This means that you would not cook with flaxseed oil, opting for naturally saturated (and therefore more heat stabile) fats like palm, coconut oil or ghee (clarified butter) instead. Flaxseed meal is an excellent addition to smoothies or for sprinkling on foods. The key is that you always stay hydrated when using flaxseed by consuming more and more liquid or water, as it can cause significant binding in a dehydrated individual. The Diet like corn, canola, soy, and peanut, all of which have several orders of magnitude more omega 6 than omega 3. Generally, a tablespoon or two of meal a day is a good dose for ensuring you are getting a physiologically significant amount. We'll leave you with some nutritional snapshots of flaxseed from the more quantitative perspective, so that it is clear how valuable it is in human nutrition simply as a source of both macronutrients and micronutrients.

Table 4: Flaxseed Fatty Acids

Fats & Fatty Acids

Amounts Per Selected Serving		%DV
Total Fat	70.8 g	109%
Saturated Fat	6.2 g	31%
Monounsaturated Fat	12.6 g	
Polyunsaturated Fat	48.3 g	
Total trans fatty acids	~	
Total trans-monoenoic fatty acids	~	
Total trans-polyenoic fatty acids	~	
Total Omega-3 fatty acids	38325 mg	
Total Omega-6 fatty acids	9931 mg	

9). Lentils (Teel):

Total Dietary Fibre is 15.6 grams of fibre per cup (cooked). Notable Nutrients are Protein, Iron, Foliate, Manganese, and Phosphorous. In addition to great fibre, lentils are backed with foliate, and are one of the top 10 high foliate foods. Foliate is essential for pregnant women, individuals with liver disease, and people on certain medications. Lentil pilaffs and soups are great way to incorporate this high fibre food into your diet. Lentils are kitchen all-stars—they take less time to cook and are more versatile than many other legumes. This recipe takes advantage of their slightly meatier taste and turns them into a juicy patty that's held together with lemon juice, cilantro, and walnuts.

10). Peas:

Total Dietary Fibre is 8.6 grams per cooked cup; majority insoluble fibre. Notable Nutrients are Vitamin C, Vitamin K, B6, Thiamine, Manganese, Foliate, Vitamin A, and Protein. The humble green pea is packed with fibre, and powerful antioxidants, anti-inflammatory properties and phytonutrients that support wellness. Frozen peas are available year round, making them ideal to incorporate into your diet. Lightly steam peas and add to soups, and salads. They add a gentle sweetness, while providing nearly 100% of your daily-recommended Vitamin C, and over 25% of Thiamine and Foliate. Pureeing veggies is a great way to squeeze extra nutrients into any meal—this recipe comes together lightning-fast and is filled with protein, omega-3s, and, of course, fibre.

11). Quinoa:

Total Dietary Fibre is 5 grams of fibre per 1 cup cooked. Notable Nutrients are Iron, B-6, Magnesium, and Potassium. Quinoa is a truly remarkable seed that eats like a grain! All grains are high in fibre, but not all of them are packed with nutrition. It is Quinoa's amazing nutritional profile and the fact that it is easier to digest and gluten-free, that pushed quinoa over the ultimate fibre food edge. Quinoa is also high in other essential nutrients such as iron, vitamin B-6, potassium and magnesium. Magnesium is one of the most underrated, yet essential vitamins that both protect the heart and helps nearly every function of the body. And many people have a magnesium deficiency, and don't even know it. So, Quinoa not only adds valuable fibre to your diet, but is a real super food for many other reasons as well.

12).Split Peas (Dal):

Total Dietary Fibre is 16.3 grams of fibre per cup (cooked). Notable Nutrients are Protein, Thiamine, Foliate, Manganese, Omega-3 fatty acids, Omega-6 fatty acids. Split pea soup may be an "old school" soup, but it should make a comeback. One serving of split peas contains a third of the Foliate recommended daily, in addition to over half of the recommended intake of dietary fibre. Spinach and Yellow Split Pea (Dal) Soup in Indian cooking form a terrific, protein-rich base for soups, stews, and dals. This South Asian recipe is the best kind of comfort food, healthy, satisfying, and super filling.

13). Black Gram (Kala chana):

Black Gram (Urad): Black Gram is also known as black lentil; it is one of the most widely consumed lentils in India. Black gram is a member of the Asiatic Vigna crop group. Black gram is clinically referred to as Phasiolus mungo and it's also popularly known as Urad in India. These are rounded black lentils, slightly elongated with a sticky texture and bland flavour. White lentil is black lentil with the black skin removed. These lentils have a very strong earthy flavour. Black Gram, whole or split is used to make daal. Boiled seed is also eaten whole or its paste is used to make dishes like dosa. It is used for making the famous 'Daal Makhani' of North India, besides other things. It can also be fried with condiments like onion and garlic for a snack.

Nutritional Value: Black Gram Nutrition Facts are that it bears a sheen black colour skin. Beneath the skin is a whitish portion which is oval in shape. Black gram has a number of nutritional benefits which makes it one of the highly prized pulses in India.

Nutrient	Amount
Moisture	10.9%
Protein	24%
Fat	1.4%
Fibre	0.9%
Minerals	3.2%
Carbohydrates	59.6%
Calcium	154mg
Phosphorous	385mg
Iron	9.1mg
Calorific value	341

Medicinal Uses: Serves as an emollient and has a comfy effect on human skin. Preferably used as a nerving tonic, due to the essential ingredients present in it. When taken with gourd juice and honey, Black Gram heals mild diabetes, if taken daily for 3-4 months. Black Gram acts as a healthy supplement for people suffering from malnutrition. Black Gram can be taken with wheat bread and honey for treating impotency. It heals a number of nervous disorders such as weakness of memory, schizophrenia, nervous weakness and hysteria. Black Gram paste, when applied on hair keeps dandruffs at bay and cures a number of hair problems at the same time lengthening the hair to a maximum level. Black Gram treats digestive disorders and is crucial in curing gastric catarrh, dysentery, dyspepsia and diarrhoea. Rheumatic pains, stiff shoulder and contracted knee can be healed with the help of the medicinal properties present in Black Gram.
1. Germinated black gram is good for mild diabetics.
2. It helps purify the system and remove toxins from the body.
3. Black gram is a very rich source of protein.
4. It helps maintain a healthy digestive system and is good for diarrhoea.
5. It is great for hair growth and reduces cholesterol to improve blood circulation.
 Health benefits of Black gram
Due to its therapeutic as well as healing qualities, Black gram is essentially utilized in Ayurvedic medication. Black gram can be purchased in the whole form with its skin on, split form with its skin on

or even split form without its skin. Soaking this particular lentil just before cooking will accelerate the cooking time.

Black Gram is probably high nutritional beans. Urad daal is healthier compared to almost every other beans available for sale. It may be consumed daily since it has numerous incredible qualities that are great for health. Followings are some health advantages of Black gram

1. Energy Booster: Black gram is really a healthy pulse since it is full of iron content. This can help increase the energy levels within the body and keeps you active. This is particularly important for women going through menstruation who've a greater possibility of an iron deficiency or a deficiency of iron. Consuming urad daal frequently boosts your energy considerably since it creates the body's iron stores.

2. Improves Digestion: The best advantage of ingesting urad daal is that it improves digestion of food due to its rich fibre content. Urad daal benefits the health since it has got both soluble and insoluble fibre that is great for digestion and in addition helps prevent constipation.

3. Boosts Heart Health: Black gram has been discovered to be useful for boosting the health of your heart. The fibre within this lentil helps to reduce cholesterol and also the potassium helps you to balance the effects of sodium, therefore helping in reducing high blood pressure levels. Nutrition just like foliate and magnesium present in this particular lentil works well for avoiding damage of the arterial walls. Magnesium raises blood circulation helping your heart function at its optimum best. Black gram helps reduce lipids and cholesterol in body and Hyperlipidemia. These types of black seeds have capability to inhibit procedure for absorption of lipids and cholesterol.

4. Improves healthy sex life and male reproductive system: Urad Daal is recognized as an all natural aphrodisiac since it treats sexual dysfunction. Soak urad Daal in water for 5-6 hours and after that fry it in ghee. Have this particular pulse to have a healthy sex life. Also, it improves milk secretion in lactating mothers.

5. Muscle building: Black gram is definitely the rich source of protein and therefore ideal for overall growth and development of the body as well as in the reinforcement and building of muscle tissue.

6. Excellent for diabetes: Black gram is quite great at the disease of diabetes and shows quite good results whenever used together with bitter gourd juice and honey. With this treatment, the unnecessary use of carbohydrates ought to be confined.

7. Nervous disorders: It is important in several nervous related problems like nervous weakness, memory weakness, schizophrenia, hysteria etc.

8. Black gram has anti-inflammatory properties: Ayurvedic medication considers black gram just as one outstanding cure for dealing with inflammation as well as joint pain because of its powerful anti-inflammatory qualities. A hot poultice of the lentil placed on the affected area may help in reducing the inflammation and also the pain related to it. Massaging the area along with oil that contains Vigna mungo is additionally useful in decreasing inflammation and pain

9. Black gram increases immunity: While being used as well-liked lentil, its use has been typical in traditional Ayurveda where it's been utilized to deal with numerous diseases. It really is typically considered to be food which boosts immunity. In the lab research along with black gram extract, researchers were able to observe its capability to encourage immunity in rat.

10. Home remedy for pain and inflammation of the joints: A decoction obtained by boiling black gram along with rock salt and sesame oil, whenever used on the affected areas is found to be valuable in decreasing inflammation and pain. This is particularly ideal for people struggling with joint pain and also arthritis.

11. Black gram for diabetic patient: Vigna mungo is a great food alternative for individuals struggling with diabetes since it is fibre rich. A diet that contains higher quantities of fibre works well for managing blood glucose levels and helps prevent spikes within these levels particularly after a meal. An excellent home cure for diabetics to keep their blood glucose levels in check is to take black gram (germinated) together with half a cup of bitter gourd once daily for around 4 months.

12. Black gram minerals good for bones: Black gram is full of proteins as well as minerals just like calcium, phosphorus and magnesium that encourage the growth and repair of healthy and strong bones. The nutrients within this lentil strengthens your bones as well as helps prevent problems just like osteoporosis, that is seen as a decrease in bone density as well as bone mass, therefore making your bones easily vulnerable to breakage as well as fractures.

13. Black gram is good for pregnant women: Pregnant women are frequently recommended to include black gram within their diet due to its higher nutritional value. Black gram is really a rich source of iron that is required for the creation of haemoglobin and increased blood flow. Additionally it is full of protein, dietary fibre as well as nutrition

just like folic acid which is not only great for the expecting mother but in addition for the foetus since it works well for avoiding birth defects.

14. Black gram is good for pregnant women: Apart from offering you a number of health advantages, black gram can work miracles for the skin and hair. It is full of minerals which will make the skin look supple and soft. Listed here are methods for you to include Black gram within your beauty routine. 1. Exfoliates your skin: Black gram can be used like an effective scrub to eliminate the dirt, grime and dead skin cells from the skin to expose a fresh as well as supple skin. 2. Heals sunburn and removes tan: Black gram features a cooling effect on the skin that can help remove the suntan. Its skin lightening qualities likewise helps to eliminate the tan. 3. Treats acne: Black gram cleanses the pores and eliminates the extra oils therefore dealing with acne. Additionally, it has natural germ killing qualities which kill the bacteria causing acne. 4. Lightens your skin tone: Black gram has natural bleaching qualities that may lighten up your skin. The pulse is additionally loaded with a number of nutrition that will help to maintain the health of the skin. 5. Reduces skin spots: Black gram has anti-bacterial qualities that may reduce age spots as well as acne scars. It may also help in skin regeneration and is also therefore a fantastic cure to keep a young skin. 6. Combats dry and frizzy hair: Black gram may also help you manage dry brittle hair. It really is full of minerals as well as fatty acids that can help to revive the lustre of your hair. It will likewise condition your hair and provide it a shiny appearance. 7. Home remedy for eliminating dandruff: Make a paste of black gram as well as green gram and make use of this mixture to wash your hair. This particular remedy works well for eliminating dandruff, strengthening your hair as well as in keeping your hair clean and soft.

Recipe of Black Gram:

1. Black Gram Flour Cake:

Ingredients
Black gram flour – 1 cup
Baking powder – 1 tsp
Sugar – 1/2 cup
Oil/ Ghee – 1/4 cup
Cocoa powder – 3 tsp
Egg – 1

Directions: Beat the egg till it gets frothy. Add sugar and beat again. Add oil/ghee mix again. Mix black gram flour, cocoa powder as well as baking powder completely and fold with the egg mixture. Add the mixture in the glass bowl, lined with butter paper in the oven for 7-8 minutes on medium power and after that grill for 3-4 minutes.

The cake is ready.

2. Black Daal:

Ingredients

3/4 cup black gram dal

1/4 cup green gram dal

1 large onion finely chopped

1 tomato finely chopped

1 tsp. ginger garlic paste

4 green chillies finely chopped

1/4 tsp. turmeric powder

1 tsp. lemon juice

Salt to taste

3 tbsp. ghee

1tsp. chopped coriander

1 tsp. each cumin & mustard seeds

2 pinches asafoetida

1 tsp. sugar

Seasoning:

1 bay leaf

4 cloves

1" cinnamon stick broken

Directions: Wash Daal and pressure cook in 2 cups water. Cool and remove from cooker. Mash very lightly using a spoon. Heat half the ghee in the deep saucepan. Add seeds, asafoetida, and seasoning. Allow to splutter. Add ginger garlic paste, fry for the minute. Add onions. Fry till light brown. Add tomatoes and green chillies. Fry for 2-3 minutes more. Add dal, bring to boil. Add turmeric, salt, sugar and lemon juice. Take in serving dish. Heat the remaining ghee in a small saucepan. Add chopped coriander to the hot ghee and pour over Daal immediately. Stir gently. Serve with hot paratha, Roti or rice.

3. Black gram laddu:

Ingredients:

1 cup – Black gram (skinned)

1 cup – jiggery, grated

1/2 cup – Ghee

Directions:

Fry the black gram. When it becomes light brown in colour, cool it and grind it to a fine powder. Mix it with grated jiggery. Slowly pour hot ghee over this mix and mix well. Make laddoos of this mixture.

4. Wheat and Black gram Dosa:

Ingredients:
1 cup – Black gram
2 cups – wheat flour
1 tsp – methi seeds
1 tbsp – cooked rice
Salt to taste
Directions: Soak black gram as well as methi together for 3-4 hours. Grind it fine along with water while adding the cooked rice. Mix it good with wheat flour adding salt. Ferment the batter like you always do for dosa by keeping it in the warm place. Make dosa the next day. It's not only low carb. But it will be additionally delicious.
5. Black Gram Puris:
Ingredients:
250 gms – Black gram
250 gms – flour (maida)
2 tbsp – hot oil
2 to 3 tbsp – oil for frying the dal paste
Enough water
Salt to taste
For Dry Roasting
2 – Cardamoms (seeds)
1 ½ tsp – coriander seeds
1 ½ tsp – cumin seeds
8 to 10 – pepper corns
1 ½ tsp – fennel seeds
6 to 8 red dry chillies
1 small stick – cinnamon
3 to 4 – cloves
Directions: Clean, wash and soak the urad Daal for around 4-6 hours. Remove the water and coarsely grind. Roast seeds, pepper corns, fennel seeds, and red dry chillies for couple of minutes on the low flame. Grind this to powder. Cool. Make stiff dough by mixing flour, 2 tbsp of hot oil, salt to taste and enough water. Knead the dough well and cover using a cloth and keep aside for around 30 minutes. In a kadhai (Frying Pan) add 2-3 tbsp of oil and fry the Daal paste until golden in colour on the low flame, stirring continuously. Remove from fire and cool completely and now add some masala (spices) powder and salt to taste. Divide the kept aside dough into 15 equal portions. Roll each portion into 3 diameter puree. Put a heaped tbsp of the urad dal mixture in the centre of the puree. Gather the outer edges of the puree and lightly roll out into small purees. Fry the purees in hot oil till

golden. Serve along with aloo (Potatoes) pethe ka sabzi (vegetable), pickle and onion kachumber.

Precaution: The excessive use of black gram can cause flatulence as well as in order to cure it, generally pepper, ginger, along with a little asafoetida is included. The people struggling with urinary calculi as well as rheumatism shouldn't take black gram mainly because it consists of oxalic acid in high quantity.

14). Mung Beans and Mung Dal (Split Mung):

Black Gram (Urad Daal)	Mung Beans	Kala Chana / savoury bean	Mung

Mung beans is a type of small, green legume in the same plant family as peas and lentils and is a high source of protein, fibre, antioxidants and phytonutrients. Although in most parts of the world they're less popular than other bean varieties, like chickpeas or black beans, Mung beans have some huge health benefits to offer!

While Mung beans may be new to most people in the U.S, they've been a part of traditional Ayurvedic diets in India for thousands of years. Mung beans are considered "one of the most cherished foods" in the ancient Indian practice that's been a traditional form of medicine since roughly 1,500 B.C.

These days, Mung beans are beginning to pop up in protein powders, canned soups and in restaurant dishes state-side. Mung beans are a high source of nutrients including: manganese, potassium, magnesium, foliated, copper, zinc and various B vitamins. They are also a very filling food, high in protein, resistant starch and dietary fibre. You can find Mung beans in dried powder form, as whole uncooked beans, "split-peeled" form (just like you'd find split green peas), as bean noodles, and also as sprouted seeds (which are the kind you'd see used on sandwiches or salads). Their dried seeds may be eaten raw, cooked (whole or split), fermented, or milled and ground into flour.

Because of their high nutrient density, Mung beans are considered useful in defending against several chronic, age-related diseases, including heart disease, cancer, diabetes and obesity. Clinical evidence continues to show that plant-derived foods have various potential health benefits, including lowering inflammation. Health experts recommend that plant-based foods make up a large portion of every person's diet, and many worldwide health organizations have recommended an increase in the intake of plant-derived foods to improve health status and to prevent chronic diseases. Among plant-based sources of protein and nutrients, Mung beans are one of the foods gathering the most attention. As you'll come to learn, Mung beans are one of the healthiest sources of plant protein there is when you consider how many other nutrients they contain in addition to amino acids (the building blocks of proteins). One cup of cooked Mung Beans Nutrition Facts is that it contains the following (percentages based on the RDAs for the average adult female):

212 calories
14 grams of protein
15 grams of fibre
1 gram of fat
4 grams of sugar
321 micrograms of foliated (100%)
97 milligrams of magnesium (36%)
0.33 milligrams of vitamin b1 thiamine (36%)
0.6 milligrams of manganese (33%)
7 milligrams of zinc (24%)
0.8 milligrams of vitamin B5 pantothenic acid (8%)
0.13 milligrams of vitamin B6 (11%)
55 milligrams of calcium (5%)

If you choose to sprout Mung beans and eat them raw, each cup will only have about 31 calories and will provide about three grams of protein and two grams of fibre.

Health Benefits of Mung Beans:

Mung beans Help Lower High Cholesterol Levels and protect against Heart Disease. Mung beans are highly effective at inhibiting LDL "bad" cholesterol oxidation. Mung beans have the ability to regulate cholesterol levels because their antioxidants act like potent free-radical scavengers, reversing damage done to blood vessels and lowering inflammation. Oxidized LDL cholesterol is one of the biggest risks of deadly cardiovascular events, such as heart attacks or stroke. LDL cholesterol can accumulate within the inner lining of blood vessels, called the endothelium, and block blood flow, triggering cardiac arrest. Mung beans are a great addition to any anti-inflammatory diet thanks to their ability to keep arteries clear and to improve circulation.

Mung beans Helps Lower High Blood Pressure. Mung beans nutrition includes the ability to fight another significant cardiovascular disease risk factor: high blood pressure. In a 2014 study published in the Chemistry Central Journal, rats that were given Mung bean sprout extracts for one month experienced significant reductions in systolic blood pressure levels.

Mung beans contain Antioxidants that fight Cancer development. High levels of amino acids, oligosaccharides and polyphenols in Mung beans are thought to be the main contributors to their antioxidant power that can fight cancer development. In clinical studies, Mung beans show anti-tumour activity and are able to protect DNA damage and dangerous cell mutation.

Mung beans can help prevent or treat Type 2 Diabetes. Strong evidence exists that Mung beans nutrition has a significant anti-diabetic effect and can naturally help prevent or treat cases of type 2 diabetes.

Mung beans provide a high source of Protein. Mung beans nutrition includes a very impressive amount of protein for a plant, with about 20–24 percent of their chemical structure being amino acids (protein. Globulin and albumin are the main storage proteins found in Mung bean seeds and make up over 85 percent of the total amino acids found in Mung beans. Mung beans nutrition is also rich in other essential amino acids, including leucine, isoleucine and valine, which can be combined with other plant sources (like whole grains or some vegetables) to make a "complete protein." Their highly absorbable protein content makes them a smart choice for vegans or vegetarians, especially considering how many other nutrients they add to someone's diet.

Mung beans boost Immunity and protects against Infections and Viruses. Mung beans nutrition contains a range of phytonutrients that are considered anti-microbial and anti-inflammatory, helping them to increase immunity and fight harmful bacteria, viruses, colds, rashes, irritations and more. Mung beans promote a healthy balance of bacteria within the digestive tract, which helps with nutrient absorption and immune defence.

Mung beans are high source of Vitamins and Minerals, Like Foliate and Magnesium. Mung beans nutrition provides a whopping 100 percent of your daily value of foliated in every one cup serving. Foliate (also known as vitamin B9) is an important vitamin for DNA synthesis, cell and tissue growth, hormonal balance, cognitive function, and even reproduction. In fact, consuming enough foliated is especially important during pregnancy because it's essential for preventing early births, neural tube defects and even termination.

Mung beans also provide about 36 percent of daily magnesium needs for the average adult woman. Many adults are actually deficient in magnesium, which is unfortunate because most people really need a substantial amount in their diet in order to control stress levels and manage pain. Magnesium is important for digestive health, proper heart beat functioning, neurotransmitter release and for repairing muscle tissue in people who are very active.

Mung beans fights Obesity and helps with Weight Loss, because Mung beans nutrition contains high levels of fibre and protein, they are one of the most filling foods there is. In a study published in the Journal of Nutrition, that a single meal with high-fibre beans produced a two-fold greater increase in the satiety hormone called cholecystokinin when compared to meals that didn't contain beans.

Mung beans help decrease PMS Symptoms. Mung beans nutrition provides B vitamins, including vitamin B6 and foliated, which are both important for controlling hormone fluctuations that can lead to PMS symptoms. B vitamins, foliated and magnesium are useful for lowering the severity and pain associated with PMS cramps, headaches, mood swings, and fatigue and muscle pains.

Mung beans are easy to digest compared to many other Beans. While some people experience gas or bloating from eating beans, Mung beans are considered one of the easiest beans to digest and can actually help with detoxification in some cases. Mung beans have many benefits for digestion due to their high fibre content, for example, they can help prevent IBS symptoms like constipation.

Soaked and sprouted Mung beans can also help reduce "antinutrients" that are naturally present within all legumes and beans, making them easier to digest and also releasing more of their nutrients. Types of carbohydrates called oligosaccharides, raff nose, stachyose and verbascose are present in raw (un-sprouted) or poorly processed legumes, which can cause uncomfortable flatulence. Some of these antinutrients are present in Mung beans, but to a lesser degree than many other beans. In addition, antinutrients found in Mung beans are soluble in water and can be eliminated by soaking, sprouting (germinating) or fermenting before eating them.

Methods to use Mung Beans in Recipes:

In order to add Mung beans into your diet without experiencing unwanted digestive effects, try first soaking and sprouting dried beans overnight and then cooking them with traditional Ayurvedic spices that can help increase digestibility. In India, they are commonly cooked with such spices as ginger, cumin, coriander and turmeric in order to help make them taste great while also helping to avoid any stomach pains.

Sprouting, or germination, is thought to improve the nutritional and medicinal qualities of Mung beans nutrition, making them easier to digest and tolerate and so always try to consume sprouted Mung beans if you can.

The sprouts of mug beans is one type that is edible after germination, which have more obvious biological activities and more plentiful beneficial metabolites than un-sprouted Mung beans do. Sprouting helps biosynthetic enzymes to become activated during the stages of germination, which means Mung beans nutrition, become more absorbable by the human body.

Mung beans, which have the scientific species name Vigna radiate, appear in cuisines around the world, mostly in India, China, the Philippines and Korea. In India, split and peeled Mung beans are traditionally used in the dish called Dal, which is a thick stew that is high in fibre and protein, yet low in calories. It's a filling meal and is considered a staple in Indian cooking that is eaten multiple times per week for most families.

In Chinese cuisine, Mung beans are also used to make pancakes or dumplings, combined with rice in stir- fries as a staple dish and even used in desserts. Whole Mung beans are used to make "Tangshui", a type of Chinese dessert which literally translates to "sugar water" because the beans are cooked with sugar, coconut milk and a little bit of ginger. They are also ground into a paste to form a popular type of ice cream and sorbet (Juice) in Hong Kong.

Mung bean sprouts are made into a processed version of starch noodles that are most common in Asian cuisine. Mung beans have a much greater carbohydrate content (about 50–60 percent) than soybeans do, so they work well as flour and noodle products. Mung beans' starch is the predominant carbohydrate in the legume and is why they are typically used for the production of starchy noodles, such as the kind called "Muk" in Korea.

Mung Bean Recipes: Thai Spring Rolls:

Total Time: 15 minutes

Serves: 6-8
Ingredients:
16 pieces of rice paper
2 cups cucumber
2 cups shredded lettuce
2 cups shredded carrots
2 red bell peppers, seeded and sliced very thin
1 cup mung bean sprouts
1 cup chopped fresh mint
1 cup chopped fresh basil
1 cup chopped fresh cilantro
1 small onion chopped
2 tablespoons balsamic vinegar
Sea salt to taste
Warm water
Directions:
Chop the vegetables and fresh herbs until they are uniform in sizei, i.e. 1/4" or smaller.
Mix in bowl with remaining spices and balsamic vinegar.
Place warm water in a bowl. Soak rice paper in the water until soft.
Lay rice paper on a flat surface.
Place approximately 1/4 cup of the mixture on one end of the rice paper.
Begin Rolling, being careful to fold in sides as you progress.
Cut in half and serve cold.
Mung beans can help restore your bowels after a bout of food poisoning. Their cooling nature reduces inflammation in the digestive tract. Mung bean's fibre and astringency can help bind up loose stools in diarrhoea. Mung bean kitchari is a restorative for those recovering from any illness. Mung Beans & Weight Loss: Mung beans are a low-calorie, natural choice to help you overcome the hardest challenge of weight loss: curbing your hunger pangs and keeping your cravings quiet.
The high fibre content in Mung beans aids in cholesterol reduction and lowers blood sugar levels.
Mung beans are a mild diuretic which helps to reduce excess water weight. They are especially useful for oedema in the lower limbs. To enhance their diuretic effect, prepare them with diuretic spices like cumin, coriander and fennel, or celery and parsley.
Nutritional Information

Mung beans contain vitamins A, C and E, folacin, phosphorous, magnesium, iron and calcium. They are also a source of phytoestrogens.

16). Jowar (Sorghum/ White millet)

High-fibre foods like Jowar may lower your risk of heart disease.

Jowar is the Indian name for Sorghum, a cereal grain native to Africa. Also known as white millet, whole Jowar kernels can be steamed, boiled, added to soups and stews or ground into flour that can be used as a substitute for wheat flour in baked goods. Jowar is a gluten-free, high-protein, cholesterol-free source of a variety of essential nutrients, including dietary fibre, iron, phosphorus and thiamine. Belonging to the millet family, the use of this grain was restricted to animal feed. However, recent research has revealed that this grain has unique health benefits for humans. When compared to rice and wheat, Sorghum has a higher content of calcium. Besides calcium, it also packed with iron, protein and fibre. The latest revelations in connection with this grain point to cardiac benefits. This benefit accrues from the presence of antioxidants in fairly large amounts. These antioxidants present in Sorghum are polyphenolic compounds. In addition to the antioxidants, the presence of sorghum wax, contributes to the cardiac benefit that this millet provides. The wax in this grain contains policosanols, which help in lowering cholesterol levels.

Dietary Fibre: A 1-cup serving of Jowar contains 12 grams of dietary fibre. This amount supplies approximately 48 percent of the Food and Nutrition Board's recommended daily allowance of fibre for the average adult. Compared to other cereal grains like barley or rice, Jowar contains a much higher concentration of fibre. According to a 2009 study published in "Nutrition Reviews," a diet rich in high-fibre foods like Jowar may lower your risk of obesity, stroke, high blood pressure, heart disease, diabetes, elevated blood cholesterol and digestive problems like diverticulitis disease, colon cancer, constipation and haemorrhoids.

Iron: Jowar contains 8.45 milligrams of iron in every cup, or nearly 47 percent of the required daily intake of iron for women and over 100 percent of the RDA for men. Iron is necessary for the body to produce red blood cells and adenosine tri-phosphate, or ATP, the main source of cellular energy. Without adequate iron, you may be more likely to develop anaemia or neurological disorders like attention-deficit hyperactivity disorder. The iron in Jowar is non-heme iron, a form of the mineral that is not absorbed as easily as the heme iron in animal-based products. You can increase the iron you absorb from Jowar by eating it with meat or a source of vitamin C. Try tossing steamed, chilled Jowar into a salad with orange segments, or serve it as a simple side dish for grilled beef or chicken.

Phosphorus: Phosphorus is required by the body to support the growth and maintenance of bones. It is also a necessary part of the structure of cell membrane phospholipids, DNA and RNA, and plays a vital role in triggering the action of a variety of hormones and enzymes. Each 1-cup serving of Jowar provides 551 milligrams of phosphorus or about 78 percent of the daily intake for adults. According to the Linus Pauling Institute, only 50 percent of the phosphorus in plant-based foods like Jowar is digestible since the mineral is in the form of phytate. Humans lack the enzymes needed to break down phytate. To increase the amount of phosphorus you get from Jowar, incorporate Jowar or Jowar flour into baked goods containing yeast.

Thiamine: Every 1-cup serving of Jowar provides men with 38 percent of their recommended daily intake of thiamine and women with 41 percent of their daily thiamine requirement. Thiamine belongs to the B family of vitamins and is also known as vitamin B-1. Your body needs adequate thiamine to support the function of the nervous and immune systems, to aid with energy metabolism and to help synthesize ATP. Eating plenty of thiamine-rich foods may lower your risk of heart failure, neurodegenerative problems such as Alzheimer's disease and eye problems like cataracts.

Health Benefits of Jowar: Jowar or sorghum is rated among the top five healthy grains in the world. Steam it, boil it, use it in a stew, make a soup out of it; well this grain can be used in multiple ways rather than just grinding it to flour.

In the initial years, this millet was used as animal feeds. However, soon jowar's exceptional health benefits came to light post which it featured in the human plate too. Jowar could easily replace staple grains such as rice and wheat making for a gluten-free alternative.

Incredible Health Values: Needless to say, Jowar is a treasure trove of nutrients such as calcium, fibre, iron, phosphorus, thiamine and protein. Consuming this whole grain millet could render many of the supplements.

The Weight Loss Effects: The fibre content in Jowar could keep hunger pangs at bay by influencing satiety. Looking for weight loss? Jowar is your friend then.

It improves Digestive System and Fights Constipation. Jowar helps to regulate the bowel movements, boosts metabolism and averts issues like cramps, bloating, gas and stomach ache owing to its rich fibre content.

It boosts Immune System: Jowar amplifies your immunity to a great extent. It contains magnesium, calcium and copper that is responsible for stronger bones and tissues. The iron content in Jowar ensures multiplication of red blood cells.

It Control of Cholesterol Level: Consuming Jowar reduces the bad cholesterol effectively. Phytochemicals and plant sterols present in Jowar have shown to have hypocholesterolemic effect. Jowar also helps in regulating the plasma LDL cholesterol concentration.

It thwarts Cardiovascular Diseases: The presence of antioxidants; in addition to nutrients like vitamin E and B, magnesium and iron, helps to avoid many cardiovascular conditions. It also prevents the clumping of platelets, thereby reducing the threat of heart attack.

Anti-diabetic: Jowar is recommended for patients with diabetes due to the nutrients which double up as antioxidants. These nutrients help impede diabetes causing factors like protein glycation. High fibre content slows down the raptness of carbohydrate, which help to regulate the sugar level in blood.

It Prevents Cancer: According to the research, 3-Deoxyanthocyanidins, a chemical composite in Jowar could have anti-cancer properties.

Essential for Cellular Membranes: Jowar contains phosphorus, which supports the growth and repair of bones. It is also essential for building the cell membrane phospholipids, DNA and RNA.

Good for Celiac Patients: Patients having celiac disease experience inflammation, digestive problems and joint pains. It is the gluten content in grains like wheat which causes this condition. As Jowar is gluten free, it is beneficial for their good health and wellbeing. Jowar is a high-end source of phosphorus, calcium, protein and fibre. The presence of iron and copper helps regulate proper blood circulation, which fuels cell growth, hair repair and enhances overall functioning of the body.

The rising incidence of Celiac disease has also led to new interest in this grain. Newer hybrid variety of this grain is being used to produce gluten free foods for such patients.

Sorghum does not contain gluten, which also happens to be the component responsible for the viscosity and elasticity of the dough. Thus, in the absence of gluten, when making food items from Sorghum flour, a batter of this flour is prepared. The batter of the flour goes into making bread, pizza base, pancakes and rotis.

Health food stores today stock the grain Sorghum as broken grain that can be made as porridges, either sweet or savoury, as one desires. The relatively bland flour made from Sorghum is also being added to other cereal flours to improve the overall nutritive value.

The superiority of this grain is not just from the point of view of well-being but also from the environmental perspective. The drought resistant nature of this grain along with its ability to produce a good yield with limited water supply is the need of the hour.

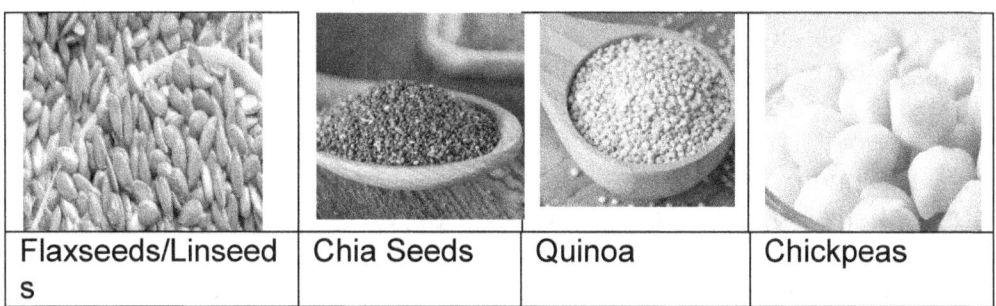

Flaxseeds/Linseeds	Chia Seeds	Quinoa	Chickpeas

17). Gram (Chana):

Kala Chana Beans are full of so much nutritious goodness that the U.S. Department of Agriculture considers them both a protein and a vegetable. Kala chana, also known as the dark chickpea, Bengal gram and is a savoury bean popular in India and very similar to the yellow chickpeas at your grocery store. Like other beans, kala chana is full of protein, fibre and iron, and makes a healthy and colourful addition to any meal.

Kala Chana Nutritional Facts: Kala chana is dark brown and smaller in size than the yellow chickpeas. One half cup of dried Kala chana has 360 calories, 5 grams of fat, 60 grams of carbs, 17 grams of fibre and 19 grams of protein. While these beans are high in protein, more than 60 percent of the calories come from carbs. It is a good source of energy for your body and brain. The amino acids in the beans contribute to making hormones, muscle and enzymes. Adults need 46 to 56 grams of protein a day, and half a cup of dried kala chana meets more than 30 percent of these needs.

Vitamins and Minerals in Kala Chana: Beans like kala chana are considered both protein and vegetable because they are a rich source of vitamins and minerals present in both food groups. These savory beans are rich in calcium and iron and can help you get more vitamin C in your diet. A half-cup serving of the uncooked bean meets 40 percent of the daily value for iron, 11 percent of the daily value for calcium and 7 percent of the daily value for vitamin C. Certain groups of people, mainly children and women, have a hard time getting enough iron and calcium in their diet, according to the Office of Dietary Supplements. Iron is essential for delivering oxygen to all the tissues in your body, and calcium is necessary for bone health. The vitamin C in the bean improves bioavailability of iron, which means it helps you absorb more.

Health Benefits of Kala Chana: People who eat more beans (Kala Chana) tend to live longer. This may be due to the fibre content in the bean, which has been shown to help improve blood sugar, prevent constipation and lower cholesterol, decreasing risk of chronic illnesses such as diabetes and heart disease. Making beans a regular part of your diet may also help with weight control, to lose more than half a pound over a six-week period.

Kala Chana Nutritional Facts: A cup of boiled kala chana contains 269 calories. It has 4 grams of total fat, with less than 1/2 gram of cholesterol-raising saturated fat. Beans are good plant-based sources of protein, and 1 cup of kala chana contains 15 grams of protein, or 30 percent of the daily value based on a 2,000-calorie diet. Each cup of cooked kala chana provides 45 grams of total carbohydrates, including 8 grams of natural sugars. Kala Chan is cholesterol-free.

Dietary Fibre: Kala chana is a good Source of Dietary Fibre. Each cup of kala chana provides 13 grams of dietary fibre. A high-fibre diet lowers your cholesterol levels and helps prevent constipation. Fibre helps regulate blood-sugar levels in individuals with diabetes. A 2,000-calorie diet should include at least 28 grams of fibre per day, but the average people consume only 12 to 18 grams of fibre per day. Kala chana and other types of beans, lentils, fruits, vegetables and whole grains are good sources of fibre.

Potassium and Sodium: Each cup of kala chana provides 477 milligrams of potassium, or 14 percent of the daily value, and 11 milligrams of sodium, or less than 1 percent of the daily value. Sodium causes your body to retain water and increases your blood pressure, while potassium helps reduce the effects of sodium, according to MayoClinic.com. A high-potassium, low-sodium diet helps prevent high blood pressure and an increased risk of stroke and kidney disease. A cup of kala chana boiled in salt water contains 399 milligrams of sodium.

Iron, Calcium and Foliate: A cup of boiled kala chana provides 4.7 milligrams of iron, or 28 percent of the daily value. Iron is a component of haemoglobin, which is the oxygen-carrying component of your red blood cells. Iron deficiency causes anaemia. Each cup of boiled kala chana provides 80 milligrams of calcium, or 8 percent of the daily value for this bone-strengthening mineral. Pregnant women need to have adequate stores of foliate for preventing neural tube birth defects, and a cup of boiled kala chana supplies 282 micrograms of foliate, or 71 percent of the daily value.

Kala Chana Uses: You can add boiled kala chana to salads to increase the protein and fibre content. Kala chana curry is a spicy Indian stew that uses kala chana, oil, turmeric and other spices, such as ginger, red chilli powder and coriander. You can limit the sodium in kala chana recipes by adding less salt for seasoning during cooking.

Kala Chana Sprouts: Calories in Chana Sprouts is 15Cal 100g or 37 Cal or 248g 1 bag. Chana sprouts are known as black gram sprouts or kala chana sprouts. Chana sprouts are a favourite topping on noodles dishes. utrition facts for Chana Sprouts (1 bag 248g): Nutrition info displayed such as percent meal value and PFC balance scales are based on a 1800 calorie diet for women between ages 18 and 29 years old weighing around 112 pounds and daily nutritional requirements.

Calories and Macronutrient Composition:

Energy	37 Cal	536~751Cal
Protein	4.96g (19.84 Cal)	15~34g
Fat	0g (0 Cal)	13~20g
Carbohydrate	6.7g (26.8 Cal)	75~105g

The calories in Chana Sprouts per 248g (1 bag) are 37 calories. Chana Sprouts is calculated to be 15Cal per 100 grams making 80Cal equivalent to 533.33g with 6.7g of mostly carbohydrates، 4.96g of protein، 0g of fat in 248g while being rich in vitamins and minerals such as Foliate and Vitamin C.

Vitamins, minerals, dietary fibre, and sodium content for 248g (1 bag) of Chana Sprouts Vitamin (Percent Meal Value):

Vitamin E	0.25mg	2.2mg
Vitamin K	7.44µg	17µg
Vitamin B1	0.1mg	0.32mg
Vitamin B2	0.15mg	0.36mg
Niacin	0.99mg	3.48mgNE
Vitamin B6	0.15mg	0.35mg
Foliate	104.16µg	80µg
Pantothenic Acid	0.84mg	1.5mg
Vitamin C	27.28mg	33mg
Sodium	14.88mg	~1000mg
Potassium	176.08mg	833mg

Calcium	37.2mg	221mg
Magnesium	27.28mg	91.8mg
Phosphorus	69.44mg	381mg
Iron	0.99mg	3.49mg
Zinc	0.99mg	3mg
Copper	0.17mg	0.24mg
Manganese	0.2mg	1.17mg
Total Dietary Fibre	3.47g	5.7g

Nutrition Information (Chana Dal (1/2 cup): Amounts per selected serving amounts per Custom Food (100g) %DV:

Protein	22.0g	44%
Vitamin A	100IU	2%
Calcium	20.0mg	2%
Iron	3.6mg	20%
Sodium	10.0mg	0%

Kala Chana	Jowar		

Lima Beans	Split Peas	Lentils (Teel)	Black Beans

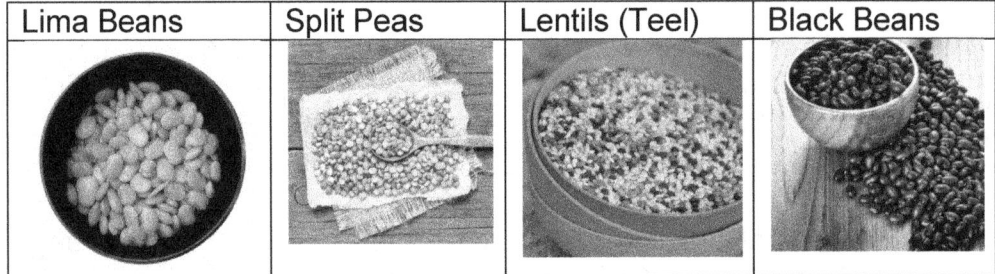

5.9   High Fibre Vegetables Diet:

Eat enough fibre-rich food like vegetables and drink adequate water, or exercise on a regular basis, keep yourself well hydrated with a good intake of water, fresh fruit juices, butter milk but avoid unhealthy artificial drinks and readymade juices or alcoholic and caffeinated beverages. Chew the food properly.

1. Acorn Squash: Total Dietary Fibre is 9 grams of fibre per cup (baked). Notable Nutrients are Vitamin C, Thiamine, Potassium, Manganese, Vitamin A, B6, Foliate, and Magnesium. Winter squash including pumpkins, butternut squash, spaghetti squash, and acorn

squashes are packed with nutrients, and fibre. The nutrient dense and brightly colour flesh is high in soluble fibre, which slows the rate at which food is digested, allowing for the absorption of nutrients. Acorn squash and other squash can be roasted in the oven and used as a substitute for white potatoes

2. Broccoli: Fibre is 5.1 grams per cup, boiled. This caveman-friendly dish is pretty simple. To make these fritters, just combine onion, garlic, broccoli, eggs, and almond meal. Once they hit the table, you'll be surprised how much broccoli gets finished in one sitting.

3. Brussels sprouts (Cabbage): Total Dietary Fibre is 7.6 grams of fibre per cup, near balance of soluble and insoluble fibre.

Notable Nutrients are Vitamins C, K, B1, B2, B6, Foliate, and Manganese. As one of the power-packed cruciferous vegetables, Brussels sprouts are one of the better high fibre foods. Rich with antioxidants and anti-inflammatory properties, Brussels sprouts support healthy detoxify, and may reduce the risk of some types of cancer. Add baked Brussels sprouts recipe to incorporate these nutrient dense vegetables into your diet.

4. Artichokes: Total Dietary Fibre is 10.3 grams of fibre per medium artichoke. Notable Nutrients are Vitamins A, C, E, B, K, Potassium, Calcium, Magnesium and Phosphorous. Low in calories, rich in fibre and essential nutrients, artichokes is a great addition to your diet. Just one medium artichoke accounts for nearly half of the recommend fibre intake for women and a third for men. In addition, artichokes are one of the top 10 high antioxidant foods.

5. Okra (Lady Finger): Total Dietary Fibre is 8.2 grams per cup. Notable Nutrients are Vitamins A, C, K, Riboflavin, Thiamine, Niacin, Calcium, Iron, Phosphorous, Zinc, and Protein. Just one cup provides for nearly a third of recommended daily fibre, and is one of the top calcium rich foods. It is packed with nutrients and is easily incorporated into soups and stews.

6. Turnips (Shalgam): Total Dietary Fibre is 4.8 grams of fibre per ½ cup. Notable Nutrients are Vitamin C, Calcium, Magnesium, and Potassium. In the U.S. turnips are underutilized. Packed with essential nutrients and a great source of fibre, turnips can be enjoyed raw, or cooked.

7. Spinach: Among the vegetables, spinach has been considered to be the most vital food for the entire digestive tract from time immemorial. Raw spinach contains the finest organic material for the cleansing, reconstruction, and regeneration of the intestinal tract. Raw spinach juice-100 ml, mixed with an equal quantity of water and taken

294

twice daily, will cure the most aggravated cases of constipation within a few days.

8. Leafy Greens (Spinach, Kale, Bok Choy and Arugula): Leafy greens are also great foods to eat while doing a colon detoxify. They are very high in dietary fibre, folic acid, calcium, vitamin k, vitamin c and magnesium, not to mention many other antioxidants, which are all essential nutrients for a healthy body. They also contain a high amount of chlorophyll, which has previously shown to be one of the best foods that detoxify the body. Spinach, Kale, Bok Choy and Arugula are just a few of the leafy greens you should add to your cleansing diet.

Acorn Squash	Spinach	Peas	Tomatoes

9. Tomatoes: Tomatoes are another food you can eat while doing a colon cleanses. There is an excellent source of Vitamin C, Vitamin A and Vitamin K, not to mention provide you with approximately 10% of your daily fibre needs. They are also very high in lycopene, an antioxidant that helps protect you from developing colon cancer and prostate cancer. Buy locally-grown, organic tomatoes, if possible.

10. Peas: Total Dietary Fibre: 8.6 grams per cooked cup; majority insoluble fibre. Notable Nutrients: Vitamin C, Vitamin K, B6, Thiamine, Manganese, Foliate, Vitamin A, Protein. The humble green pea is packed with fibre, and powerful antioxidants, anti-inflammatory properties and phytonutrients that support wellness. Frozen peas are available year round, making them ideal to incorporate into your diet. Lightly steam peas and add to soups, and salads. They add a gentle sweetness, while providing nearly 100% of your daily-recommended Vitamin C, and over 25% of Thiamine and Foliate.

11. Turnips: Total Dietary Fibre is 4.8 grams of fibre per ½ cup. Notable Nutrients are Vitamin C, Calcium, Magnesium and Potassium. Packed with essential nutrients and a great source of fibre, turnips can be enjoyed raw, or cooked. Try my Turnip Fries recipe; the taste and texture will delight you.

Cabbage	Turnips		
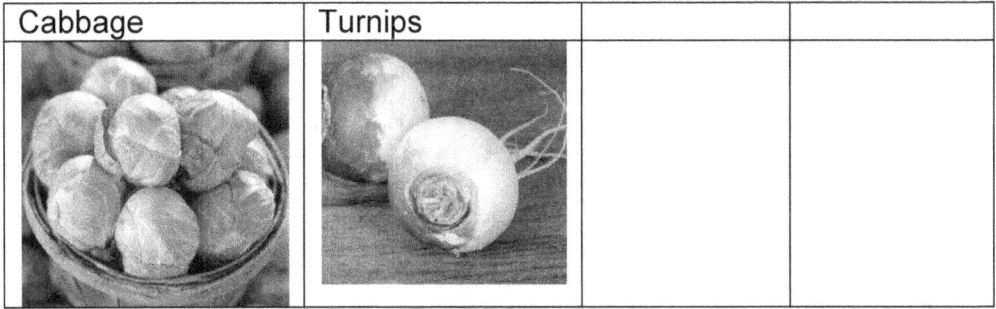			

5.10 Fresh Fruits Fibre Diet to prevent Constipation and Colon Cleanse

You can get the nutrient from fresh fruits and dry fruits like, Bale, Pear, Guava, Grapes, Prang, Papaya, Apple, Banana, Kiwi, Berries, Pears, Plums, Banana and apples, vegetables, nuts, and beans. Simplified, if you are eating a lot of live fibrous foods such as bananas, broccoli, apples, carrots, then is sure to drink lots of water. If you excessively consume fruits and vegetables high in fibre, and you are drinking liquid which dehydrate you further and it altogether lead to soft and easy to pass stools resulting in relieving constipation. Eating lots of organic, raw fruits and vegetables that are high in fibre are important for overall colon health, but especially important during cleanse. Here is a list of ten foods you can eat while doing a colon cleanses:

1. Constipation Treatment using Bale Fruit: Generally all fruits, except banana and jack fruit are beneficial in the treatment of constipation. Certain fruits are, however, more effective. Bale fruit is regarded as the best of all laxatives. It cleans and tones up the intestines. Its regular use for two or three months throws out even the old accumulated faecal matter. It should be preferably taken in its original form and before dinner. About sixty grams of the fruit are sufficient for an adult.

2. Constipation Treatment using Berries: Raspberry Total Dietary Fibre: 8 grams of fibre per cup
Raspberry Notable Nutrients: Vitamin A, Vitamin C, Vitamin E, Vitamin K, Foliate, Total Blackberry Dietary Fibre: 7.6 grams of fibre per cup. Blackberry Notable Nutrients: Vitamin C, Vitamin K, Omega 3 fatty acids, Potassium, Magnesium, Potassium, Manganese. Blackberries are high in Vitamin K that is associated with boosting

of bone density; while the raspberry's high manganese levels help to support healthy bones, skin, and blood sugar levels. All of these benefits, in addition to providing a great tasting way to add fibre to your diet. Try my easy Blackberry Sorbet recipe; frozen raspberries, or a combination of the two would work well too.

Bale	Pear	Guava	Grapes

3. Constipation Treatment using Guava: Guava is another effective remedy for constipation. When eaten with seeds, it provides roughage to the diet and helps in the normal evacuation of the bowels. One or two guavas should be taken every day.

4. Constipation Treatment using Grapes: Grapes have proved very beneficial in overcoming constipation. The combination of the properties of the cellulose, sugar, and organic acid in grapes make them a laxative food. Their field of action is not limited to clearing the bowels only. They also tone up the stomach and intestines and relieve the most chronic constipation. One should take at least 350 gm of this fruit daily to achieve the desired results.

5. Constipation Treatment using Orange: Oranges are known for their high in fibre, calcium, vitamin A and high concentration of Vitamin C. One orange will provide you with approximately 12-15% of your daily recommended fibre. It is recommended you eat the whole orange, as the juice doesn't contain the necessary fibre to assist a cleansing program. Orange is beneficial in the treatment of constipation. Taking one or two oranges at bedtime and again on rising in the morning is an excellent way of stimulating the bowels. The general stimulating influence of orange juice excites peristaltic activity and helps prevent the accumulation of food residue in the colon.

6. Constipation Treatment using Papaya: Other fruits specific for constipation are papaya and figs. Half a medium-sized papaya should be eaten at breakfast for it to act as a laxative.

7. Constipation Treatment using Apples: Apples are a great food to eat while doing a colon cleanse. Not only are they high in fibre, but they are also very low in calories and fat. One apple, with the skin still on it, will give you approximately 20-25% of your daily recommended fibre. They are a great food for anyone to eat, especially if they are trying to lose weight. Apples are usually high in pesticide residue, so be sure to buy organic, if possible. Drinking freshly-squeezed apple juice is another great addition to a cleansing diet, but stay away from juices that are high in sugar.

8. Constipation Treatment using Bananas: Bananas are another food that is great to consume, whether you're following a cleansing program or not. They are easy to carry around. Contain about 15-20% of your daily fibre needs. They are very high in potassium, which will help restore valuable electrolytes back to your intestinal tract. Bananas also contain a natural compound called fructo oligosaccharide, which can help encourage beneficial bacteria in your intestinal tract. Bananas provide constipation relief, as well as regulate healthy bowel movements. Other health sources state that bananas cause constipation. Final result tells us that Bananas both cause and relieve constipation. Obviously, this can be confusing. Whether you are suffering from constipation or not, bananas are great for the body. Let's start with several key nutritional facts about bananas.

- Very low in saturated fat, cholesterol and sodium
- A good source of dietary fiber. Bananas contain about 15-20% of your daily fiber needs.
- A good source of Vitamins C, A and B6
- Rich in dietary minerals, mainly in Potassium, Manganese, Calcium, Iron, Magnesium, and Phosphorus

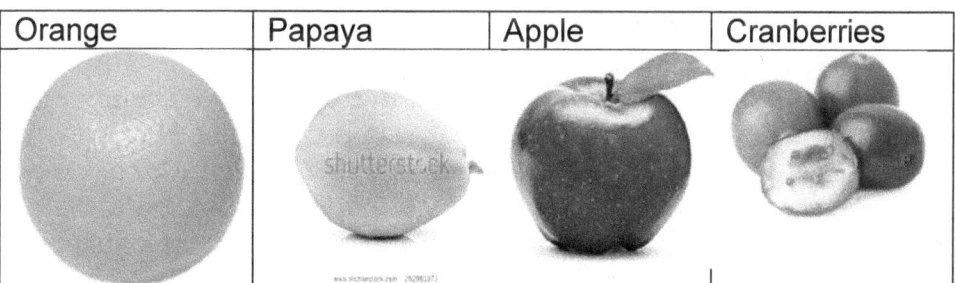

Orange	Papaya	Apple	Cranberries

Since bananas are high in potassium, eating a banana a day will help restore valuable electrolytes to your intestinal tract. Additionally, they contain a natural compound called fructooligosaccharide, which can help encourage beneficial bacteria in your intestinal tract.

Let's revert back to the nutritional facts section for bananas above, and concentrate on the minerals part of the banana. Bananas are rich in dietary minerals mainly in Potassium, Manganese, Calcium, Iron, Magnesium, and Phosphorus. Each of these minerals, when taken in appropriate portions, plays an important role in our overall health. Iron, is one of fifteen minerals essential to health, known for transporting oxygen. Iron deficiency can result in anaemia, which can produce symptoms such as depression, irritability, fatigue, loss of attention span, and insomnia. However, Iron taken excessively can be very harsh on the digestive tract and is known to cause constipation. Therefore, I recommend a safe level of daily iron to be in the 15-30mg range. 1 banana contains about .5mg of iron

Since bananas are rich in dietary fibre and other minerals, I recommend adding 2 organic bananas a day to your balanced diet 20 minutes before meals. A Banana a Day Helps Keep the Doctor Away.

The report that bananas helps provide constipation relief and regulate bowel movement are correct. The sources that state bananas cause constipation are somewhat correct, with an adjustment that eating bananas excessively without proper hydration can cause constipation for reasons explained above. In general, should you choose to eat more fibrous foods to help relieve and prevent constipation, whether bananas, apples, carrots, broccoli, raw nuts, etc., be conscious of consuming such foods in balanced proportions, and hydrate your body by increasing your water intake.

9. Constipation Treatment using Cranberries: Highly regarded for their ability to treat and prevent urinary tract infections, fresh cranberries are another food that helps promote optimal gastrointestinal health. They contain plenty of vitamin c, vitamin k and dietary fibre, but it's the natural robotic effect that makes them such a valuable colon cleansing food. Eat an abundance of fresh berries or drink cranberry juice while doing a colon cleanse.

10. Constipation Treatment using Asian Pears: Total Dietary Fibre is 9.9 grams of fibre per medium fruit, skin on. Notable Nutrients are Vitamin C, Vitamin K, Omega 6 fatty acids, Potassium. Crisp, sweet, and delicious, Asian Pears contain high levels of fibre, but also are rich in Omega-6 fatty acids (149 mg per serving) associated with healthy cells, brain and nerve function.

11. Constipation Treatment using Avocados: Avocados are one of the best foods you can add to your diet, whether you doing a colon cleanse or not. Avocados are packed with many nutrients, including vitamin k, potassium, foliate, and dietary fibre. In fact, one avocado will provide you will approximately 30% of your daily fibre needs. Total Dietary Fibre is 10.5 grams per cup (sliced). Notable Nutrients are Vitamin C, Vitamin E, Vitamin B6, Foliate, Vitamin K, and Potassium.

The fibre content of avocados varies depending on the type. There is a difference in fibre content and makeup between the between the bright green, smooth skinned avocados (Florida avocados) and the smaller darker and dimpled variety (California avocados). Florida avocados have significantly more insoluble fibre than California avocados. In addition to the fibre, avocados are packed with healthy fats that help to lower cholesterol and reduce the risk of heart disease. Start incorporating fresh avocado into your diet with some of these avocado recipes.

12. Constipation Treatment using Berries: Total Dietary Fibre in Raspberry is 8 grams of fibre per cup. Raspberry Notable Nutrients are Vitamin A, Vitamin C, Vitamin E, Vitamin K, and Foliate.

Avocados	Asian Pears	Berries	Coconut

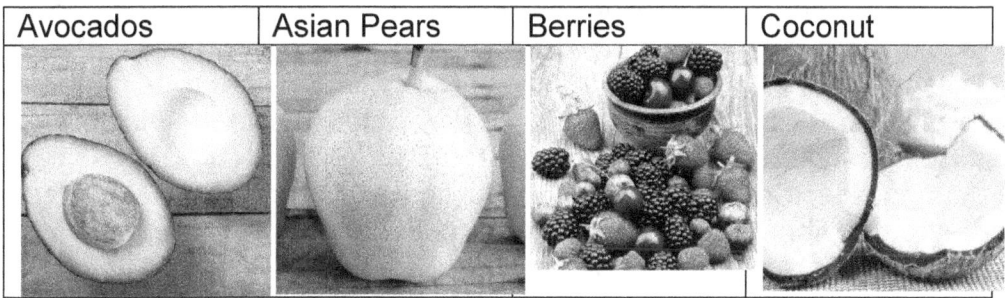

13. Constipation Treatment using Blackberries: Total Dietary Fibre in Blackberry is 7.6 grams of fibre per cup. Blackberry Notable Nutrients are Vitamin C, Vitamin K, Omega 6 fatty acids, Potassium, Magnesium, Potassium, and Manganese. Blackberries are high in Vitamin K that is associated with boosting of bone density; while the raspberry's high manganese levels help to support healthy bones, skin, and blood sugar levels. All of these benefits, in addition to providing a great tasting way to add fibre to your diet. Successfully mixing sweet and savoury isn't for the faint of heart, but the salad makes use of blackberries, lemon, scallions, and dill to great effect.

14. Constipation Treatment using Coconut: Total Dietary Fibre is 7.2 grams per cup. Notable Nutrients are Manganese, Omega-6 fatty acids, Foliate, and Selenium. Coconut products are growing in popularity, with good reason. Coconut has low glycemic index, and is easy to incorporate into your diet; with 4 to 6 times the amount of fibre as oat bran, coconut flour and grated coconut is a great way to add a healthy natural fibre to your diet. In countries where coconut is a dietary staple, there are fewer incidents of high cholesterol and heart disease. For most baking recipes, you can substitute up to 20% coconut flour for other flours.

15. Constipation Treatment using Raspberries: Fibre is 8 grams per cup, raw. Raspberries aren't a hard sell—they're basically nature's candy. With the help of coconut, oatmeal, and vanilla, they make a relatively healthy dessert that pleases any palate.

5.11 High Fibre Dry Fruits Diet to prevent Constipation:

1. Constipation Treatment using Almonds: Almonds Total Dietary Fibre is 0.6 grams of fibre per 6 almonds. Almond Notable Nutrients are Protein, Vitamin E, Manganese, Magnesium, Riboflavin, Omega-6 fatty acids, Riboflavin. Almonds are lower in calories and fats than walnuts, while higher in potassium and protein.

2. Constipation Treatment using Figs: Both fresh and dry figs have a laxative effect. Four or five dry figs should be soaked overnight in a little water and eaten in the morning. Total Dietary Fibre is 14.6 grams of fibre in 1 cup dried figs, evenly distributed between soluble and insoluble fibre. Notable Nutrients are Pantothenic acid, Potassium, Manganese, Copper, and B6. Dried figs and fresh figs are a great source of fibre. Unlike many other foods, figs have a near perfect balance of soluble and insoluble fibre. Figs are associated with lower blood pressure and protection against macular degeneration, in addition to the benefits of the fibre. Even if you don't like dried figs, fresh figs are delicious and can be enjoyed on top of cereals, salads, and even stuffed with goat cheese and honey for a special dessert.

3. Constipation Treatment using Walnut: Walnut Total Dietary Fibre is 1.9 grams of fibre per 1 ounce by weight. Walnut Notable Nutrients are Protein, Manganese, Copper, Omega-6 fatty acids, Omega-3 fatty acids, Foliate, Vitamin B6, and Phosphorus. Walnuts however have been shown to improve verbal reasoning, memory, and mood and are believed to support good neurologic function.

Figs	Prune	Walnuts	Raisins
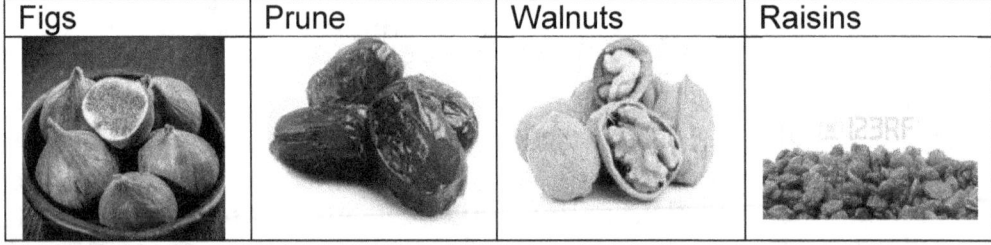			

4. Constipation Treatment using Prunes: Commonly considered "Nature's Laxative", prunes are another great addition to any colon cleansing diet. Prunes are packed with antioxidants, vitamin A, potassium and dietary fibre. Not only do prunes help provide the necessary fibre for a healthy colon, but they also improve your overall transit time and provide beneficial bacteria to the intestines.

5. Constipation Treatment using raw nuts (Almonds, Brazil nuts, Walnuts and hazelnuts): Raw nuts are a great way to get loads of energy during a colon cleanse. They are high in protein, minerals and monounsaturated fat, all of which will help keep our heart healthy and our cholesterol low. The best raw nuts to eat during a cleansing program include – almonds, Brazil nuts, cashews, pistachios, walnuts and hazelnuts.

6. Constipation Treatment using Raisins: Raisins, soaked in water, can be used. Raisins should be soaked for twenty-four to forty-eight hours. This will make them swell to the original size of the grapes. They should be eaten early in the morning, along with the water in which they have been soaked.

5.12 Other High Fibre diets to prevent Constipation

1. Constipation Treatment using Butter milk: A glass of hot water, with half a teaspoon of salt or Butter milk is also an effective remedy for constipation. Drinking water which has been kept overnight in a copper vessel, first thing in the morning, brings good results.

2. Constipation Treatment using Physical activity: Physical activity is known to help reduce the risk of constipation and yoga is particularly noteworthy as a physical fitness regime in this regard. Yoga comprises of a variety of postures and movements, many of which stimulate and encourage the bowel functions. Practicing yoga or walking can thereby enhance your digestive systems functioning and eliminate or at least reduce the occurrence of digestive disorders like constipation.

3. Constipation Treatment using pure olive Oil: Pure olive oil helps to relieve constipation. It stimulates your digestive system, which helps get things moving through your colon, and taken regularly it can prevent constipation as well. You will need - 1 tablespoon of olive oil and -1 teaspoon of lemon juice (optional). In the morning consume one tablespoon of olive oil. It works best on an empty stomach, so have it before you eat anything else. You can mix it with a little bit of lemon juice if you like to lighten the flavour (lemon juice also acts as a natural aid for constipation).

Olive is a natural stool softener, which helps in treating constipation. Constipation is a condition in which the frequency of the elimination of faeces is reduced to even lesser than thrice a week. The faeces are hard, difficult to eliminate and black in colour. Ideally, a person should have at least one or two bowel movements per day. Not eliminating the faeces on a daily basis, can lead to accumulation of wastes in the body. Accumulated wastes produces such toxins that can have harmful effects on the whole body system. There are many medicines that are available in the market to treat constipation, but majority of people prefer to treat it at home using various home remedies or alternative herbal medicines. The reason behind this is that long term usage of over-the-counter laxatives, can make the person dependent on them. In order to avoid this, people prefer home remedies such as olive oil to relieve constipation. Olive oil for constipation can be quite effective.

Benefits of Olive Oil for constipation: Olive oil is rich in iron, vitamin E, vitamin K, antioxidants, omega 3 and omega 6 essential fatty acids which improves the overall health of the body. It is very helpful in keeping the gastrointestinal tract in a healthy condition. It stimulates the gallbladder to release more bile juice which helps in the digestion of fat. Olive oil also protects the mucous lining of the colon which may get stressed during the excretion of hard stool. Following are some of the most important benefits of olive oil for constipation.

It softens the Faeces: The faeces become very hard in constipation. The person is not able to eliminate them easily. Regularly taking olive oil propels muscle contractions in the intestines, thereby stimulating the bile flow and thus, softening the faeces in the process. Soft faces, unlike the hard ones are easily eliminated and hence, constipation is cured.

It reduces Intestinal Dilation: Olive oil is extremely effective for constipation, particularly in babies. It is often seen that babies are not able to eliminate faces easily, resulting in accumulation of stools in the intestines. When this happens, the intestines dilate, causing stomach pain in the babies. Due to this pain, babies hold back faeces to avoid the pain. Regularly, massaging olive oil on the baby's stomach helps in relieving his pain and thus, he is able to eliminate stool.

There are no Side-effects: Olive oil does not have any side-effects. Long term usage of medicines can aggravate constipation, but olive oil is natural oil which is extracted from the fruits of the olive tree, hence, even if it is not able to cure severe cases of constipation, it will not aggravate the situation.

Method to use Olive Oil:

When you wake up in the morning, take one tablespoon of pure, extra-virgin, high quality, raw olive oil. You can continue this for a few days. If you still feel constipated, you may start taking one tablespoon of olive oil, in the evening, one hour before dinner.

Another way to take olive oil is to eat it with some fibre rich fruit such as orange, apple, etc. Take one tablespoon of olive oil in the morning, followed by an orange or whatever fibrous fruit you have. Repeat the same in the evening with perhaps a fibre rich vegetable, such as, a broccoli.

Use olive oil in salad. Mix olive oil with fresh lemon and use it in place of other sauces. This will not only help you in constipation but will also give your body a healthy treat.

You can prepare a cocktail of olive oil and orange juice. Mix a tablespoon of olive oil in a glass of orange juice and have it every morning on empty stomach. This will lubricate your digestive system and will relieve constipation.

Olive oil can be used to relieve mild cases of constipation. But if prolonged use of olive oil is still unable to give you relief from constipation, then consult a doctor for further treatment, as constipation can also be a result of serious conditions like colour cancer, lupus, etc. Hence it is always better to consult a doctor in the initial stage itself.

Olive oil alone cannot treat constipation. It has to be complemented with a lot of other lifestyle changes such as a high fibre diet, lots of fluid, regular exercising, etc. Hence it is very important to take care of things which may contribute to constipation.

4. Constipation Treatment using fresh lemon Juice: The citric acid in lemon juice acts as a stimulant for your digestive system, and can also help flush out toxins and undigested material that may have built up along the walls of the colon. Mixing the juice with water not only lessens the intensity of the lemon flavour, but helps get you the fluids you need to get everything moving normally again. You will need - 1 fresh lemon and -1 cup of warm water. Squeeze the juice of 1 lemon into 1 cup of warm water. Drink or sip until finished completely.

5. Constipation Treatment using Molasses: Blackstrap molasses has been a sweet saviour for more than a few sufferers of constipation, be it chronic or occasional. The reason blackstrap molasses works so well is because of how it is made. Regular molasses is essentially pure cane sugar juice boiled to concentrate and crystallize the sugar. The boiling results in blackstrap molasses, which is crystallized but contains significant amounts of vitamins and minerals, specifically magnesium, which is what helps the constipation. You will need -1 teaspoon of blackstrap molasses and - warm water. Consume one teaspoon of blackstrap molasses and add it to a cup of warm water to dilute the taste. If you find that a teaspoon has not been effective, you can go as high as 1-2 tablespoons, but try less at first.

6. Constipation Treatment using Walking/Exercises: If you want stuff to move through your body, you need to move too. Our lifestyle these days not only involves dietary changes that increase constipation, but we're often sitting much more than we're active. The scientific reason is that lack of exercise is linked with getting clogged up, and so moving the body helps get the smooth muscle in the colon moving as well. Keep in mind, however, that you should wait an hour after big meals before exercising. There are also specific stretches and workouts that are supposed to help with getting good old stool out the door.

7. Constipation Treatment using Flaxseed oil: Flaxseed oil is a pretty simple home remedy for constipation. It sort of coats the walls of the intestine, as well as stool, and increases the number of bowel movements you are having. Enjoying your oil with orange juice is a double whammy when it comes to constipation, since oranges have a good amount of fibre in them (make sure to get orange juice with pulp, which is what has most of the fibre). You will need -1 glass of orange juice with pulp (8 oz.) and -1 tablespoon of flaxseed oil.

Mix 1 tablespoon of flaxseed oil with 1 glass of orange juice. Drink as needed, but give it time (up to 5 hours) to start working so you don't overdo it.

8. Constipation Treatment using Pure Aloe Vera gel from the plant: Aloe Vera gel is known to soothe minor cuts and burns, but it can also soothe your tummy. It's best to use pure Aloe Vera Gel from the plant. The gel straight from the plant is more concentrated than commercial aloe juice so don't use more than 2 tablespoons. If you don't have an aloe plant, than drinking aloe juice can accomplish similar results. You will need -2 tablespoons of pure aloe gel or 1 cup of aloe Vera juice and – 1 fruit juice or -1 cup warm water and drink in the morning.

9. Constipation Treatment using routine of Bath Room: Maintain a Potty schedules, they're a great way to relieve and prevent constipation in humans too. Regulating the timing of when you go to the bathroom will regulate your bowel movements as well. Set aside about 15 minutes anywhere from 1-3 times a day, and take your time, even if nothing happens. Make sure you stay relaxed, and eventually your body will catch on.

10. Constipation Treatment using Baking Soda: Baking soda lies at the heart of home remedies. It's is so incredibly versatile, and it pretty much does its job 95% of the time. It works incredibly well for constipation (and tummy aches in general) because it is a bicarbonate, which will encourage air to come out of you one way or another, and relieve pain from pressure. It also re-alkalizes the stomach, neutralizing the acid a little bit and helping things pass through your gut. You will need -1 teaspoon baking soda and -1/4 cup warm water. Mix a teaspoon of baking soda with ¼ cup of warm water. Drink all of the mixture-the quicker you finish it, the better it seems to work.

11. Constipation Treatment using virgin & natural Coconut oil: Eating coconut oil is the best natural laxative that helps to relieve difficulty in constipation, pooping or infrequent bowel movements. Some people mistakenly thought that coconut oil causes constipation. It actually cures constipation instead. Coconut oil contains medium-chain fatty acids (MCFAs), which is the secret for constipation relief. That's because MCFAs provide quick energy for your intestinal cells that boost their metabolism and hence, stimulate your bowel movements. MCFAs help to soften your stool too. Not only acute sufferers get to effectively relieve their constipation, chronic sufferers find eating coconut oil good for their chronic condition too. However, you have to be cautious about its dosage because suddenly taking too much dose can over loosen your bowels and cause the reverse diarrhoea-like symptoms. To make matters worse, there's no best dosage for different individuals. Some people after taking 1 teaspoon already can feel the bowel-loosening effect while others require at least 2 tablespoons daily. That said, how much you need for treating constipation depends on how your body reacts to the MCFAs in coconut oil and how serious your constipation is. If this is the first time you use coconut oil for constipation treatment, I suggest that you take 1/2 tablespoon in the morning and 1/2 tablespoon at dinner (simply add to your meals) and see how it goes. For first-timer, you should never consume more than 2 tablespoons per day for fear it might give you the runs. If you're a chronic case, you might want to start with 1 tablespoon of coconut oil and add it into your breakfast plus 1/2 tablespoon at dinner time. If you don't feel much impact, then increase to 1 tablespoon in morning and 1 tablespoon at night the following day. Gradually up your intake until you find the best dose for relieving your constipation problem. Virgin coconut oil Recognition:

Virgin coconut oil should possess a natural coconut scent in itself. It could be subtly mild or strong, depending on its country of origin and how it is being extracted etc. But if it smells or tastes like pork lard, cheese or it simply stinks, you might be getting a rancid virgin coconut oil. If it tastes or smells smoky or appears yellowish (or brownish), it is a refined coconut oil in disguise. So, beware.

5.13 Bulk-forming laxatives Diet to prevent Constipation

Sometimes these are known as fibre supplements. These increase the bulk of your stools in a similar way to fibre. They can have some effect within 12-24 hours but their full effect may take several days to develop. There are four main groups of Laxatives that work in different ways:

- Bulk-forming laxatives.
- Stimulant laxatives.
- Osmotic laxatives.
- Faecal softener laxatives.

Bulk-forming laxatives include Bran, ispaghula (psyllium), methylcellulose, sterculia, wheat dextrin, inulin fibre and whole linseeds (soaked in water).

Table: Different types of Fibre and their Health Benefits

Types of Fibre	Soluble or Insoluble	Sources	Health Benefits
Wheat bran	insoluble	It is natural farm product of whole wheat. Bran is the hard outer shell of the wheat plant	It is "Nature's laxative" and reduces constipation. It aids digestion, adds bulk to stools and prevents constipation.
Oat bran	insoluble	Oat bran is the outer layer of the oat grain, just beneath the inedible husk. While it is part of oat grouts and steel-cut oats and found at health food stores.	Oat bran is "Nature's laxative" and is high in fibres and contains a good amount of vitamins B2, E, Magnesium, Potassium, iron, zinc, pantothenic acid and

		Oats bran helps to lower cholesterol, regulate digestive system.	copper and contains of protein and fibres.
Rice bran	insoluble	Rice is a plant. The outer layer of the grain rice is called Rice bran and contains various antioxidants, oil, vitamin E, gamma-oryzano, beta-sitosterol; high fibres, and ferulic acid.	It is "Nature's laxative", reduces constipation, and contains over 100 known vitamins, minerals and antioxidants, including gamma oryzanol,
Cellulose, some hemicelluloses	Insoluble	Naturally found in nuts, whole wheat, whole grains, bran, seeds, edible brown rice, and skins of produce.	"Nature's laxative": Reduces constipation, lowers risk of diverticulitis, can help with weight loss.
Inulin oligofructose	Soluble	Naturally found in onions and by-products of sugar production from beets or chicory root. Add to foods to boost fibre.	May increase "good" bacteria in the gut and enhance immune function.
Lignin	Insoluble	Found naturally in flax seed, rye, some vegetables.	Good for heart health and possibly immune function. Use caution if you have celiac disease or are gluten intolerant.
Mucilage, beta-glucans	Soluble	Naturally found in oats, oat bran, beans, peas, barley, flaxseed, berries, soybeans, bananas,	Helps lower bad LDL cholesterol, reduces risk of coronary heart disease and type 2 diabetes. Use caution

		oranges, apples, carrots.	if you have celiac disease or are gluten intolerant.
Pectin and gums	Soluble (some pectin can be insoluble)	Naturally found in fruits, berries, and seeds, citrus peel and other plants boost fibre in adding in foods.	Slows the passage of food through the intestinal GI tract, helps lower blood cholesterol.
Polydextr ose polyols	Soluble	Added to processed foods as a bulking agent and sugar substitute. Made from dextrose, sorbitol, and citric acid.	Adds bulk to stools, helps prevent constipation. May cause bloating or gas.
Psyllium	Soluble	Extracted from crushed seeds or husks of plantago ovata plant. Used in supplements, fibre drinks, and added to foods.	Helps lower cholesterol and prevent constipation.
Resistant starch	Soluble	Starch in plant cell walls naturally found in un-ripened bananas, oatmeal, and legumes. Also extracted and added to processed foods to boost fibre.	May help manage weight by increasing fullness; helps control blood sugars. It increases insulin sensitivity and reduces the risk of diabetes.
Wheat dextrin	Soluble	Extracted from wheat starch, and widely used to add fibre in processed foods.	Helps lower cholesterol (LDL and total cholesterol), reduces risks of coronary heart disease and type 2 diabetes. May lower blood sugar and reduce risk for heart disease; more research is

			needed. Avoid if you have celiac disease or are gluten intolerant.

1). Wheat Bran:

It is natural farm product. Unprocessed bran is a cheap fibre supplement. If you take bran, it is best to build up the amount gradually. Start with two teaspoons a day and double the amount every five days until you reach about 1-3 tablespoons per day. You can sprinkle bran on breakfast cereals, or mix it with fruit juices, milk, stews, soups, crumbles, pastries, scones, etc.

Bran is the hard outer shell of the wheat plant. As the insoluble wheat bran passes through your system, it aids digestion, adds bulk to stools and prevents constipation. To benefit from the nutrition and fibre provided by wheat bran, food products should be made from 100 percent whole-wheat flour because the process that produces white flour removes the bran. According to University of Michigan Integrative Medicine, wheat bran loses vitamins and fibre during processing. Wheat bran can be purchased in bulk but must be kept cool as it can quickly turn rancid.

Wheat bran is well known for providing a significant source of dietary fibre, but it is also a great source of minerals and some vitamins. Harvard University's "Nutrition Source" indicates that a high intake of cereal fibre and whole grains such as wheat bran is linked to a reduced risk of heart disease and metabolic syndrome.

Basic Nutrition: This food is low in Saturated Fat, and very low in Cholesterol and Sodium. It is also a good source of Protein, Thiamine, Riboflavin and Potassium, and a very good source of Dietary Fibre, Niacin, Vitamin B6, Iron, Magnesium, Phosphorus, Zinc, Copper, Manganese and Selenium.

Table: Nutrition (Amounts per 1 cup (58g) %DV:

Calorie	125; (523 kJ) 6%	
From Carbohydrate	88.2 (369 kJ)	
From Fat	20.6 (86.2 kJ)	
From Protein	16.4 (68.7 kJ)	
From Alcohol	0.0 (0.0 kJ)	

Total Calories	125; (523 kJ)	6% DV
Total Carbohydrate	37.4g	12%

Dietary Fibre	24.8g	99%
Sugars	0.2g	
Fats & Fatty Acids:		
Total Fat	2.5g	4%
Saturated Fat	0.4g	2%
Monounsaturated Fat	0.4g	
Polyunsaturated Fat	1.3g	
Total Omega-3 fatty acids	96.9mg	
Total Omega-6 fatty acids	1183mg	
Protein & Amino Acids:		
Protein	9.0g	18%
Vitamins:		
Vitamin A	5.2IU	
Vitamin C	0.0mg	
Vitamin E	0.9mg	4%
Vitamin K	1.1mcg	1%
Thiamine	0.3mg	20%
Riboflavin	0.3mg	20%
Niacin	7.9mg	39%
Vitamin B6	0.8mg	38%
Foliate	45.8mcg	11%
Vitamin B12	0.0mcg	0%
Pantothenic Acid	1.3mg	13%
Choline	43.1mg	
Minerals:		
Calcium	42.3mg	4%
Iron	6.1mg	34%
Magnesium	354mg	89%
Phosphorus	588mg	59%
Potassium	686mg	20%
Sodium	1.2mg	0%
Zinc	4.2mg	28%
Copper	0.6mg	29%
Manganese	6.7mg	333%
Selenium	45.0mcg	64%
Sterols:		
Cholesterol	0.0mg	0%
Alcohol	0.0g	0%
Water	5.7g	
Ash	3.4g	

Percent Daily Values (%DV) are for adults or children aged 4 or older, and are based on a 2,000 calorie reference diet. Your daily values may be higher or lower based on your individual needs.

2). Oat Bran:

If you are concerned about your cholesterol, heart disease or other chronic disease, consider adding oat bran to your diet. Oat bran is a high-fibre food that can lower your cholesterol and provide a number of other health benefits. To get the most health benefits from oat bran, make it a part of your daily diet.

Cholesterol: One major benefit of oat bran is its ability to lower cholesterol. Beta-glucan, the main soluble fibre in oat bran was shown to significantly lower total cholesterol and LDL or "bad" cholesterol. The fibre in oat bran binds with cholesterol-rich bile to increase the amount of cholesterol that is excreted. Oat bran also helps to reduce the amount of cholesterol absorbed from the foods you eat. Reducing cholesterol can help to prevent the build-up of dangerous plaque in your arteries.

Cardiovascular Disease

A second benefit of oat bran is the prevention of cardiovascular disease. In a study of patients with an increased risk for coronary heart disease, Berg et al found that oat bran reduced total and low-density lipoprotein cholesterol. High levels of cholesterol can result in plaque build-up in your arteries and lead to high blood pressure and heart disease, which may result in a heart attack or stroke. Oat bran has been shown to lower these risks.

Diabetes: A third benefit of oat bran is its ability to produce long-term improvements in your blood sugar following a meal, as demonstrated in a study reported in the "Journal of the American Dietetic Association." Oat bran helps to keep blood sugar levels from getting too high after a meal by slowing down the digestion of carbohydrates and reducing the rate at which sugar enters your bloodstream. It may also improve blood sugar levels by increasing sensitivity to insulin, which helps to clear sugar from the blood.

Weight Loss: If you are trying to lose weight, eating oat bran might help. According nutrition expert at the University of Minnesota, fibre may help to promote weight loss by absorbing water as food passes through the gut, causing an increase in bulk and creating a sense of fullness. Fibre also delays digestion and absorption of food, thus delaying hunger. As a result, you may consume fewer calories, which could aid in weight loss.

Constipation: The fibre in oat bran can keep you from becoming constipated by increasing the bulk of your stool and helping to keep it soft. In a Canadian study, researchers found that adding oat bran biscuits to the daily diet of patients produced a marked improvement in bowel frequency and consistency. You can become constipated if your diet is lacking in fibre. Not drinking enough fluid on a high-fibre diet could also lead to constipation. On the other hand, adding oat bran to meals and snacks and drinking lots of fluids can help to prevent constipation by keeping your stool soft and easy to move.

Difference between Oat Bran & Whole Grain Oats

Oats: Oats are one of the most popular grains worldwide. They're nutritious, provide numerous health benefits and are a versatile cooking ingredient. Oat bran and whole grain oats both begin as oat groats; the product that results after oat grain is cleaned, toasted and hulled. Bran and whole oats contain much of the nutrition as the original oat groat, but they are processed in different ways. Oatmeal, or rolled oats, are processed further, losing some of the nutrition whole oats contain.

Whole Grain Oats

The whole grain of the oat is often referred to as Scotch, Irish or steel-cut oats. These result when oat groats are cut by steel blades into small, light-brown pieces. The oats take about the same time to cook as oat grouts, anywhere from 45 minutes to one hour. Many people soak the oats overnight to speed up cooking in the morning. These whole-grain oats include the oat bran.

Oat Bran: Oat bran is the outer layer of the oat grain, just beneath the inedible husk. While it is part of oat grouts and steel-cut oats, you'll also find it sold separately at health food stores or in the bulk foods section of your local grocery. Use oat bran in the same way you would wheat germ, the outer layer of the wheat grain, by sprinkling it over your cereal or in soups and stews.

Nutrition: Both oat bran and whole oats are high in vitamin B1 and contain a good amount of vitamins B2 and E. Both varieties of oats also are a good source of magnesium and also contain potassium, iron, zinc, pantothenic acid and copper. They are low in fat and contain no cholesterol. Oat bran contains about 5.4 grams of protein in a 1 ounce serving, while whole grain oats contain 4 grams of protein.

Fibre: The large amount of insoluble fibre in oats helps to lower your cholesterol and regulate your digestive system. Both types of oats contain lots of fibre, with 6 grams for whole grain oats and 4.9 grams

313

in a third-cup serving for oat bran. On the other hand, highly processed oat cereals, while still a healthy breakfast choice, contain 1.2 grams of fibre in a third-cup serving.

3). Rice Bran:

Rice is a plant. The outer layer of the grain is called bran and the oil made from the bran is used for medicine. Rice bran oil is popular as "healthy oil" in Japan, Asia, and particularly India. Be careful not to confuse rice bran with other forms of bran such as oat and wheat bran.

Rice bran is used for treating diabetes, high blood pressure, high cholesterol, alcoholism, obesity, and AIDS; for preventing stomach and colon cancer; for preventing heart and blood vessel (cardiovascular) disease; for strengthening the immune system; for increasing energy and improving athletic performance; for improving liver function; and as an antioxidant. Rice bran oil is also used for high cholesterol. Some people apply rice bran directly to the skin for an allergic skin rash called eczema (ectopic dermatitis).

Rice bran might help lower cholesterol because the oil it contains has substances that might decrease cholesterol absorption and increase cholesterol elimination. One of the substances in rice bran might decrease calcium absorption; this might help reduce the formation of certain types of kidney stones.

Bran, also known as miller's bran, is the hard outer layers of cereal grain. It consists of the combined aleurone and pericarp.

Along with germ, it is an integral part of whole grains, and is often produced as a by-product of milling in the production of refined grains. When bran is removed from grains, the grains lose a portion of their nutritional value. Bran is present in and may be in any cereal grain, including rice, corn (maize), wheat, oats, barley, rye and millet. Bran is not the same as chaff, coarser scaly material surrounding the grain but not forming part of the grain itself.

Bran is particularly rich in dietary fibre and essential fatty acids and contains significant quantities of starch, protein, vitamins, and dietary minerals. It is also a source of phytic acid, an antinutrient that prevents nutrient absorption.

The high oil content of bran makes it subject to rancidification, one of the reasons that it is often separated from the grain before storage or further processing. Bran is often heat-treated to increase its longevity.

Rice bran is a by-product of the rice milling process (the conversion of brown rice to white rice), and it contains various antioxidants that impart beneficial effects on human health.

Table: Nutrition Composition

Nutrients (%)	Wheat	Rye	Oat	Rice	Barley
Carbohydrates w/o starch	45–50	50–70	16–34	18–23	70–80
starch	13–18	12–15	18–45	18–30	8–11
proteins	15–18	8–9	13–20	15–18	11–15
fats	4–5	4–5	6–11	18–23	1–2

A major rice bran fraction contains 12%-13% oil and highly unsaponifiable components (4.3%). This fraction contains tocotrienols (a form of vitamin E), gamma-oryzanol and beta-sitosterol; all these constituents may contribute to the lowering of the plasma levels of the various parameters of the lipid profile. Rice bran also contains a high level of dietary fibres (beta-glucan, pectin and gum). In addition, it also contains ferulic acid, which is also a component of the structure of nonlignified cell walls. However, some research suggests there are levels of inorganic arsenic (a toxin and carcinogen) present in rice bran. One study found the levels to be 20% higher than in drinking water. Other types of bran (derived from wheat, oat or barley) contain less arsenic than rice bran, and are just as nutrient-rich.

Uses: Bran is often used to enrich breads (notably muffins) and breakfast cereals, especially for the benefit of those wishing to increase their intake of dietary fibre.

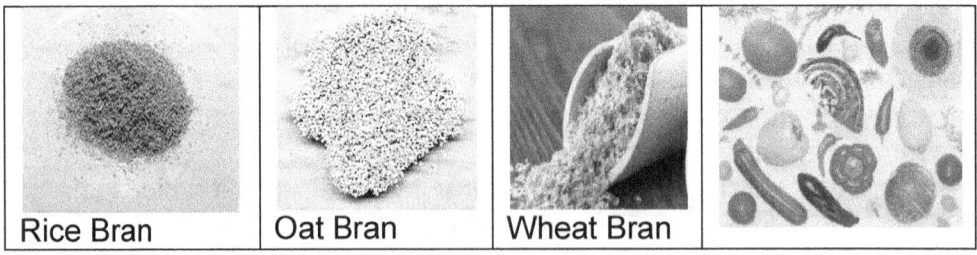

Rice Bran | Oat Bran | Wheat Bran

Rice Bran may also be used for pickling (nukazuke) as in the tsukemono of Japan. Bran is also used in preparing bors soup.

Table: Rice Bran Nutrition Value (Amounts per 1 cup - 118g)

Calorie Information:	Vitamins:
Calories-373 (1562 kJ) 19%	Vitamin E-5.8mg 29%
From: Carbohydrate- 138 (578 kJ)	Vitamin K-2.2mcg 3%
	Thiamin3.2mg 217%
From Fat-206 (862 kJ)	Riboflavin-0.3mg 20%
From Protein-28.7 (120 kJ)	Niacin-40.1mg 201%
From Alcohol-0.0 (0.0 kJ)	Vitamin B6-4.8mg 240%
Carbohydrates:	Folate-74.3mcg19%
Total Carbohydrate-58.6g 20%	Vitamin B12-0.0mcg 0%
Dietary Fibre- 24.8g 99%	Pantothenic Acid-8.7mg 87%
Starch- ~	Choline-38.0mg
Sugars- 1.1g	Minerals:
Fats & Fatty Acids:	Calcium-67.3mg 7%
Total Fat- 24.6g 38%	Iron-21.9mg 122%
Saturated Fat- 4.9g 25%	Magnesium-922mg 230%
Monounsaturated Fat- 8.9g	Phosphorus-1979mg 198%
Polyunsaturated Fat-8.8g	Potassium-1753mg 50%
Total Omega-3 fatty acids-373mg	Sodium-5.9mg 0%
	Zinc-7.1mg 48%
Total Omega-6 fatty acids-8428mg	Copper-0.9mg 43%
	Manganese-16.8mg 838%
Protein & Amino Acids:	Selenium-18.4mcg 26%
Protein-15.8g 32%	
Vitamins:	
Vitamin A-0.0IU 0%	
Vitamin C-0.0mg 0%	

Rice bran in particular finds many uses in Japan, where it is known as nuka. Besides using it for pickling, Japanese people also add it to the water when boiling bamboo shoots. In Kitakyushu City, it is called jinda and used for stewing fish, such as sardine. Rice bran and rice bran oil are also widely used in Japan as a natural beauty treatment. The high levels of oleic acid makes it particularly well absorbed by human skin, and it contains over 100 known vitamins, minerals and antioxidants, including gamma oryzanol, which is believed to impact pigment development.

In Myanmar, rice bran, called phwei-bya, is mixed with ash and used as a traditional detergent for washing dishes. Rice bran is also stuck to commercial ice blocks to hinder them from melting. It is also burned for fuel for rice mills in the rice growing regions of the Irrawaddy delta. Bran oil may be also extracted for use by itself for industrial purposes (such as in the paint industry), or as a cooking oil, such as rice bran oil. Japan has considered rice bran to a valuable resource since ages and extracted oil out of it and it is popularly known as heart oil. Also it is emerging as popular cooking oil in Asian countries, especially for shallow and deep frying application.

4). Ispaghula (Psyllium) Benefits and Nutrition Facts:

Psyllium is the common name used for several members of the plant genus Plantago whose seeds are used commercially for the production of mucilage. Psyllium is mainly used as a dietary fibre to relieve symptoms of both constipation and mild diarrhoea and occasionally as a food thickener. Research has also shown benefits in reducing cholesterol levels. The plant from which the seeds are extracted tolerates dry and cool climates and is mainly cultivated in northern India.

Psyllium is mainly used as a dietary fibre, which is not absorbed by the small intestine. The purely mechanical action of psyllium mucilage is to absorb excess water while stimulating normal bowel elimination. Although its main use has been as a bulk laxative, it is more appropriately termed a true dietary fibre and as such can help reduce the symptoms of both constipation and mild diarrhoea. The laxative properties of psyllium are attributed to the fibre absorbing water and subsequently softening the stool. It is also one of the few laxatives that do not promote flatulence.

Adverse effects: Since psyllium husk-containing products are sometimes used as a source of dietary fibre, the intake of dietary fibre could hinder the absorption of vitamins, minerals, and proteins. Psyllium fibre has been shown in studies to lower blood cholesterol and glucose levels while another common fibre, methylcellulose, has not shown these benefits. Gas or stomach cramping may also occur. It is recommended that this product be taken with a full glass of water to avoid it swelling in the throat and causing choking. Serious allergic reaction to this drug is rare. However, seek medical attention if any signs of anaphylaxis arise, such as a rash, itching/swelling, dizziness or difficulty breathing.

Choking is a hazard if psyllium is taken without adequate water as it thickens in the throat. Cases of allergic reaction to psyllium-containing cereal have also been documented.

The soluble fibre in psyllium is arabinoxylan, hemicelluloses. Psyllium is produced mainly for its mucilage content. The term mucilage describes a group of clear, colourless, gelling agents derived from plants. The mucilage obtained from psyllium comes from the seed coat. Mucilage is obtained by mechanical milling (i.e. grinding) of the outer layer of the seed. Mucilage yield amounts to about 25% (by weight) of the total seed yield. Plantago-seed mucilage is often referred to as husk, or psyllium husk. The milled seed mucilage is a white fibrous material that is hydrophilic, meaning that its molecular structure causes it to attract and bind to water. Upon absorbing water, the clear, colourless, mucilaginous gel that forms increases in volume by tenfold or more.

Fibrous secondary roots: A large number of flowering shoots arise from the base of the plant. Flowers are numerous, small, and white. Plants flower about 60 days after planting. The seeds are enclosed in capsules that open at maturity.

The fields are generally irrigated prior to seeding to achieve ideal soil moisture, to enhance seed soil contact, and to avoid burying the seed too deeply as a result of later irrigations or rainfall. Maximum germination occurs at a seeding depth of 6 mm (1/4 in). Emerging seedlings are frost sensitive; therefore, planting should be delayed until conditions are expected to remain frost free. Seed is broadcast at 5.5 to 8.25 kg/hectare (5 to 7.5 lb/acre) in India. In Arizona trials, seeding rates of 22 to 27.5 kg/ha (20 to 25 lb/acre) resulted in stands of 1 plant/25mm (1 inch) in 15 cm (6 inch) rows produced excellent yields. Weed control is normally achieved by one or two hand weeding early in the growing season. Control of weeds by pre-plant irrigation that germinates weed seeds followed by shallow tillage may be effective on fields with minimal weed pressure.

P. ovate has small seeds; 1,000 seeds weigh less than 2 grams. Under ideal conditions of adequate moisture and low temperature 10 to 20 °C (50 to 68 °F), 30% of seeds germinate in 5 to 8 days. The seed shows some innate dormancy (3 months) following harvest. Attempts to eliminate this dormancy period by scarification, or by exposure to wet or dry heat, cold, ethylene, or carbon dioxide, are ineffective. Post-dormancy seeds show reliable germination in excess of 90% at 29 °C (84 °F), with lower rates of germination as temperature is increased.

The use of psyllium husk as a normalizing agent for bowel function was discovered by Melvin A. Barbera.

Psyllium is a form of fibre made from the husks of the Plantago ovata plant's seeds. It sometimes goes by the name ispaghula.

It's most commonly known as a laxative. However, research shows that taking psyllium is beneficial to many parts of the human body, including the heart and the pancreas.

Psyllium is a bulk-forming laxative. This means it soaks up water in your gut and makes bowel movements much easier. It also helps promote regularity without increasing flatulence. It can be used as a one-off to ease constipation, or it can be added to your diet to help promote regularity and overall digestive health.

People with irritable bowel syndrome and Crohn's disease are all too familiar with the banes of the bathroom. The results of studies on psyllium's effectiveness in treating these conditions are still mixed.

Besides keeping your bowel movements regular and managing a chronic condition, psyllium has the ability to soften your stool. This can come in handy with short-term ailments, such as constipation. Used in this way, it can prevent complications of constipation, such as haemorrhoids and anal fissures.

Preliminary research shows that psyllium may help the painful symptoms associated with these conditions. Since there is no real scientific consensus, talk to your doctor to see if psyllium could help you.

Heart health: Research has shown that taking soluble fibre can help people manage their cholesterol levels. Proper cholesterol regulation is important for everyone, but vital for people over the age of 50. One study shows that at least 6 weeks of daily psyllium intake is an effective way for people who are obese or overweight to lower their cholesterol with very few side effects.

If you've been told that you need to watch your cholesterol, ask your doctor if adding psyllium to a low-fat, low-cholesterol diet will help you.

High cholesterol is merely one way a bad diet can affect your heart. Numerous studies have shown that fibre like psyllium, taken as part of a healthy diet, can help lower a person's risk of heart disease. Psyllium can affect your heart by lowering blood pressure, improving lipid levels, and strengthening heart muscle.

Maintaining a healthy weight is a concern for many people, especially those with a chronic condition like diabetes. Besides being good for your heart and blood sugar levels, psyllium may help you lose weight.

Because psyllium absorbs liquid in your body, it can help give you a feeling of being full. This can help you control the amount of food you eat. Talk to your doctor about the possibility of taking psyllium if they have suggested you lose weight.

Diabetes: People with diabetes are constantly watching their diet to maintain a healthy balance of insulin and blood sugar (glucose). Some research has suggested that fibres like psyllium can help people maintain a healthy glycemic balance.

One study found that taking 5 grams of psyllium twice a day can help patients with type 2 diabetes controls their blood sugar. Another study of men with type 2 diabetes found similar results, but stressed that psyllium therapy should be tailored to the individual.

Psyllium is most commonly consumed in powder or wafer form. It is also available in capsules, granules, and in liquid form. It is the main ingredient in many over-the-counter laxatives, including:

- Metamucil
- Fibre
- Cilium
- Maalox Daily Fibre Therapy
- Uni-Laxative

Benefits: Psyllium is the common word used to refer to fibres taken from the plant known as Plantago ovate (Plantago psyllium); the fibre is characterized by being water soluble (hydrophilic) and gel forming, while possessing low ferment ability. It is commonly known by the brand name Metamucil.

Psyllium is used clinically as a bulk laxative, an agent that has laxative effects but secondary to increasing faecal size; a gentler laxative relative to chemical agents like Caffeine or Senna alexandrina. This bulk occurs due to water and gas absorption in the small intestines and colon to give chyme (made from digested food) more size and softness. This bulk is retained in the colon despite microflora as psyllium is poorly fermented (highly fermented fibres may be metabolized by bacteria in the colon, and water retaining properties with the fibre would be lost in this scenario).

Psyllium is proven to increase faecal size and moisture, and the most common characteristics of stool following supplementation of psyllium are 'soft, sleek, and easily passable.' Relative to other sources of dietary fibre, psyllium appears to be more effective at forming faeces and appears to be one of the few fibre sources not associated with excessive flatulence.

Beyond the faecal properties, psyllium appears to be able to reduce total cholesterol and LDL cholesterol in persons with high cholesterol (secondary to the gel forming properties leeching bile acids, and cholesterol being used up to replace hepatic bile acids) and there is a slight reduction of HDL as well. This is common to all dietary fibres and is not unique to psyllium.

There appears to be some glucose reducing properties associated with psyllium supplementation that may benefit diabetics. These are not overly potent, but appear reliable as long as psyllium is taken; cessation of psyllium usage is associated with a loss of the glucose reduction, and this may be common to all soluble dietary fibres rather than just psyllium.

Psyllium may reduce appetite slightly when taken in high doses, but does not appear to be potent or reliable; long term studies using psyllium in the doses for faecal management have failed to find weight reducing properties of psyllium suggesting it is not a good weight management intervention.

On the lower end of dosing, 5g of psyllium is taken once with meals alongside some form of liquid (200mL of water or more) and can be taken at every meal if desired.

Acute doses of up to 30g appear to be well tolerated assuming enough water (in these instances, around 500mL or so) is also co ingested.

If using psyllium for the faecal forming properties, a daily dose of 15g (thrice daily dosing of 5g) is a good starting point and then the dose can be titrated up or down depending on its effects on faecal formation.

5). Methyl cellulose Benefits and Nutrition Facts:

Methyl cellulose (or methylcellulose) is a chemical compound derived from cellulose. It is a hydrophilic white powder in pure form and dissolves in cold (but not in hot) water, forming a clear viscous solution or gel. It is sold under a variety of trade names and is used as a thickener and emulsifier in various food and cosmetic products, and also as a treatment of constipation. Like cellulose, it is not digestible, not toxic, and not an allergen. Methyl cellulose does not occur naturally and is synthetically.

6).Sterculia Benefits and Nutrition Facts:

Sterculia is a genus of flowering plants in the mallow family, Malvaceae. Sterculia species are used as food plants by the larvae of some Lepidoptera species including the leaf miner Bucculatrix xenaula, which feeds exclusively on the genus. Gum karaya is extracted from Sterculia species, and is used as a thickener and emulsifier in foods, as a laxative, and as a denture adhesive.

7). Inulin Benefits and Nutrition Facts:

Inulin is a plant and improves gut, heart and metabolic health as well. Onions and garlic are excellent natural sources of dietary inulin. The Jerusalem artichoke, or sun choke, is a good source of inulin. Inulin is produced by plants such as spring onions. The chicory plant, the most common and concentrated source of inulin, has chemical similarities to the sugar beet plant that's often used to derive sugar. Inulin acts like an insoluble fibre because they're not able to be broken down or absorbed once they enter the human digestive tract. This part is what provides many health benefits. Inulin has 6 proven benefits, such as; inulin is a soluble plant fibre and is considered a functional plant-based ingredient that effectively boosts digestion and other processes. Dietary fibres have been used for hundreds of years to improve bowel functions and gut health, curb appetite, and help maintain heart health, all completely naturally. Other plants that naturally contain inulin include wheat, onions, bananas, garlic, asparagus and Jerusalem artichokes plants that are sometimes called prebiotics. There is more than one type of inulin fibre sold as a dietary supplement, most of which are commonly derived from the chicory plant. Inulin is present inside the roots of plants as a means of storing energy and regulating the plant's internal temperature. It has osmotically active properties (a benefit to plants because this helps them resist cold temperatures and survive), a high molecular weight, the ability to absorb a high amount of liquid and a natural resistance to enzymes produced by humans. Inulin occupies in the digestive tract once eaten, helping to make you feel fuller; absorbs water, which helps to form stool; clings to cholesterol to help prevent metabolic syndrome; and allows you to go to the bathroom more easily. Benefits of inulin: There are among the top six benefits of inulin, such as, 1). Reduces Constipation; 2). When inulin is mixed with liquid it forms a creamy gel that's ideal for naturally relieving constipation. When gelled, inulin has a structure similar to lipids (fats) that also help lubricate the digestive system and lessen risk for things like haemorrhoids. Inulin increases faecal biomass, water content of stool, improves bowel habits, positively affect gastrointestinal functions and rapidly ferment in the colon to produce healthy bacteria. Chicory Root Inulin, taking daily 15 grams, improves constipation and quality of life in an elderly population with constipation; 3). It improves Gut Health by acting like a Prebiotic. Insulin and its other frucan fibres product can help improve gut health. This has very far-reaching benefits like improved immune functioning, protection from heart disease and diabetes, better weight management, improved nutrient absorption, healing leaky gut syndrome, and much more. Oligofructose acts like a prebiotic that impacts the lining of the gut and colon, changing the profile of organisms present and modulating the endocrine and immune functions. Fermentation of Inulin-type fructans in the large bowel stimulates bacteria to grow, which causes significant positive changes in the composition of the gut micro flora and significant decreases in the number of potentially harmful yeast, parasites and bacterial species living in the body that trigger inflammation. This is why inulin-type fructans have been found to reduce the risk of colon carcinogenesis and improve management of inflammatory bowel diseases; 4). Inulin Curb Appetite: Dieticians recommend that people looking to lose weight eat plenty of fibre in order to feel more satisfied and deal with fewer blood sugar fluctuations. When combined with water, inulin bulks up and forms a gel-like substance that expands in the digestive tract. This can help decrease appetite and cravings that potentially helping with weight loss because it slows the process of food emptying from the stomach and takes up more volume, which decreases appetite hormones. The result is that you feel full for longer after eating and deal with fewer hunger pangs. That's why consuming fibre leads to satiety. The addition of 6 grams inulin to a commercially available yogurt diet affects feelings of appetite, but not energy intake, which helps reducing weight; 5). Inulin boosts Heart Health and Lowers Metabolic Syndrome Risk factors. When it passes through the digestive system unabsorbed by digestive enzymes, inulin takes with it toxins, waste, fat and cholesterol particles. This is exactly the reason a high-fibre diet has been tied to heart health; 6) Another benefit of inulin is the fact that it doesn't cause insulin to be secreted and won't raise blood sugar since its carbohydrates/sugars cannot be broken down. Foods with Inulin: The best way to get inulin is through natural foods. Some of the best food sources of inulin include: ground chicory root (the most common source of inulin due to its extremely high concentration); dandelion root; asparagus; leeks and onions; bananas and plantains (especially when they're slightly green); sprouted wheat (such as the kind used in Ezekiel bread); garlic; artichokes; fresh herbs; yams; burdock root; camas root; coneflower, also called Echinacea; jicama; and yacon root. People around the world are believed to consume inulin every single day in the form of natural plant foods and some packaged products.

8). Wheat dextrin:

There are several types of fibre. Each works differently in your body and gives you distinct health perks. You may be familiar with the terms "soluble fibre" and "insoluble fibre," but within each of those labels are many different kinds of the nutrient. All types of soluble fibres slow digestion, so it takes longer for your body to absorb sugar (glucose) from the foods you eat. This helps prevent quick spikes in your blood sugar levels which is an important part of managing diabetes. Soluble fibres also bind with fatty acids, flushing them out of the body and helping to lower LDL (bad) cholesterol.

Insoluble fibres help hydrate and move waste through your intestines. That's one thing it does that helps prevent constipation and keeps you regular. Most of us get both types of fibre from foods and supplements. You can get the nutrient from fruits, vegetables, nuts, beans, and grains. "Functional" fibre is extracted from its natural sources, and then added to supplements or fortified foods and drinks to boost their fibre content. Most nutritionists say to get fibre from whole foods because they're healthy in other ways, too. But if you don't get enough from your diet, fibre supplements can help fill in the gap. And evidence shows that most of us aren't getting enough. The average person only gets about half of the fibre needed daily. Women 50 and younger should try to get 25 grams a day, and men should shoot for 38 grams.

Wheat bran, wheat dextrin and psyllium may be helpful for improving digestive health. Wheat bran consists of mainly insoluble fibre, which is helpful for making your stool more bulky so it passes through your digestive tract quickly. It can help treat digestive issues, such as diverticulitis, constipation and haemorrhoids. Psyllium, on the other hand, consists of mainly soluble fibre, which soaks up water and forms a gel. This gel slows down the emptying of the stomach and the digestive process. It can also help make stools firmer during diarrhoea. Psyllium swells when it soaks up water, so it may help with constipation and is often used as a laxative. Wheat dextrin is a soluble fibre supplement, and as such may help increase the absorption of micronutrients and regulate your digestive system. Potential Considerations: Drink plenty of water when increasing your fibre intake. This is especially important with psyllium, which can cause choking if you don't drink it mixed with plenty of water. Increase the fibre in your diet slowly to allow your body to get used to the added fibre. This will minimize any digestive side effects, such as gas, bloating and diarrhoea. Fibre may also interact with supplements, including medications for diabetes, depression, high cholesterol and seizures, causing these medications to be more or less effective and increasing the risk of side effects, so talk to your doctor before taking fibre supplements to make sure these are safe for you.

Wheat dextrin can also help make stools firmer during diarrhoea. Psyllium swells when it soaks up water, so it may help with constipation and is often used as a laxative. Wheat dextrin is a soluble fibre supplement, and as such may help increase the absorption of micronutrients and regulate your digestive system.

5.14 Stimulant laxatives to prevent Constipation

Stimulant laxatives: These stimulate the nerves in the large bowel (the colon and rectum). This then causes the muscle in the wall of the large bowel to squeeze harder than usual. This pushes the stools along and out. Their effect is usually within 8-12 hours; accordingly, it is better to have it as bedtime dose so you are likely to feel the urge to go to the toilet sometime the following morning. Possible side-effects from stimulant laxatives include abdominal cramps, and long-term use can lead to a bowel that is less active on its own (without laxatives). Stimulant laxatives include: Senna bisacodyl, docusate sodium, and glycerol and sodium pyrosulphate.

1). Senna Leave Benefits and Nutrition Facts:

Senna leave is a natural medicine containing sennosides that are derived from the leaves of the senna plant. Sennosides irritate the lining of the bowel causing a laxative effect. Senna has been used in alternative medicine as a Stimulant Laxative and an aid to treat constipation. Senna is often sold as an herbal supplement. Do not use this product for longer than 1 or 2 days. It is not safe for you to use senna if you have: a bowel disorder such as Crohn's disease or ulcerative colitis; heart disease; or stomach pain, nausea, or vomiting. It is used to treat constipation and to clear the bowel before diagnostic tests such as colonoscopy. Senna is also used for irritable bowel syndrome (IBS), haemorrhoids, and weight loss. Senna is the most effective medicinal plant (Cassia angustifolia and Cassia acutifolia) in relieving constipation. When compared with placebos and other remedies, an oral preparation of Senna at bedtime proved to be the most effective in eliminating the constipation problem within 24 hours.

While senna has always been effective at relieving constipation, it can have some minimal self-limited side effects. Since it is quite powerful, it may also cause diarrhoea, abdominal pain, heartburn, and/or nausea. By combining other herbs with senna you can often counteract its minor side effects. The following is a combination herbal tea very often used to relieve constipation.

Bring one quart of water to a boil and turn off the heat. Then, add ½ teaspoon of each of the following: caraway seeds, fennel seeds, peppermint leaves, and senna leaves. Let the mixture sit for 15 minutes and then filter the residue using cheesecloth or other method. Having one cup in the morning and another at night is the recommended dosage to relieve

Senna is a natural medicine containing sennosides that are derived from the leaves of the senna plant. Sennosides irritate the lining of the bowel causing a laxative effect.

Senna has been used in alternative medicine as a laxative and an aid to treat constipation.

Not all uses for senna have been approved by the FDA. It should not be used in place of medication prescribed for you by your doctor.

Senna is often sold as an herbal supplement. There are no regulated manufacturing standards in place for many herbal compounds and some marketed supplements have been found to be contaminated with toxic metals or other drugs. Herbal/health supplements should be purchased from a reliable source to minimize the risk of contamination.

Important information

Not all uses for senna have been approved by the FDA. Senna should not be used in place of medication prescribed for you by your doctor.

When considering the use of herbal supplements, seek the advice of your doctor. You may also consider consulting a practitioner who is trained in the use of herbal/health supplements.

If you choose to use senna, use it as directed on the package or as directed by your doctor, pharmacist, or other healthcare provider. Do not use more of this product than is recommended on the label. Senna is usually taken before bed to produce a bowel.

Method for taking Senna: If you choose to use senna, use it as directed on the package or as directed by your doctor. Do not use more of this product than is recommended on the label. Senna is usually taken before bed to produce a bowel movement 6 to 12 hours later when you wake up.

Senna side effects: Senna has an allergic reaction. Get emergency medical help if you have any of these signs of an allergic reaction to senna:

- It hives;
- difficulty breathing;
- Swelling of your face, lips, tongue, or throat.
- Call your healthcare provider at once if you have a serious side effect such as:
- severe stomach pain,
- severe diarrhoea,
- watery diarrhoea;
- weight loss;
- worsening constipation after you stop taking senna;
- enlargement of your fingers and toes;
- low potassium (confusion, uneven heart rate, extreme thirst, increased urination, leg discomfort, muscle weakness or limp feeling); or
- Nausea, upper stomach pain, itching, loss of appetite, dark urine, clay-colour stools, jaundice (yellowing of the skin or eyes).
- stomach cramps, bloating, gas, mild diarrhoea;
- numbness or tingly feeling;
- joint pain; or
- Discoloured urine.

Other Side effects of Senna include: Abdominal discomfort, nausea, mild cramps, griping, faintness, gastrointestinal side effects, Hypersensitivity, mediated asthma and rhino-conjunctivitis, and Musculoskeletal side effects. Do not take senna if you are using any of the following medications: digoxin (Lanoxin); a diuretic (water pill); or a blood thinner such as warfarin (Coumadin, Jantoven).

Tips to prevent Constipation

Use these all-natural alternatives as below:

- Zylitol
- Raw honey
- Green tea,
- Pomegranate juice,
- Homemade organic fruit juices,

Green tea is packed full of antioxidants to help flush out toxins.

Avoid any fast foods, fried foods, fatty meat & fast foods like french-fries, chips, hamburgers, beef, pork, pizza, hot dogs, and foods high in saturated fats, low in fibre. These foods, when consumed, will considerably slow down your digestive process and cause constipation that cause constipation. This works great at targeting the source of the problem. Every single day, your body absorbs millions of toxins from genetically modified foods, pesticides, meat, dairy, soy, white flour, table salt, monosodium glutamate (MSG), microwave foods, refined sugar, and artificial sweeteners. You also receive toxins from caffeine, alcohol, electromagnetic radiation, heavy metals, industrial chemicals, and prescription drugs. These impurities contaminate nearly everything we eat, drink, touch, or breathe and they are the root cause of constipation and disease. On the other hand, good fat and great sources of protein can be found in avocado, egg whites, lean poultry (chicken and turkey), fish and fish oil, unrefined raw organic vegetable oils like olive oil and coconut oil, raw nuts (almonds), raw seeds, and natural nut butters, just to name a few. Beans, peas, and legumes are low in fat and cholesterol. Beans and legumes are high in fibre and protein, and are a great substitute for meat. Dairy Foods like milk, frozen yogurt, ice cream, sour cream, and cheeses, including cottage cheese, can cause constipation. Dairy foods, in general lack in fibre, with the exception of natural yogurt products made with "probiotics". These types of yogurt made with probiotics may help relieve constipation. Simply put, probiotics are living microorganisms that assist your body's natural balance. They can be delivered in a number of ways, but most often are found in live fruits and vegetables, liquid or capsule forms. One of their most popular functions is the promotion of intestinal balance and general digestive health, which means they also make a great compliment to your colon cleansing routine.

Avoid Constipating Foods and Drinks: Constipating foods and drinks include white flour, cheese, fried and fatty foods, sweets, salt, beef, pasteurized milk, all junk food, carbonated drinks, caffeine, and alcohol, just to name a few.

Chewing your food properly, and having meals at unusual times like at late night

Do not drink dehydrating colas, coffee and especially alcohol. Not only can they all may harm the development of the baby, but they may also cause you to become constipated.

Don't fight the urge to go to the bathroom. If you feel like you need to go, and then go immediately. Try to get on a regular routine for bowel movements.

Drink Fifteen Glasses of Water a Day: Now where have you heard that one before, right! Water is vital to your body, and makes up approximately 80 percent of your body weight. Every system in your body depends on water. For example, water flushes toxins out of vital organs, carries nutrients to your cells and provides a moist environment for ear, nose and throat tissues. Water will also help moisten the intestines, so that the bowels will move easily.

- Eat Plenty of Apples – The high pectin levels in apples stimulate the bowels and also provide bulk for bowel movements. One of the best natural laxative foods is organic apple cider vinegar. Just pour a small amount into a glass of purified water and drink it in the morning.
- Eat Plenty of Bananas – High in fibre and a natural bulk-producing agent, bananas are great for promoting easy digestion.
- Eat Plenty of Beans, Peas & Legumes – Low in fat and cholesterol, beans and legumes are high in fibre and protein. They make for a great substitute for meat.
- Eat Plenty of Bran Cereals – High fibre cereals are a great addition to your diet and a healthful way to start your day. Usually low in preservatives and sugars, bran cereals are a great source of dietary fibre.
- Eat Plenty of Broccolis – Very high in fibre and an excellent natural antibiotic, broccoli has also demonstrated some cancer-fighting potential.
- Eat Plenty of Carrots – A rich source of Beta-Carotene, carrots are natural body detoxifiers. Also high in pectin, carrots add bulk to stool and can stimulate bowel contractions.
- Eat Plenty of Cherries – A natural blood stimulant, cherries have been used for centuries to detoxify the kidneys. Cherries also have the anti-cancer compound, ellagic acid, and are very effective at relieving constipation.
- Eat Plenty of Cinnamon – Cinnamon stimulates intestinal peristalsis (the wave-like contractions) and also triggers the release of bile for digestion.
- Eat Plenty of Dried Fruit – When dried organically, dried fruit keeps much of the nutritional properties of the raw variety. Dried figs, prunes, and apricots are great intestinal movers.
- Eat Plenty of Green Vegetables – Leafy green vegetables like spinach, kale, and turnip greens are very high in vitamins and minerals.
- Eat Plenty of High Fibre Foods: By increasing your intake of foods high in fibre, you will greatly reduce your chances of developing any symptoms of constipation, as well as prevent many other colon-related health problems. Below is a list of high fibre foods

you should add to your diet. Eat plenty of these foods throughout your day. If possible, always buy organic fruits and vegetables.

- Eat plenty of other natural foods for relieving constipation: tamarind, dates, prunes, coconut, and Brussels sprouts. Fresh berries such as strawberries, raspberries and blackberries are also great at preventing constipation.
- Eat Plenty of Raw Nuts & Seeds – Raw almonds, sunflower seeds, chia seeds, hazelnuts, and chestnuts lead the way as the best choices, because they are high in fibre, protein, vitamin E and calcium. Nuts and seeds are also very filling, so you don't have to eat many before feeling satisfied. Chew thoroughly for easier digestion.
- Engage in plenty of exercise to tone your body and sweat out as many potential toxins as you can. Exercise regularly. Implementing a regular exercise routine into your schedule will nourish your blood and oxygenate your system. It stimulates the nerves in the large bowel (the colon and rectum). The more you move, the more your bowels will move. Exercise does not have to be a rigorous work out! Here is the best part – exercise is cost friendly, and will also help reduce your stress. You can start with walking three times a week for 30 minutes per walk.
- Get plenty of rest at night. Try to wind down and relax after a long day. Get plenty of sleep. If your sleep schedule has been rough, try taking little breaks throughout the day
- Make delicious drinks with organic fruits and vegetables that are both nutritious and high in fibre and antioxidants, that will help relieve constipation rather than aggravate it.
- Reduce consumption of dairy and meat products.

Reduce your Stress:

Easier said than done, I'm sure. But isn't everything else? Take time out occasionally and treat yourself to some fun and relaxation. Paint, dance, play music, write poetry, laugh, whatever it is you've always wanted to do and somehow stored your creative passions in your inner treasure chest somewhere. Perhaps, it can be as simple as taking a weekend and just resting, or visiting a friend you haven't seen in over 10 years. You're entitled to your escape. As hard as it may seem, reducing your overall levels of stress will go a long way towards a happy and healthy pregnancy. Take it, and add the "oxygen of living life" to your health, instead of stress. Enjoy life because you deserve it, and because you can! What is your choice?

Avoid refined and processed Foods: Foods containing white flour and white sugar, including but not limited to white bread, breads containing bleached flour, white pasta, white rice, cookies, pastries, cakes, pies, and junk foods in general can cause constipation, because they lack in fibre

Stay well hydrated by drinking plenty of purified water throughout the day. It is wise to drink at least 6-8 glasses every day.

Enjoy more – when was the last time you took some time off and did something you enjoy, whether fishing, camping, painting, dancing?

Take a Probiotic Supplement – Probiotics will help introduce beneficial bacteria to your colon, which will.

5.15   Detoxify the Body

It may shock you to know that the average person has about 300 or more toxic chemicals within their blood stream. While the body has the ability to process a moderate amount of toxins, 300 toxic chemicals is too much for anyone to have to bear. For this reason, more and more people are suffering from chronic illnesses and diseases related to toxic overload.

Currently, our fast-paced, mass-produced environment leaves people little time to focus on their health. Toxic overload can come from the air we breathe, the chemicals in our cleaning and beauty products, highly-processed or chemically-sprayed food products, as well as the wide array of consumer products dipped in flame-retardant chemical treatment baths.

Oxygen based Colon Cleansers:

Oxy-Powder released oxygen over 18 hours in testing. Oxy-Powder® is the leader, and has an aggressive, fast electromotive power of 2.4 or above.

Most companies claiming to produce oxygen based colon cleansers fail. These companies do not employ a scientific method for attaching and stabilizing oxygen correctly. Moreover, many of these companies merely use or mix combinations of magnesium oxides with magnesium peroxide and sell their products as oxygen releasing compounds, but this is not accurate and correct.

Magnesium oxide holds oxygen but does not release oxygen very well unless properly assisted. You must pick the proper combination of vectors to hold and deliver oxygen effectively. The magnesium acts as a carrier of the oxygen to transport it through the intestinal lining, kidneys, bladder and out through the intestines. You do not want a form of magnesium that can be completely assimilated; that is not the purpose. The purpose of stabilizing oxygen is to deliver monatomic oxygen using a timed-release process. There is a big misconception that the gut is home to all anaerobic organisms. Digestive disease actually starts with the misuse of antibiotics, which kills friendly bacteria in addition to harmful organisms. In actuality, friendly bacteria are facultative strains mostly anaerobic (without oxygen) but will also flourish in an aerobic condition. The friendly bacteria in the bowel secrete hydrogen peroxide as a by-product and can live in a high spectrum of oxygen exposure. They will also fight for the receptor sites of the bad bacteria or the bad organisms concentrating themselves in the bowel.

Each bug or harmful organism picks its own environmental pH to live in. What the body wants is a good colony of Probiotics thriving from the stomach all the way down through the colon. Ideally, the friendly bacteria should fight the unfriendly bacteria and secrete hydrogen peroxide as a by-product within the bowel.

By taking oxygen based colon cleansers every other evening before bed, we will feed the friendly bacteria with the oxygen needed to create a stable bowel environment. Oxygen will also oxidize and clean the entire bowel, relieving constipation and compaction. When you take oxygen based colon cleansers, you raise the level of ORS (Oxygen Reactive Species), which causes a stimulation of lymphocytes to produce T-cells. This process promotes a strengthened immune system.

You shouldn't take oxygen based colon cleansers every day but you should take a good Probiotic and enzyme formula to enhance the effectiveness of the cleanser you are using. Increasing your antioxidant intake is also recommended.

Women and men are starting to develop a condition called progressive constipation. Progressive constipation is developed when you don't go to the bathroom as soon as you feel the urge. This reduces the contraction of the muscles in the bowel, resulting in progressive constipation and a lazy bowel. Make sure you pay attention to the urge to go to the bathroom. As soon as you feel an urge, get up and go! Waiting can cause the bowel muscles to lose their effectiveness over time. When looking at oxygen based colon cleansers one must determine the following.

Titration test Oxygen based colon cleansers: This is determined using a titration test, which shows that whether oxygen is really being released. Titration will show if oxygen is being released and for how long it is released. Oxy-Powder® released oxygen over 18 hours in testing. How aggressively is the oxygen being released? This is measured with electromotive force. The majority of the products claiming oxygen delivery have an electromotive force of 1.23 or below, which is not good. Oxy-Powder® is the leader, and has an aggressive, fast electromotive power of 2.4 or above.

Be aware of so-called oxygen based colon cleansers containing the ingredient ascorbic acid. Ascorbic acid is a strong antioxidant, which will neutralize any benefits of oxygen release.

On the other hand it must be kept in mind that ascorbic acid can also act as a pro-oxidant, especially in the presence of iron and copper.

Following a body detoxify helps your system re-set itself from a chemical overload. Through detoxing, you can help get rid of some of the garbage the body is processing, as well as eventually bring the system back into balance.

1. Ward off Future Diseases: If you are doing a body detoxify, it will help you ward of any future diseases. There is nothing better for prevention than getting rid of toxins in the body. Many of today's common diseases are related to environmental pollutants. By detoxifying, the body can let go of these harmful chemicals, thus increasing the immune system's ability to function properly.

2. Cleaning of Colon: Following a body detoxify program will help remove excessive mucus and waste from your digestive tract and clean your colon. As soon as you begin a body detoxify, you will notice lightness in your intestinal tract. Your bowel movements will also begin to improve and you will be relieved of excess bloating and gas. A body detoxify will help clean out the excessive waste in the colon, thus increasing the absorption rate of vitamins and minerals in the food we eat.

3. Lose Weight: Detoxing can also help you let go of any extra weight you are carrying. The body has a natural fat-burning mechanism. Oftentimes, toxins lodged in the system can actually block the body's natural ability of removing fats.

4. Reduce Pain: Crystallized toxins are one of the most common causes of pain. Getting these toxins out of your body, will help reduce the amount of pain you may be experiencing.

5. Eliminate Some Medications: Many of our common ailments are directly related to toxins in the blood. By removing them, it's not uncommon for many people to of these common complaints, such as headaches, migraines, cramps, etc., no longer needed pharmaceutical treatment.

6. Naturally Boost Your Metabolism: Following a body detoxify program will help help increase metabolism in your body. Once you start losing weight and cleaning out your intestinal tract, your body will

be able to digest foods at a more efficient pace. You metabolism will naturally rise.

7. Aligns us with Natural Rhythms of the Earth: Most animal species go for months in a state of fasting and purging. This process helps to keep our system functioning at optimal levels. This is why animals in the wild never have chronic diseases.

8. Increases Absorption of Nutrients: When your digestive tract is clogged with excessive waste, it can be hard for all of the nutrients in your food to be absorbed. A body detoxify will help clean out the excessive waste in the colon, thus increasing the absorption rate of vitamins and minerals in the food we eat.

9. Eliminates Body Waste: We all eat, therefore we all produce some sort of waste. A colon detoxify will help clear out all the excessive waste that may be trapped in your intestinal tract, or other areas of your body.

10. Boosts Vitality & Energy Levels: Everyone who detoxifies notices a feeling of lightness. They get more energy which allows them to complete everyday errands with renewed enthusiasm.

11. Purifies the Liver: The liver is where dangerous toxins are metabolized. With 300 different chemicals rushing to the liver, it is no wonder that this is the organ that suffers the most. Doing a body detoxify can help ease the amount of work the Liver has to do. There are also many ways to detoxify your liver.

12. Increases Mental Clarity: After completing a body detoxify, many people feel as if "a fog has lifted". Not only do you get more energy after detoxify, but you also think faster and keep their focus for longer.

13. Gives Skin a Healthy Glow: It's a well known fact that the skin is the largest organ. Beautiful, radiant skin is the first sign that you have removed toxins from your system. After completing a body detoxify, you will notice your skin clear up, and blemishes start to fade away.

14. Add Years to Your Life: Studies have shown that toxic residues in the system can increase your chances of getting cancer, obesity, and much other disease that can lead to an earlier death. If you get those chemicals out of your body, you can literally add years to your life.

15. Slows the Process of Age-Degeneration: As the body removes toxins from the system, cells can get more nourishment. The more nourished our cells, the more we appear young and vibrant.

16. Boosts the Immune System: Detoxing boosts the immune system, helping protect us from everything from the common cold to cancer.

17. Helps you sleep better: Once you get all the dangerous toxins out of your body, you will start to notice a drop in many negative symptoms you may be experiencing. This will help you get a better

nights rest, and allow your body the necessary sleep it needs to start the next day off strong.

18. Improves Your Hair: After completing a full body detoxify, you will notice the hair become shiner and healthier. Just like the improvements in your skin, you will notice an improvement in your hair.

19. Positive Healing Effect on the Emotions: Many people believe that detoxing your body gives you the opportunity to "go within" and heal many emotional issues that may be on your mind. Not only will you notice improvements in the way your body feels, but you may also feel a renewed sense of clarity.

20. Reduces Bad Breath: If your intestinal tract has excessive waste, or you frequently experience constipation, then it's very possible that you may sometimes have bad breath. This is because sometimes bad aromas could be lingering in your digestive system. Following a colon detoxify is just one of many bad breath remedies.

5.16 Prevent Constipation in Pregnancy

More than 50% of all pregnant women suffer some degree of constipation. As you may already know, suffering from symptoms of constipation alone can be uncomfortable, painful, embarrassing, and frustrating all at the same time. Now imagine having to go through the pains of constipation during pregnancy.

Generally, a woman's body goes through many changes during pregnancy that can make her uncomfortable, such as extreme tiredness, tender/swollen breasts, swollen ankles, skin blemishes, upset stomach (morning sickness), cravings or distaste for certain foods, mood swings, headaches, weight gain or loss, and the urge to urinate more often, just to name a few. When constipation is added to the list of aches and pains, it can make her feel worse. There are minimum four causes of Constipation for Pregnant Women. Constipation in early pregnancy can sometimes cause many other symptoms, such as bloating, excess gas, heartburn, and back pain. Constipation tends to be more pronounced during pregnancy and the reasons are:

1. Change in Hormones (especially during early pregnancy): When a woman becomes pregnant, her body puts out special hormones for softening her ligaments and muscles. One of these hormones is called progesterone, which acts by relaxing muscles. On the positive side, this aids in the birthing process by allowing foods consumed to

stay longer for both mother and child to absorb nutrients. On the challenging side, relaxed intestinal muscles mean less frequent bowel contractions, thereby causing food and waste to move slower through your digestive system. The longer the stool sits in the large intestine, the harder and drier it gets, which means constipation.

2. Prenatal Vitamins: Prenatal Vitamins, particularly those containing iron, can potentially cause or possibly aggravate constipation for pregnant women. Although iron can help keep pregnant women from becoming anaemic, know that iron can also be very harsh on the digestive tract and is known to cause constipation. Consuming the right amount of nutrients is important for the development of your baby, so be sure to talk to your doctor about the best prenatal vitamins you can take.

3. Pressure of the Baby on the Intestines: Pregnant women may become constipated when their uterus expands due to the weight of the baby pushing down on the bowel and intestines, making it difficult for faecal matter to pass through. In the event she is experiencing pain from laceration, she might be afraid to have bowel movements. As a result, consciously or unconsciously, she will find herself holding the waste in to avoid excruciating pains, which in turn worsens the constipation.

4. Loss of Bladder Control (Incontinence): Generally, most pregnant women experience loss of bladder control in the third trimester, when the baby has grown so much, that the baby's weight is pressed up against the mother's bladder. As a result of added pressure on it, the amount of urine the bladder can hold is reduced, causing the mom to potentially lose control of her bladder and wanting to urinate more often. Now add constipation to loss of bladder control during pregnancy. Pregnant women who are constipated may develop a more aggravated, intense and problematic bladder control problem. In addition to the baby's weight bearing down on the bladder, the added pressure of a backed up bowel can cause urinary incontinence from the intestinal discomfort. On the flip side, some women may experience the opposite where the added weight on the bladder makes it more difficult for them to urinate.

Other causes of constipation in pregnant women may include:

Not drinking enough water

Not exercising regularly

Irregular Eating Habits

Stress, Worry and Anxiety

Inadequate consumption of dietary fibre

Develop an organic diet with plenty of raw fibrous vegetables and

5.17 Sufficient Intake of Liquid to prevent Constipation

An adequate fluid intake is important to help prevent constipation and help regulate body temperature. If you don't take enough fluid, this can result in dehydration, which can lead to irritability. The recommended intake of fluid is 12 to 18 glasses of non–sugar drinks; this includes water, soup and fresh fruit juice prepared in. The best choice is water. Fruit juices are a good source of vitamin C.

Some older people have a decreased sense of thirst and go for a long time without fluid. You may need to think more carefully about taking enough water during the day. If you are concerned about using the toilet more often, you may find it helpful to drink the majority of your fluids earlier in the day, so your body has enough time to process the fluid before you go to bed.

It is far better, if you switched to a liquid diet for a while, it helps my constipation. While dehydration can cause constipation, it is rare for this to be a chronic cause in an otherwise healthy person. The gastrointestinal tract secretes a substantial amount of fluid into early part of the tract, and then reabsorbs it in the later part. Adequate fluid intake is important.

Extra fluids help keep the stool soft and easy to pass. Fruit and vegetable juices, clear soups, and herbal teas are also good sources of fluids. Stay away from alcohol. It is a diuretic, which gets rid of water from your body and leads to dehydration. Caffeinated drinks like coffee, tea, and colas are also diuretics and cause dehydration.

Lack of sufficient water intake stimulates the colon to reabsorb the water from stool in the colon to maintain the water balance leading to dry, hard stool. Hence drink at least five litres of water and other fluids a day unless restricted by your physician for some other medical condition. If you are a sort of person wandering in daylights, of course this baseline has to be increased to suit your needs. Liquids such as coffee and soft drinks that contain caffeine tend to have a dehydrating effect and needs to be avoided until your bowel habits return to normal or even some people may need to avoid milk and milk products, as dairy products can be the catalysts for constipation for them. Try one litre of warm water in the morning and before bed to bring that urge and prevent constipation.

So take care of the two major players, fibre and water; fibre and water help the colon pass stool. Fluids that can help relieve constipation include pear and prune juice. However, it's important not to drink too much at a time as these fruit juices can cause cramping. A small glass, 4 or 5 ounces, once daily is a good starting point -- or as much as your doctor recommends. Drinking extra water does not relieve constipation in people who are not dehydrated, but staying well hydrated is important to prevent constipation from worsening.

5.18 Probiotic Foods to prevent Constipation and treat Irritable Bowel Syndrome:

Probiotic is a Good Bacteria or Body healthy Acid food made of natural live fruit or vegetable, which is very good to prevent Constipation and to Conquer Irritable Bowel Syndrome. Study showed that probiotics are great. There are numerous health benefits consuming probiotics. Your gut health is closely linked to the overall health, so feeding your gut with good bacteria in the form of probiotics makes perfect sense. But you must aim to eat a wide variety of probiotic rich foods such as sauerkraut (make sure it's raw unpasteurized sauerkraut. I love the Sauerkraut from Vegetables, kombucha, kimchi & kefir. Probiotics (Body healthy Acid) is a: Fresh fruit and vegetable-Probiotics and is a natural Colon Cleanser. Healthy stomach acid is the key to creating the proper bowel speed. It all starts with the acid level, which is a first line body defence that destroys pathogens, toxins, and starts the digestive process through the intestines.

There is much importance of stomach acid in curing chronic constipation. A more effective and holistic approach to healing chronic constipation is to first repair and rebuild your body's ability to effectively produce stomach acid. Also known as hydrochloric acid (HCL), stomach acid is arguably the most important factor in regulating digestive health, and a lack of it may be the reason why you are constipated. HCL, after all, is essential for breaking down food and eliminating waste from the small intestine. "Stomach acid is a digestive fluid formed in your stomach to break down food". A serious but common problem is that because low stomach acid leads to impaired digestion, it is often misdiagnosed as having too much stomach acid. This is because when the stomach does not empty correctly, partly digested carbohydrates and proteins that have started to ferment in the stomach will back up into the esophagus -- an uncomfortable problem that is interpreted by uninformed individuals and physicians as too much stomach acid."

The aim of the present study was to investigate the effect of a probiotic beverage on gastrointestinal symptoms in patients with chronic constipation. There is much importance of bacterial balance in alleviating chronic constipation. Once you get your stomach acid in check, the next step is to support your inner ecosystem with living probiotics. Cultured vegetables, kombucha tea, yogurt, raw milk, and kefir are a few examples of probiotic-rich foods that will help populate your gut with the bacteria needed to break down food and eliminate toxins, including heavy metals like mercury that can become impacted in the gut.

Lactobacillus Casei Diet:

Lactobacillus casei is a type of bacteria that's found naturally in the human gut, as well as in fermented foods such as yogurt. While people often think of bacteria as being the cause of health problems, Lactobacillus casei or L. casei, as it is often abbreviated—is what's known as "probiotic" bacteria, one that has a positive effect on human health. The makeup of bacteria in the human gut can influence metabolic factors such as weight and insulin levels. A study showed that the Lactobacillus casei strain Shirota altered the makeup of gut bacteria in obese mice in a way that led to improved insulin resistance and could alleviate symptoms of rheumatoid arthritis and lower inflammation markers in women with the disease. Lactobacillus Casei contains stomach acid, hydrochloric acid and lucid acid IBS-C can easily be the result of slow digestion. As I said above, there are a number of things that can slow digestion down like stress, emotions, and toxins (to name a few more). But if the structural components that govern the speed are broken, then all other treatments are only going to be marginally effective.

Diet is one of the most common dietary sources of Lactobacillus casei is "Yogurt". When yogurt is made in a certain way, it retains live bacteria cultures, such as Lactobacillus casei and Lactobacillus acidophilus. "Live and Active Cultures" seal. Lactobacillus casei can also be found in probiotic supplements, such as, Yakult, which is a probiotic dairy product made by fermenting a mixture of skimmed milk with a special strain of the bacterium Lactobacillus casei Shirota. In our digestive system, there lives a diverse and large population of bacteria. Our poop is mostly made of bacteria so it is important to support the good bacteria that make perfect poops possible. There are a couple ways of getting more good bacteria in your life. The first, like our ancestors did, is to eat fermented foods on a regular basis. The second way is to take probiotic pills which contain known strains of good bacteria that will help. When I started taking probiotics I immediately saw an improvement in my bowel movements. I also saw good results eating SCD legal yogurt (a lactose-free fermented food) on a regular basis. So, I would recommend picking one or the other to get started. Try either fermented foods. However, avoid Yakult, Probiotic Drinks, because it is very harmfulbecause of the reasons as below:

1). Lactic acid (Vegetable Pickles):

Throughout history and across the globe, pickled vegetables have been a means of preserving food for winter. Lactic acid plays a key role in the fermentation process that produces kimchi (Cabbage Pickle), sauerkraut and Cucumbers (pickle). Lactic acid fermentation begins with beneficial bacteria. These lactic acid bacteria, such as Lactobacillus, convert carbohydrates into lactic acid without the need of oxygen. As a result, the "Pickled Vegetable" retains most of its composition, is preserved and has a distinctive taste. The lactic acid bacteria are desirable in fermentation because they produce a high acidity level and inhibit the growth of other bacteria. Lactic acid is effective in preventing the spoilage of olives, gherkins, pearl onions and other vegetables preserved in brine. There are many reasons to eat fresh unpasteurized Sauerkraut. Sauerkraut combines the anti-carcinogenic properties of cabbage, cauliflower or cucumber, with the benefits of lactic acid fermentation. Lactic acid is naturally present in many foodstuffs. It is formed by natural fermentation in products such as cheese, yogurt, soy sauce, sourdough, meat products and pickled vegetables (Cabbage, Cauliflower, Cucumber etc). Lactic acid is also used in a wide range of food applications such as bakery products, beverages, salads, dressings, ready meals, etc. Lactic acid in food products usually serves as either as a pH regulator or as a preservative. It is also used as a flavouring agent.

2). Lactic acid (Sauerkraut):

Sauerkraut is high content of the antioxidants lute in and zeaxanthin, both associated with preserving ocular health. Other nutrients in sauerkraut include calcium, potassium, magnesium, and vitamins C and K. To reap the benefits of sauerkraut, it's not necessary to eat a lot of it. A few tablespoons daily, taken as a side dish with meals or added to salads are easy to incorporate into the diet. Sauerkraut is high in digestive enzymes. Enzyme rich foods help support the pancreas and increase digestive strength. It is also one of the best ways to establish various beneficial lactobacilli cultures in the digestive tract. Sauerkraut is very high in naturally occurring lactic acid which helps maintain a healthy acidity in the large intestine, thus creating an environment that is hostile to parasites and yeast but comfortable for good bacteria. Among its other attributes, Sauerkraut is very high in vitamin C, a powerful antioxidant.

3). Lactic acid (Salads & dressings):

Lactic acid may be also used as a preservative in salads and dressings, resulting in products with a milder flavour while maintaining microbial stability and safety.

4). Lactic acid (Wine):

The fermentation of grapes into wine involves yeast and lactic acid bacteria. Malolactic fermentation is one means of adding complexity to a wine. Following the primary fermentation of the sugar in the grapes to alcohol, bacteria convert the grape acids into malic acid and lactic acid. Lactic acid is less sour than malic acid. It adds to the complexity and flavour to a good wine.

5). Yogurt:

Yogurt is one of the best sources of probiotics, which are friendly bacteria that can improve your health. Yogurt is made from milk that has been fermented by friendly bacteria, mainly lactic acid bacteria and bifid bacteria. Eating yogurt has been associated with many health benefits, including improved bone health. It is also beneficial for people with high blood pressure. In children, yogurt may help reduce the diarrhoea caused by antibiotics. It can even help relieve the symptoms of irritable bowel syndrome. Additionally, yogurt may be better than milk for people with lactose intolerance. This is because the bacteria turn some of the lactose into lactic acid, which is also why yogurt tastes sour.

However, keep in mind that not all yogurts contain live probiotics. In some cases, the live bacteria have been killed during processing. For this reason, make sure to make yogurt in your house with active or live cultures. Probiotic yogurt is linked to a number of health benefits. It may also be more suitable than milk for people with lactose intolerance. Make sure to choose yogurt that has active or live cultures.

6). Kefir:

Kefir is a fermented probiotic milk drink. It is made by adding kefir grains to cow's or goat's milk. Kefir grains are not cereal grains, but rather cultures of lactic acid bacteria and yeast that look a bit like cauliflower. The word kefir allegedly comes from the Turkish word key if, which means "feeling good" after eating. In fact, kefir has been linked to various health benefits. It may improve bone health, help with some digestive problems and protect against infections. While yogurt is probably the best known probiotic food in the Western diet, kefir is actually a better source. Kefir contains several major strains of friendly bacteria and yeast, making it a diverse and potent probiotic. Like yogurt, kefir is generally well-tolerated by people who are lactose intolerant. Kefir is a fermented milk drink. It is a better source of probiotics than yogurt, and people with lactose intolerance can often eat kefir with no problems.

7). Sauerkraut:

Sauerkraut is finely shredded cabbage that has been fermented by lactic acid bacteria. It is one of the oldest traditional foods and is popular in many countries, especially in Europe. Sauerkraut is often used on top of sausages or as a side dish. It has a sour, salty taste and can be stored for months in an airtight container.

In addition to its probiotic qualities, sauerkraut is rich in fibre, as well as vitamins C, B and K. It is also high in sodium and contains iron and manganese. Sauerkraut also contains the antioxidants lute in and zeaxanthin, which are important for eye health. However, make sure to choose unpasteurized sauerkraut. Pasteurization kills the live and active bacteria. Sauerkraut is finely cut, fermented cabbage. It is rich in vitamins, minerals and antioxidants. Make sure to choose unpasteurized brands that contain live bacteria.

8). Tempeh:

Tempeh is a fermented soybean product. It forms a firm patty, and people have described the flavour as nutty, earthy or similar to a mushroom. Tempeh is originally from Indonesia, but has become popular all over the world as a high-protein meat substitute. The fermentation process actually has some surprising effects on its nutritional profile. Soybeans are typically high in phytic acid, a plant compound that impairs the absorption of minerals like iron and zinc. However, the fermentation process lowers the amount of phytic acid, which may increase the amount of minerals the body is able to absorb from tempeh. Another interesting by-product of this process is that the bacteria produce some vitamin B12, a nutrient that soybeans do not contain. Vitamin B12 is mainly found in animal foods, such as meat, fish, dairy products and eggs. This makes tempeh an overall great choice for vegetarians, as well as anyone looking to add a nutritious probiotic to their diet. Tempeh is a fermented soybean product. It is a popular, high-protein substitute for meat. It also contains a decent amount of vitamin B12, a nutrient found mainly in animal products.

9). Kimchi:

Kimchi is a fermented, spicy Korean side dish. Cabbage is usually the main ingredient, but it can also be made from other vegetables. A mix of seasonings is used for flavour, such as red chilli pepper flakes, garlic, ginger, scallion and salt. Kimchi contains the lactic acid bacteria Lactobacillus kimchii, as well as other lactic acid bacteria that may benefit digestive health. Kimchi made from cabbage is high in some vitamins and minerals, including vitamin K, riboflavin (vitamin B2) and iron. Kimchi is a spicy Korean side dish, usually made from fermented cabbage. It contains lactic acid bacteria, which may benefit digestive health.

10). Miso:

Miso is a Japanese seasoning. It is traditionally made by fermenting soybeans with salt and a type of fungus called koji. Miso can also be made by mixing soybeans with other ingredients, like barley, rice and rye. This paste is most often used in miso soup, a popular breakfast food in Japan. Miso is typically salty, and you can buy it in many varieties, such as white, yellow, red and brown.

Miso is a good source of protein and fibre. It is also high in various vitamins, minerals and phytonutrients, including vitamin K, manganese and copper. Miso has also been linked to some health benefits. One study reported that frequent miso soup consumption was associated with a lower risk of breast cancer in middle-aged Japanese women. Another study found that women who ate a lot of miso soup had a reduced risk of stroke. Miso is a fermented soybean paste and a popular Japanese seasoning. It is rich in several important nutrients and may reduce the risk of cancer and stroke, especially in women.

11). Kombucha:

Kombucha is a fermented black or green tea drink. This popular tea is fermented by a friendly colony of bacteria and yeast. It is consumed in many parts of the world, especially Asia. On the internet, there are many claims about the potential health effects of kombucha tea. However, high-quality evidence on kombucha is lacking. The studies that exist are animal and test tube studies and the results may not apply to humans. Yet, because kombucha is fermented with bacteria and yeast, it does probably have health benefits related to its probiotic properties. Kombucha is a fermented tea drink. It is claimed to have a wide range of health benefits, but human evidence for these claims is currently lacking.

12). Pickles:

Pickles (also known as gherkins) are cucumbers that have been pickled in a solution of salt and water. They are left to ferment for some time, using their own naturally present lactic acid bacteria. This process is what makes them sour. Pickled cucumbers are a great source of healthy probiotic bacteria, which may improve digestive health. They are low in calories and a good source of vitamin K, an essential nutrient for blood clotting. Pickles also tend to be high in sodium. It is important to note that pickles made with vinegar do not contain live probiotics. Pickles are cucumbers that have been pickled in salty water and fermented. They are low in calories and high in vitamin K. However, pickles made using vinegar do not have probiotic effects.

13). Traditional Buttermilk:

The term buttermilk actually refers to a range of fermented dairy drinks. However, there are two main types of buttermilk: traditional and cultured. Traditional buttermilk is simply the leftover liquid from making butter. Only this version contains probiotics, and it is sometimes called Grandma's probiotic. Traditional buttermilk is mainly consumed in India, Nepal and Pakistan. Cultured buttermilk, commonly found in American supermarkets, and generally does not have any probiotic benefits. Buttermilk is low in fat and calories, but contains several important vitamins and minerals, such as vitamin B12, riboflavin, calcium and phosphorus. Bottom Line: Traditional buttermilk is a fermented dairy drink mainly consumed in India, Nepal and Pakistan. Cultured buttermilk, found in American supermarkets, does not have any probiotic benefits.

14). Natto:

Natto is another fermented soybean product, like tempeh and miso. It contains a bacterial strain called Bacillus subtilis. Natto is a staple in Japanese kitchens. It is typically mixed with rice and served with breakfast. It has a distinctive smell, slimy texture and strong flavour. Natto is rich in protein and vitamin K2, which is important for bone health and cardiovascular health. A study in older Japanese men found that consuming natto on a regular basis was associated with higher bone mineral density. This is attributed to the high vitamin K2 content of natto. Natto is fermented soybeans. Natto is a traditional Japanese food made with soybeans fermented with

Bacillus subtilis var (known also as the hay bacillus or grass bacillus). Other studies suggest that natto may help prevent osteoporosis in women. Natto is a fermented soy product that is a staple in Japanese kitchens. It contains a high amount of vitamin K2, which may help prevent osteoporosis and heart attacks.

15). Naturally Fermented Foods

If you're like me, you pay attention to food trends, like growth in the popularity and availability of naturally fermented foods. I'm talking about live cultured foods, naturally fermented the way our ancestors have done it for centuries. For them, it was a method of preservation. It was also a secret to good health, and it's making a serious comeback.

The traditional cultures around the world have made their own naturally fermented sodas and ale, as well as fermented dairy products, vegetables, fruits and even meats. Japanese cuisine features fermented pickles, natto and miso. In Germany, sauerkraut is a traditional dish. In other parts of Europe, sourdough bread is made from naturally fermented dough. In Korea, people eat kimchi made from live cultured cabbage.

A strong immune system depends on a healthy digestive tract. If digestive health is not up to par, chances are neither is the immune system. Healthy bacteria are the key. That's where fermented foods come in. They contain probiotics (friendly bacteria) that colonize our digestive track, keeping our bacterial flora balanced. Because of our culture's reliance on pasteurized foods, we've eliminated most sources of these important probiotics that we used to consume on a regular basis. To make sure your diet contains these valuable live foods, consider adding the following:

Live cultured pickles, sauerkraut, vegetables, kimchi (made from live cultured cabbage), Cheese made from raw milk, Unpasteurized miso (which has not been heated), Tempeh, made from fermented soybeans, Fermented drinks and tea such as kombucha, Yogurt and kefir made with live cultures (not all commercially sold yogurt or frozen yogurt, but live cultures). Non-dairy yogurt varieties may also contain live cultures.

Homemade Raw Sauerkraut:

Make your own raw sauerkraut. You have to ferment the veggies. In fact, it's surprisingly easy to make and is cheaper than buying the store-bought stuff. You'll have more fresh and house made sauerkraut when you'll know how to do with. It's loaded with friendly bacteria for your gut, which has been shown to improve digestion and the absorption of vitamins and minerals. So, eat your fermented veggies.

Making Raw Sauerkraut:

Ingredients: 1 Head green or purple cabbage, 2 Tablespoons sea salt, and 3 spring or distilled water, as needed.

Tools: Wood cutting board, Sharp knife, Glass jar, large glass or metal bowl, Metal Tongs, and Ziploc bag (if needed for added weight).

Methods: Step 1 (Sterilization tools and containers): Sterilize or sanitize your tools, if you want to start with really clean tools. Sanitize or sterilize your jar, knife, cutting board, tongs and glass bowl with boiling water or better, with bleach in the standard mixture with water. Use only Clorox brand bleach as it is the only bleach certified for sterilization. Use a 10% solution of Clorox, soak all utensils for 10 minutes, and then rinse with tap, R.O., DI, or distilled water. This is the ONLY way to assure that all bacteria are killed before beginning. This is the process that kill off any lurking bad bacteria and that's why, every beer maker has always used and works properly. Even pouring boiling water over something does not necessarily kill adverse bacteria. This is essential, if we want only the good kind growing in our veggies. Step 2: Prepare your cabbage for Sauerkraut. Rinse cabbage well, and remove the large outer leaves. (You may save these for later use). Using a sharp knife simply shred the cabbage and transfers it to a large glass bowl. Add about 2 Tablespoons of salt, then, using tongs or clean hands, massage the cabbage until it starts to break down from the salt. It will release moisture and reduce in size. Step 3: Transfer to a jar. Transfer the massaged cabbage to a clean glass jar, preferably one that is large enough to fit your hand through the top. The most important part of making fermented veggies is that you remove all the air in the jar so you want to pack the cabbage tightly, leaving no gaps. I used my fist to punch it down, but a clean wooden spoon would work, too. Step 4: Cover with water and reserved cabbage leaves. Like I mentioned above, the key to properly fermented sauerkraut is making sure there is no air remaining in the shredded cabbage. While there is already plenty of moisture released from the cabbage to make the brine, I like to add a little extra spring water (do not use tap water) to make sure the liquid level is completely ABOVE the shredded cabbage. Once you've added the water, use the reserved cabbage leaves to press down the shredded cabbage keeping it submerged under the liquid. Ideally, you'd fill up the jar all the way to the top, but mine didn't work out that way. If that's the case for you, too, simply fill a plastic bag with salt water (in case it bursts in the jar, you want it to be salt water) to use as a "weight." Place the salt water bag on top of the large cabbage leaf layer, and seal the jar. You should be able to see the liquid layer above the shredded cabbage line. Step 5: Store in an insulated bag for 3-7 days. If your house is a too warm or too cold, the insulated bag ensures that the fermentation process is kept at an even temperature. My sauerkraut took a full week to reach the classic "tangy" flavour this time around, but it may take less time in warmer climates. You can start checking on it after 3 days, just make sure the liquid level is high enough each time you re-seal the jar. Once the sauerkraut has fermented to your liking, remove the weight and outer leaves and discard. This is not uncommon for a layer of mould to develop on the outer leaves. This doesn't mean your sauerkraut is ruined. Simply discard the layer of mould, and everything underneath the brine should be safe. As always, use your best judgement if it smells off, don't eat it. Step 6: Store in the fridge and enjoy. I've had raw food teachers tell me that raw sauerkraut can last almost indefinitely in the fridge, but hopefully you'll eat it all before you can test that theory. It will definitely last for months in the fridge, so feel free to make a BIG batch.

Once you're comfortable making your own sauerkraut, feel free to get creative with the veggies you add to it, like, Ginger, beets, carrots, garlic, and lemon juice all make tasty additions.

Homemade Raw Sauerkraut

Ingredients:

- 1 head green or purple cabbage
- 2 Tablespoons sea salt
- 3. Spring or distilled water, as needed

Instructions: Start with really clean tools. Sanitize your jar, knife, cutting board, tongs and glass bowl with boiling water, which should kill off any lurking bad bacteria. We only want the good kind growing in our veggies. Rinse cabbage well, and remove the large outer leaves. Using a sharp knife shred the cabbage and transfers it to a large glass bowl. Add about 2 Tablespoons of salt, then, using tongs or clean hands, massage the cabbage until it starts to break down from the salt. It will release moisture and reduce in size.

Transfer the massaged cabbage to a clean glass jar, preferably one that is large enough to fit your hand through the top. The most important part of making fermented veggies is that you remove all the air in the jar and so you want to pack the cabbage tightly, leaving no gaps. I used my fist to punch it down, but a clean wooden spoon would work, too. While there is already plenty of moisture released from the cabbage to make the brine, I like to add a little extra spring water (do not use tap water) to make sure the liquid level is completely above the shredded cabbage.

Once you've added the water, use the reserved cabbage leaves to press down the shredded cabbage, keeping it submerged under the liquid. Ideally, you'd fill up the jar all the way to the top or simply fill a plastic bag with salt water (in case it bursts in the jar, you want it to be salt water) to use as a "weight." Place the salt water bag on top of the large cabbage leaf layer, and seal the jar. You should be able to see the liquid layer above the shredded cabbage line.

Store the sealed jar in an insulated bag for 3-7 days. You can start checking on it after 3 days, just make sure the liquid level is high enough each time you re-seal the jar. Once the sauerkraut has fermented to your liking, remove the weight and outer leaves and discard. Note: It's not uncommon for a layer of mould to develop on the outer leaves. This doesn't mean your sauerkraut is ruined! Simply discard the layer of mould, and everything underneath the brine should be safe. As always, use your best judgement-- if it smells off, don't eat it.

Store in the fridge and enjoy. The sauerkraut will last for months in the fridge, so feel free to make a BIG batch. Note: Once you're comfortable making your own sauerkraut, feel free to get creative with the veggies you add to it, Ginger, beets, carrots, garlic, and lemon juice all make tasty additions.

We've been making huge (as in 200 quarts) batches of sauerkraut for about 30 years. We make it in crocks, letting it ferment for about 2 months. If you "stomp" the cabbage until the juice flows, there is no need to add water (which will seriously dilute the flavour). This is a 2-times-a-year family tradition for us- once to make it and once to can it.

Benefit of Probiotic Foods that are super healthy: There are numerous health benefits consuming probiotics. There are many reasons that Probiotic Foods are super healthy.

- Probiotics are live microorganisms that have health benefits when consumed.
- These are usually beneficial bacteria that serve some function in the body.
- Probiotics have all sorts of powerful benefits for your body and brain.
- They may improve digestive health, reduce depression and promote heart health.
- Some evidence even suggests that they may give you better looking skin.

- Getting probiotics from supplements is popular, but you can also get them from foods that are prepared by bacterial fermentation (fermented foods).
- It helps to maintain the acid/base balance of the body, especially useful for toxic, acidic conditions.
- It is highly recommended for healing candidacies (Candida Yeast overgrowth).
- It is high in acetylcholine, a compound known to regulate the bowels, calm the nervous system, improve sleep patterns, and lower blood presser, indoles and sulphur, all of which are recommended by the National Cancer Institute for cancer prevention; supplies the body with easily assimilated, pre-digested nutrients. Most people who ordinarily experience difficulty digesting cabbage or other raw vegetables, have no trouble eating small amounts of unpasteurized sauerkraut.
- Helps to regulate blood sugar levels making it useful for hypoglycaemic and diabetics.

5.19 Healing IBS-C with Stomach Acid, hydrochloric acid and lucid acid naturally

Healthy stomach acid, called hydrochloric acid (HCL) is the key to creating the proper digestion and bowel speed. HCL starts the digestive process through the intestines and is also a first line body defence that destroys pathogens and toxins.

HCL is essential to protein digestion and the assimilation of B12, foliate and 15 minerals. Many people with low stomach acid (hypochlorhydria) or no stomach acid (achlorhydria) often complain of bloating, belching, a feeling of heaviness in the stomach after eating, or feeling full after eating only a small amount of food. People with low stomach acid may experience constipation, while others have diarrheal, depending on which pathogens have overgrown. And then, there are those with little or no stomach acid who experience absolutely no symptoms at all.

But HCL deficiency can also result in bad breath, asthma, allergies, food intolerance, anaemia, arthritis, parasites, depression, diabetes, hormonal imbalances (such as thyroid dysfunction, elevated cortical or adrenal fatigue), broken capillaries, weight gain, osteoporosis, lupus and other auto-immune conditions and chronic headaches, etc.

Consider this – your second brain is through the gut. Over two-thirds of neurotransmitters are made in the gut. Over 90% of serotonin, our happy neurotransmitter is made in the gut, and not the brain. If your gut is inflamed or not functioning optimally, production of serotonin will be impaired and the end result can be depression. Bear in mind that an inflamed gut = an inflamed brain = increased risk of depression and dementia.

To support digestion, drink water with fresh lemon or lime juice few minutes after your meals. (Drinking water during meals dilutes HCL and weakens digestion.) You can also take digestive bitters, a tablespoon of organic apple cider vinegar before food, pure sea salt and zinc supplements to boost HCL production. Eat slowly and chew well (try to count and chew 15 times). In some cases, supplementing with digestive enzymes may also be necessary.

You will experience a miraculously improved digestion with less bloating, better bowel habits and less heartburn! Your energy, strength, endurance and sleep will also improve, and even your athletic performance, as a result of better absorption of amino acids from protein, of minerals and other important nutrients. Low stomach acid leads to a cascade of digestive problems further south in the digestion process, such as bloating, gas and constipation. Fortunately, it is an option to heal low stomach acid naturally and ameliorate the chain affect of digestive problems.

Why is it so important to heal low stomach acid? Let's start with the all-to-common consequences of low stomach acid.

Consequences of Low Stomach Acid

Low stomach acid cannot properly break down proteins into amino acids. Lack of amino acids in the bloodstream means less available neurotransmitters which can mean mood disorders like depression. Additionally, protein maldigestion leads to hair loss and brittle nails.

Low stomach acid fosters imbalanced gut flora. Pathogenic and food borne bacteria, usually killed by the low stomach pH, can make their way into the intestines. Further, lack of acidity in the stomach makes it more hospitable to bacterial growth (and the stomach should be relatively sterile).

Low stomach acid leads to nutrient mal-absorption. Specifically, when proteins aren't fully broken down, B12 absorption is disrupted. Foliate and nonhuman iron absorption is also affected by low stomach acid.

Low stomach acid leads to heartburn/GERD/reflux. I discuss the details below.

Low stomach acid often means constipation, bloating, gas and belching. With inadequate acid, food sits in the stomach and putrefies instead of being properly digested.

Low stomach acid may cause a leaky gut and therefore create food allergies. Improperly digested starches provide little "holes" between the cells of the intestinal lining. These starches also feed pathogenic bacteria that create these leaky spaces. Then, undigested proteins and other food particles leak into the bloodstream and the body reacts by creating antibodies to these foreign particles in the blood.

The Lower Oesophageal Sphincter (LES) separates the esophagus and the stomach. Proper stomach acid levels signal the LES to close tightly. With low stomach acid levels, the LES loosens and acidic stomach fluid escapes into the lower part of the esophagus causing a burning sensation. LES malfunction is also influenced by other variables like food allergies, overeating, and certain drugs.

The pyloric sphincter separates the stomach from the small intestine. The body resists opening this sphincter, however, when the contents of the stomach are not properly acidified. The body innately knows the undigested food will cause problems further south. As a result, food sits in the stomach and putrefies, producing gas and pressure which makes the LES leak open (causing heartburn as discussed above).

Natural healing of Low Stomach Acid

We understand the cascade of detrimental digestive woes that can occur due to low stomach acid. We can heal "Low Stomach Acid" naturally and effectively:

1. Take Honey for Low Stomach Acid: Manuka honey is produced in New Zealand and Australia from bees pollinating the manuka tree. It has a naturally occurring peroxide content which makes it a potent anti-bacterial agent. This therapeutic honey has been widely used to heal stomach lining and to help address h. pylori overgrowth. I took 1 tsp. of this honey twice a day when I was first healing my stomach lining. Recently, I read from one source manuka honey should not be used internally because it has a naturally occurring genotoxin. I don't know what to think about this, however, since so many people take manuka honey and experience only vastly positive results. You can weigh the pros and cons for yourself.

Honey also has the potent antibacterial properties of manuka honey without the genotoxic component. Also, regular RAW honey is less antibacterial than these two famous "powerhouse" honeys but it is still very useful in healing the stomach lining. Only purchase raw honey, preferably from a local beekeeper– never purchase regular supermarket honey.

2. Take Vitamin U for Low Stomach Acid: I've heard of A, B, C, D, E, and K, but not U. That's because it's not a real vitamin, just a label for a powerful healing enzyme found in cabbage.

Cabbage	Raw Apple Cider Vinegar	Sauerkraut	

It is applauded for its anti-ulcer abilities and quickly cures stomach ulcers and heals the stomach lining. When stomach acid has been chronically low for years, the stomach lining may be inflamed and unable to tolerate acid supplementation. In this case, vitamin U is useful in soothing an inflamed stomach lining and correcting low stomach acid.

Many studies have been conducted where the participants drank raw cabbage juice and experienced quick ulcer healing. Large amounts of cabbage juice, however, can suppress thyroid activity due to the high amounts of goitrogens. So while a daily dose of raw cabbage juice may be a great option for some folks, others may find it both more suitable and more convenient to take a vitamin u supplement. I have had great success with Gastrazyme and I highly recommend it. 5 tablets before bed and 5 upon rising is a good place to start for a potent, short-term therapy.

3. Take Sea Salt (Raw Salt) for Low Stomach Acid: Eat plenty of unrefined sea salt with meals, such as Real Salt. This provides chloride, the building block of stomach acid (sodium chloride and hydrochloric acid).

4. Raw Apple Cider Vinegar for Low Stomach Acid: There are a few theories regarding just why apple cider vinegar improves digestion and low stomach acid. First, the vinegar is acidic and will slightly lower the pH in the stomach. Frequent doses of raw apple cider vinegar are also purportedly effective in correcting candida overgrowth, and candida problems can contribute to low stomach acid production. It is very effective as a quick solution when one is experiencing heartburn, perhaps because the acidity signals the LES to close tightly.

Upon waking, drink 1/2-1 tsp. raw apple cider vinegar (it must be raw) in 1/2 cup warm water. Take this concoction before each meal and, if needed, after meals to stop heartburn.

5. Take an apple in snack for Low Stomach Acid: Hydrochloric Acid with Pepsin supplements are an important tool in treating low stomach acid. It is only part of the solution in healing low stomach acid naturally and is a temporary step.

5.20 Magnesium Supplements-Healthy Colon hydrotherapy

Magnesium Phos is also known under the following names, spellings and abbreviations: Magnesia Phosphorus, Magnesia Phosphorica, Magnesia Phos, Magnesium Phosphate, Magnesium Phosphorus, Mag Phos, Mg Ph. Magnesium Phos is one of the 12 Homeopathic Cell Salts also termed Tissue Salts or Biochemic Salts. Cell Salts means minerals for cell health. Biochemistry developed by Dr. Schuster is use of minerals in homeopathic potency. Cell Salts are used successfully because minerals are the foundational nutrition for the body's enzyme activities and energy cycles and Cell Salts are instantly bio available.

This is a wonderful Healthy Colon hydrotherapy or Remedy for muscle spasms, cramps, pain and inflammation is "Mag Phos (Magnesia Phosphorica) Magnesium Phosphate 6x or 12x". This is an amazing antispasmodic remedy and helps those:

- Person suffers constantly from emotional ups & downs
- Helpful for spasms that affect the connective muscles, intestines, retinas, & blood vessels; dizziness; migraines; & nausea & cold sweats
- People who need this remedy tend to look thin & weak, have nutritional or allergy problems, & are plagued by cramps & nervousness
- Needed by the brain, heart, & muscles to relax
- Helpful if symptoms improve with heat & pressure, pain moves from place to place & is recurrent
- Pain may show up in head, stomach & bowels, & even in the ovaries & limbs -Good for toothaches
- Recommended for most kinds of cramps, including stomach cramps with flatulence
- Can cure stubborn cases of hiccups

- Helpful for chest pains
- Soothes arthritis & rheumatism -Good for vomiting & watery diarrhoea
- Helps with forgetfulness & lack of concentration -Relieves menstrual cramps
- Good for person with a thirst for cold drinks & sugar, & an aversion to coffee & a feeling of drowsiness
- Good for excruciating pain & extreme exhaustion
- Magnesium Phos is the best remedy for muscle spasms-back, leg, abdomen or calf. Use Magnesium Phos in the evening for a peaceful night sleep without muscle cramps or charley horses. Relax tight back muscles.
- Supports intestinal health and beneficial for abdominal spasms and intestinal problems such as colitis or constipation.
- Magnesium Phos calms agitated nerves for pain relief of headache, writer's cramp, sciatica, neuralgia.
- Use before and after dental work to calm tooth pain.
- Spasmodic is a key symptom and Magnesium Phos calms spasmodic coughs, hiccups, menstrual cramps.
- Magnesium helps with abdominal pains improved by eating.
- Magnesium Phos is homeopathic Magnesium phosphate.
- Lactose free formula.
- Liquid dilution for quick absorption.
- Beneficial for those who are lactose intolerant or have a dairy allergy.

Magnesium Phos is from magnesium, an important mineral that is involved in over 300 enzyme reactions in the body. "Homeopathic Magnesium Phos" goes quickly into the system for prompt relief. Studies have shown that most adults are deficient in the mineral magnesium. Refined foods, pollution, non-absorption and insufficient ability of the body to utilize magnesium in the body are some of the causes. It is especially recommended that diabetics, individuals with heart disease and those with high blood pressure have their magnesium levels checked. Magnesium Phos, especially in low potency 6x or 12X, can help your body utilize magnesium in the body and from food and is completely safe (unlike 500 mg supplements that can cause bowel overload with resulting diarrhoea). Cell Salts can improve the body's ability to absorb Magnesium. If lacking in Magnesium Phos, nerves are on edge with the inability to relax emotionally (showing as anxiety, nervous disorders, depression) and physically (showing as muscle problems, fibromyalgia-worse with even a light touch, nerve sensitivity-even the skin may feel overly sensitive). Deficiency symptoms include stress, pain, anxiety, depression, muscle spasms, migraine headaches, PMS headaches, agitation, irritability, constipation, fatigue. Person may feel pain is better from warmth, gentle pressure. Person may feel pain is worse with cold air, drafts. Magnesium Phos is found inside the cells of muscles, nerves, bones, the brain and spine. Deficiency affects muscle fibres and nerve endings. Magnesium is one of the trios including Potassium and Calcium involved in muscle function. Magnesium deficiency has been linked with CFS, Chronic Fatigue Syndrome. Consider Magnesium Phos when there has been nerve injury or damage. Speed injury recovery with Magnesium Phos.

- Magnesium Phos is indicated when nerve pain is shooting, darting, or spasmodic. Couple this with magnesium's presence in the brain and you'll see Magnesium Phos importance in neuralgias and   headaches.
  Magnesium Phos is the #1 mineral used within the cells for nerve pain.
- Indicated for migraines,
- fatigue,
- hearing disorders,
- Meniere's disease,
- Neuralgia,   panic   attacks.
  Works successfully with other therapies.
- Absorbs instantly, great for people with digestion difficulties.
- Abdominal: Helpful for intestinal problems, calm spasmodic abdominal cramping.
- Colic: Useful for colic with much gas and belching, without relief.
- Menstrual cramps: Helpful for menstrual cramps that are relieved by onset of flow.
- Shooting, darting pains.
- Muscle spasms: Useful for leg cramps and writer's cramp Pain: Helpful for pain with sharp, cutting, shooting, and constricting sensation.
- PMS: Useful for irritability, intestinal symptoms, anxiety, PMS headaches.
- Cell Salts are used successfully because they are the foundational nutrition for the body's enzyme activities and energy cycles. Cell Salts are instantly bio available.

- Use suggested dose is 3 sprays at one time and repeated 3 times a day for treatment of symptoms. Use fewer doses as symptoms improve. But for general health use 3 sprays daily.

There are much benefits of magnesium, colon hydrotherapy in mitigating chronic constipation. For many people, a simple lack of dietary magnesium is responsible for chronic constipation. The Standard American Diet (SAD) is dominated by processed meat, dairy, and grain products, but lacks significantly in foods that contain magnesium. An important mineral for healthy bowel function, magnesium is required by your digestive muscles to process and move food.

"Magnesium normalizes tension on colon walls allowing for a normal peristaltic action," explains the website for Natural Vitality's Natural Calm magnesium supplement. "Also, magnesium attracts water and allows you to bring in more water into your colon." Colonics, and specifically colon hydrotherapy, is another option for maintaining regularity. Colon hydrotherapy involves cleansing the colon with an enema of water, or in some cases, coffee -- you can learn more about the benefits of coffee enemas for the purpose of flushing out impacted faecal matter and other waste that can clog the digestive tract and cause constipation.

Magnesium Dosage for Constipation

Magnesium is used to treat constipation and IBS. However, it needs to be taken in right dose. This article deals with the dosage and the benefits of magnesium for treating constipation. Constipation is one of the most discomfort causing conditions. If you too suffer from constipation, you may be looking for different methods to get rid of it. A large number of medications are available in the market for treating constipation. People may even recommend you to use home remedies for getting rid of constipation. You must have also heard about the use of magnesium for treating constipation. Let us first take a look at the benefits of taking magnesium for treating constipation.

Magnesium is a widely used laxative as it works in two different ways for treating constipation. Firstly, magnesium helps in drawing in water which increases the amount of water in the colon. The increased amount of water in the colon helps in softening stools, and makes them easy to pass from the intestines. Secondly, magnesium helps in relaxing the muscles of the colon or the intestine, which makes easier movement of the stools. Magnesium citrate, milk of magnesia, magnesium oxide is all helpful in treating constipation.

Magnesium Dosage

Magnesium supplements are easily available in the market and do not require any prescription. If you are wondering what should be the dosage of magnesium for treating constipation, then note that 400-500 milligrams of magnesium citrate per day is usually the ideal dose for treating constipation. However, note that there are several factors that need to be taken into consideration when taking these magnesium supplements for constipation, e.g., the dosage of magnesium for constipation in children varies from that of adults. Children, teenagers and young adults require a lesser dose. On the other hand, the dosage of magnesium for constipation during pregnancy should only be determined on consulting the doctor. Similarly, people suffering from a chronic disorder or taking drugs for hypoglycaemia, etc., should consult the doctor as magnesium can affect the function of these drugs. In short, one should note that even though these supplements are obtained without a prescription, it is recommended that one should consult the doctor before taking these supplements as laxatives on daily basis. Although magnesium supplements are effective in treating constipation, it is essential to find out the cause of constipation and try to correct it. As mentioned above, in most of the cases, constipation is caused due to having an improper diet. Therefore, one should make changes in the diet and have fibre rich food (fruits, vegetables, whole grains, etc.). Lack of activity throughout the day can also lead to chronic constipation. Therefore, one should exercise regularly to loosen up the bowels and prevent constipation. Lastly, if it is found that constipation is caused due to some underlying medical condition, one should consult the doctor immediately and try to get the condition treated as soon as possible. Lastly, we can conclude by saying that, magnesium dosage for treating constipation depends on several factors like the age of the person, the severity of the condition, the overall health of the person, etc. Therefore, one should take these laxatives only after consulting the doctor.

5.21 Colon cleansing

The need for colon cleansing is based on the theory that undigested meat and other foods, medications, and chemical or substances that we ingest cause a build-up of mucus in the colon. Over time, this accumulation of mucus produces toxins which circulate throughout the body through the bloodstream, ultimately poisoning the body. Colon cleansing is also sometimes needed before some medical procedures and for some medical conditions, such as before a colonoscopy or some surgeries. No matter what reason you want a colon cleanse, there are some ways to make one at home. You can improve your health and avoid serious health problems that develop from having a toxic colon. The good news is, there are some really excellent and simple ways you can protect your colon to be toxic.

The first step is learning about the benefits of colon cleansing and how keeping your elimination system strong, and in optimal working order, is vital to living a long, healthy life.

Our digestive systems are never designed to handle this type of food, not to mention all the fats, sugar, and preservatives commonly found within most every product on our grocery store shelves.

Obviously, we aren't going to stop eating. But even if you're careful with your diet, watching what you eat all the time; it's almost inevitably that our digestive tracts, and particularly your colon, can become compromised. Over time your colon can become partially blocked, terribly distorted, or dysfunctional through years of poor eating habits, stress, alcohol or drug use.

The end result can be dehydration causing chronic constipation, or alternating bouts of diarrhoea and poor general health.

In fact, many people who are not particularly overweight or obese may be carrying around 10 to 25 pounds of dried faecal matter in their colons. Overweight, over stressed, or people with severe allergies could easily have even more than that. Children are not exempt either, and poor eating habits may lead to a lifetime of digestive disorders, if ignored.

Accumulated waste built up in your colon can lead to colon toxicity which is responsible for many body imbalances, and could be the underlying cause of many of the weight and health problems we see people struggling with every day.

The first step to a truly successful weight loss program, may involve cleansing your colon and a visit to your local colon hydro therapist.

Maintaining a healthy colon is vital to helping you maintain a healthy body, and essential to regaining optimum health. If you want to prevent colon toxicity, chronic disease and premature aging, cleansing your colon is essential.

If you are carrying around toxic metabolic waste in your colon day after day, for weeks or even months at a time, you cannot possibly maintain a healthy body. This unwanted build-up adheres to the walls of your colon and can interfere with natural peristalsis, the wave-like muscle contractions which move waste deposits along the approximate 5½ feet of your colon, and ultimate elimination.

- This colon dysfunction, along with inadequate daily water consumption, can be a primary contributor to chronic constipation.

- When large amounts of the colon's surface become coated with impermeable dried faecal matter and lumps of mucous, 7 things can happen:
- Delays in expelling faecal matter increase the amount of toxins absorbed into your body.
- The absorption of nutrients that your body needs is severely restricted.
- Water within the colon, that would normally be filtered back into the bloodstream, cannot be reabsorbed which leads to dehydration and autointoxication.
- You may experience low energy levels, general muscle weakness, daily fatigue at work, and restless sleeping habits at night.
- This toxic environment is the perfect breeding ground for harmful bacteria and parasites.
- Chronic problems with constipation, irritable bowel syndrome and diarrhoea.

Unexplained weight gains, and an inability to control or lose the excess weight, even though you eat a moderate, balanced diet.

Left untreated, a toxic colon can prevent you from metabolizing food, fat and absorbing the nutrients from the food you eat. Eventually your body and your health deteriorate further, leading to disease and in extreme cases, death.

But this is entirely preventable. Colon cleansing is the best defence against colon toxicity developing, as well as maintaining a healthy diet and active lifestyle. Don't let an unhealthy colon become a breeding ground for toxic poisons, parasites, disease and death. Cleanse your colon today using a natural colon cleanser and visit a colon hydro therapist if one is available in your area.

Many people suffer from chronic constipation, irritable bowel syndrome, leaky gut and other issues with the digestive system. Because the colon has an important job of eliminating waste, it's critical that you keep it running smoothly. Fortunately, there are things you can do to help alleviate discomfort associated with toxins and digestion issues in the body, such as a homemade colon cleanse.

I have shared details about why a colon cleanse is important, but what's great is that you don't need to see a doctor about it and can make your own colon cleanser right at home. A homemade colon cleanse can help flush out some of the toxins in your body that could be contributing to your discomfort and also offer natural relief from constipation. Just plan a day when you do not need to leave home so that you are able to adjust to the colon cleansing changes in your body and the elimination of waste as you begin the detoxify and internal cleansing process.

Apple, Sea Salt, Ginger and Lemon Colon Cleanse

Let's get started making this great homemade colon cleanse. You will need a tall glass and a spoon. To start, place 3.5 ounces of purified water in a pan. You want to warm the water, not boil it, so that you can drink the water at a safe temperature.

Once it is warm, pour it into your glass. Then add the sea salt, often part of salt water flush, and stir. The sea salt will help release toxins, pushing waste through the body and ultimately improving digestion.

Now, add the apple juice, ginger juice and fresh lemon juice. Stir. Where do you think an apple a day keeps the doctor away came from? Well, maybe it is not specific to the colon but it did come from the idea that whole foods, such as the nutrition-rich apple, brings good health and a healthy colon definitely yields good health. In fact, a study shows that those who ate an apple a day had less visits to the doctor and fewer prescription medications.

Ginger is great because it reduces bloating while stimulating the colon, keeping it free from wastes and harmful toxins. Lemon juice aids in digestion, detoxification and is high in vitamin C, making it a great antioxidant, that's why it plays such a key role in my "Secret Deter drink."

Cleanse Method: Drink this first thing in the morning on an empty stomach. Then have this mixture again just before a light lunch, preferably of steamed vegetables and baked salmon, and again mid-afternoon.

Have 6–8 glasses of room temperature water throughout the day. It may be best to slow down the consumption of liquids after 5 p.m. so that you are not awakened in the night, with having to go to the bathroom.

Precaution: Performing this type of colon cleanse should not present any problems; however, it is always good to check with your doctor if you are pregnant, have a disease, suffer from allergies or are taking any prescriptions medications prior to any new activity.

Homemade Colon Cleanse

Juice: Total Time- 5 minutes
Serves: 1 serving
Ingredients:
½ cup 100 percent pure organic apple juice
2 tablespoons fresh lemon juice

1 teaspoon ginger juice
½ teaspoon sea salt
½ cup warm purified water

Directions: Start with a tall glass and a spoon. Place 3.5 ounces of purified water in a pan. You want to warm the water, not boil it, so that you can drink the water at a safe temperature. Once it is warm, pour it into your glass. Then add the sea salt and stir. Add the apple juice, ginger juice and fresh lemon juice. Stir. Drink first thing in the morning on an empty stomach. Then have this mixture again just before a light lunch, and again mid-afternoon. However, with the help of colon cleansing, you can easily get rid of harmful toxins and promote healthy intestinal bacteria. It will also help increase your energy and improve the body's absorption of vitamins and nutrients. There are many treatments available for colon cleansing. But for many people, the best options are simple, natural home remedies.

Here are the top 10 home remedies for colon cleansing. Before starting any colon cleansing program, consult your doctor for proper guidance, especially if you are taking any medications or suffering from any health condition.

1. Pure Water: For colon cleansing, the best thing you can do is drink plenty of water. It is essential to drink at least 10 to 12 glasses of water in a day. Regular consumption of water will give your body the liquid and lubrication required to flush out the harmful toxins and waste from the body in a natural manner. Drinking plenty of water will also stimulate the natural peristaltic action, helping the food to move through the digestive system. Also, water is essential to keep your body well hydrated. Along with water, you can also drink fresh fruit and vegetable juices.

2. Apple Juice: Fresh apple juice is one of the best home remedies for colon cleansing. Drinking apple juice regularly encourages bowel movements, breaks down toxins and improves the health of liver as well as the digestive system. Freshly squeezed apple juice provides the best results, but if it is not available, you can use packaged organic apple juice. Start your day with one glass of unfiltered apple juice. After 30 minutes, drink one glass of water. Repeat this routine several times throughout the day and continue for three days. In between, you can also drink one glass of prune juice. When following this remedy, it is advisable to avoid solid foods.

3. Lemon Juice: Lemon has antioxidant properties and its high vitamin C content is good for the digestive system. Hence, lemon juice can be used for colon cleansing. Mix the juice of one lemon, a pinch of sea salt and a little honey in a glass of lukewarm water. Drink this solution on an empty stomach in the morning. This will help you to enjoy more energy, better bowel movement and better skin condition. Add two tablespoons of fresh-squeezed lemon juice to a glass of apple juice. Drink it three or four times a day. This will thin out the mucous in the bowel. Follow either of these remedies for a few days.

4. Raw Vegetable Juice: For colon cleansing, it is essential to keep away from processed and cooked food for one or two days. Instead of solid food, drink fresh vegetable juice several times a day. Green vegetables, in particular contain chlorophyll that helps remove toxins. Also, the vitamins, minerals, amino acids, and enzymes present in it will keep your body healthy and well energized. You can also drink herbal teas. It is advisable not to use ready-made vegetable juices as they do not contain the effective enzymes that help your body break down and remove waste products. You can easily make fresh vegetable juice from carrots, beets, corn, squash, spinach, kale, etc. at home using a juicer or blender.

5. Fibre-rich Foods: Eating foods rich in fibre will help cleanse the colon of the harmful toxins. Fibre helps keep the stools soft and improve the bowel movement, which ultimately encourages the body to expel waste products. At the same time, fibre-rich foods will also help get rid of any kind of intestinal problems? You can add a lot of fibre into your diet by eating fresh fruits like raspberries, pears and apples, as well as fresh vegetables like artichokes, peas and broccoli. Cereals, whole grains, nuts, beans and seeds also contain a good amount of fibre.

6. Yogurt: Eating fresh yogurt on a regular basis is a good way to keep the colon healthy. Being a probiotic food, yogurt, especially the one with live and active cultures, will introduce "good" bacteria into the gut that promote digestion. It will also combat inflammatory bowel diseases. Plus, it contains a good amount of calcium that discourages the growth of cells lining the colon. The intestine-friendly yogurt also solves various stomach problems such as indigestion, flatulence, irregular bowel movements and lots more. You can eat yogurt as it is or add some fresh fruit such as apples, limes, bananas and berries.

Vegetable and Fruit based Colon Cleanses

1. Pick the right ingredients: For natural, food based cleanses, you need to pick the right foods. Vegetables contain fibre that is essential for healthy and frequent bowel movements. Pick the freshest fruit you can, and try to buy organic is possible. You want to be ingesting as many nutrients as possible with no additives. Make sure all vegetables and fruits are raw when you use them in the cleanse. Good produce to include is:

- Spinach
- Asparagus
- Brussels sprouts
- Cabbage
- Celery
- Collard greens
- Leeks
- Peas
- Swiss chard
- Mustard greens
- Dark green lettuces
- Wheatgrass
- Kale
- Bok Choy
- Parsley
- Cilantro
- Cucumber
- Beets and beet greens

2. Prepare the ingredients: The best ways to use fresh produce for a colon cleanse is to use a juicer or to make them as smoothes in a blender. The juices will kick start your colon and also give you added energy, and the edible skins give you added fibre. You can also add organic apple juice as needed to the juice to make it thin enough to drink easily. Apple juice contains pectin, a kind of fibre which is very helpful in achieving complete bowel movement.

You can mix and match vegetables to your own taste, but you should add enough to have three eight ounce glasses every day for five to seven days. Add some fruit to improve the taste. Use bananas, oranges, cherries, berries, plums, or apples. If you leave the edible skins on the fruit, it will give you an added boost of fibre.

3. Try a green cleanse: If you aren't sure what kind of recipe to start with, try a green cleanse recipe. Chop two apples, four stalks of celery without the leaves, one cucumber, six kale leaves and add it to a blender or juicer. Add one tablespoon of finely chopped fresh ginger root and lemon juice. Blend or juice and enjoy.

If this mixture is too bitter, try adding one teaspoon of honey to sweeten it.

4. Mix a leafy fruit cleanse: If you don't like straight greens, try a recipe with more fruit. Mix two peeled oranges, one quartered and cored apple, two tablespoons of lemon juice, 1 cup of spinach, and one kale leaf in a juicer or blender. Once smooth or juiced, drink and enjoy. You can add a little apple juice if this mixture isn't thin enough for you. You can also add some baby carrots for some extra colour, fibre, and sweetness.

5. Make an aloe Vera juice cleanse: For a more nutrient packed cleanse, try an aloe Vera juice based cleanse. Add together one cup aloe Vera juice, ½ cup of rolled oats, one cup spinach, two kale leaves, five Swiss chard leaves, one peeled banana, ½ a medium cucumber, ½ cup of blueberries, and one teaspoon of cinnamon. You can either put it through a juicer or mix it in a blender. Once smooth or juiced, drink and enjoy. You can add some honey if it isn't sweet enough.

Making a Mineral Cleanse

1. Learn about betonies clay: One popular cleanse for colon health is a psyllium and betonies clay cleanse. Betonies clay is a mixture of mineral salts, which includes calcium betonies and sodium betonies. This clay absorbs many times its weight in water as well as minerals, toxins, and organic substances. This ability makes betonies clay useful in cleanses. It is commonly used by natural health professionals and has found a place in mainstream medicine to safely treat various types of poisonings and overdoses.

Betonies clay and psyllium husks, a naturally derived fibre-heavy powder, can be purchased online or at your local health food store.

2. Make the cleanse: To make this cleanse, add one rounded teaspoon psyllium husk, which can be dark yellow or brown husks, to one teaspoon of betonies clay powder to an empty glass. Add eight ounces water or pure, organic apple juice to the glass, stirring briskly to dissolve the powder. Drink it quickly before it has time to thicken.

This should immediately be followed by another eight ounces of water or apple juice. You can also get betonies clay in liquid form.

5.22   Heal Your Solar Plexus Chakra:

Healing the solar plexus chakra is a simple process, but it may take some practice. Most people have built up a blockage over many years, so chakra balancing will take time. There are some solar plexus chakra healing exercises that are easy to practice every day.

The chakra colour associated with Manipura is yellow, which means that bananas, sunflower seeds, yellow peppers and cheeses are good solar plexus chakra healing food. Spices for the solar plexus chakra are ginger, chamomile, mint, and cumin.

Meditation can help with opening Manipura. A simple exercise is to simply envision a brilliant yellow sunflower over your solar plexus chakra. This can be even more effective with the use of chakra stones. Solar plexus chakra healing stones include yellow stones like citrine, amber, yellow tourmaline and tiger's eye.

Aromatherapy can also be helpful for Manipura chakra healing. It can be used while meditating or doing yoga, or by itself at any time. Citrusy essential oils like orange and grapefruit are good for healing the solar plexus chakra, as are chamomile, mint and ginger.

Regular yoga practice is ideal for chakra balancing. Asanas that focus on core strength are perfect for Manipura healing. Warrior Pose is the easiest yoga asana for opening Manipura. Holding it for a few minutes every morning will begin to open your solar plexus. Other helpful asanas are Boat Pose (Navasana), which strengthens the core, and Sun Salutations (Surya Namaskar). Engaging in structured risk-taking during your yoga practice, like doing a challenging pose or gently pushing yourself a bit more, can also help balance Manipura.

Finally, since the solar plexus chakra is associated with the sun and fire, simply getting outside can help. Meditating or doing yoga outdoors on sunny days will maximize your healing practice, but simply going outside for a walk or doing a little sunbathing will help open your solar plexus chakra.

The Solar Plexus Chakra, or Manipura, rules lessons involving fear of rejection, your self esteem, and sensitivity to criticism, a distorted self image, and fear of you're "secrets being found out". The wisdom of the Solar Plexus involves your sense of personal power and knowing, your personality and your sense of belonging. An imbalance in the Manipura might manifest as poor decisions, poor concentration, trouble taking action and getting things done, and an inability to judge a situation accurately. Imbalances in this Chakra can create feelings that you are more, or less, than other people. Emotional memories are stored within the Manipura, and it is where your 'gut feelings' originate, it is the centre of your emotional life, and many are naturally connected to the environment through the Solar Plexus chakra.

The Third Chakra is right above your belly button, at the centre of your solar plexus. Its colour is yellow. It is connected to the mental layer of the aura. The mental layer of the aura vibrates with, and is formed by, our thoughts, and is a fine, bright yellow energy. It pulsates and thickens when we concentrate and focus our minds.

Third Chakra foods are grains, pasta, bread, granola, cereal, flax seed, rice, sunflower seeds. Dairy foods like milk, yogurt and cheese, and spices such as ginger, mint, chamomile, cumin, turmeric and fennel.

Perhaps the most direct way to awaken the vibrant, personal power within your Solar Plexus is through sound; just 27 minutes with a pair of headphones and our Alpha Level Binaural Beats can deliver the ego boost you need! Cutting edge sound healing techniques combined with ancient Chakra balancing traditions, this program features Tibetan Singing Bowls tuned to the 3rd Chakra, and the Binaural Beats utilize a Solfeggio frequency of 528 Hz. The sound progresses along Earth Resonant frequencies to a low of 7.83 Hz (Schumann Resonance) and ramps back up to an Earth Resonance of 14.1 Hz. This deeply relaxing and releasing meditation will not only help to balance your Solar Plexus Chakra, it will also balance your mind and spirit to the frequencies of our Mother Earth.

Begin healing now. Balance your Solar Plexus Chakra with healing sound, colour and words.

Solar Plexus is the pit of the stomach and is one of the great autonomic plexuses of the body in which the nerve fibres of the sympathetic system and the parasympathetic system combine. It is a dense cluster of nerve cells and supporting tissue. It is also known as the celiac plexus. Through branches, it controls many vital functions such as adrenal secretion and intestinal contraction etc. It circulates energy to the entire body and plays an important role in the development, circulation and control of human life. It is also known as the second brain of our body. There is a strong relationship between navel and brain. As humans are becoming more and more modern and materialistic, the stress is also increasing, which causes the Solar Plexus (Navel) imbalance. In Hindi it is called "Naavi Utarna". Any fear arising inside the human brain directly affects the navel.

There is no treatment of Solar Plexus (Navel) imbalance in Allopathic except in Ayurveda, Unani and Tibb Arabi systems of medicine. A balanced and healthy navel centre increases physical energy, brightens the aura of the body, enhances physical attraction and beauty. It keeps the person, active and energetic, stress free, makes the nerves and muscles active, increases the memory and produces healthy semen. Navel is deeply related to our digestive system; hence any imbalance in navel leads to sour belches, indigestion, constipation, loose motions etc. and causes

sudden weight gains and losses. There is frequent misalignment of
the navel and stomach muscles, which occur just like a misalignment
within the spinal cord. Normally the displacement of the navel has
relation to weakening of ligaments related to large intestine. There are
several reasons for this imbalance, like lifting heavy weights, while
playing, eating very spicy food, when the person loses control while
walking due to some obstruction or holes on the road, or some
physical action which is done carelessly, and also emotional
disturbance, jumping or landing on one leg or pressure falling on one
leg, picking up heavy objects, a sudden twisting or bending
movement, sexual activity. The displacement is directly connected
with the nervous system, stomach and muscles and will affect each of
these in some manner. Unhealthy navel causes impotency too. The
displacement is said to occur more in women and may produce
unaccountable menstrual pain and excessive or scanty bleeding.
Allopathic medicines don't work because it is due to the displacement
of a nerve from its usual place in the body.

Imbalance in navel causes sudden weight gains and losses, which
affects the physical structure and look of the person. Balanced
navel is necessary for healthy mind, body and soul. Balanced
navel prevents stomach related problems. A healthy navel centre
increases physical energy and brightens the aura of the body.
The physical attraction and beauty get enhanced. A balanced and
healthy navel centre balances the mind and brain and keeps
the person stress free and increases the memory. A person with
healthy navel centre remains active and energetic. Navel
displacement is the condition when the navel Centre shifts upward,
downward, left side or right side of Navel centre. It is also called shift
in solar plexus. Sometimes Solar Plexus shifts are confused with
hiatus hernias due to wrong diagnosis. The centre shifts upward or
downward when excess weight is lifted, or when there is severe gas
trouble. In such cases, the throbbing will not be noticed somewhere
around the navel. The upward shifting of the solar plexus leads to
constipation, and the downward shifting brings more motions every
time there is a pressure or diarrhoea. If a person has cancer of the
colon, there is chronic constipation and it has been found out that the
solar plexus has moved upwards.

Solar Plexus Imbalance Indications:
To check the navel position there are various methods:

(i) Join both your palms together and try to match the lines of both palms and base of the little fingers with each other. If the top lines do not match, it indicates imbalance in solar plexus.

(ii) Let the patient lie down on a flat surface and join the toes of both the feet together. If there is imbalance of Solar Plexus, then one of the toes will be taller than the other.

(iii) In the morning, before taking any food, place the thumb on the navel. If you feel vibrations or pulsations like the heart beating, the navel is at its correct place.

(iv) Lie on your back. Put both arms at the side of the body and both big toes together. If both the big toes are parallel, it is an indication that the navel is central, otherwise slippage is indicated. (v) Put both hands out straight in front so that the palms touch on the sides. Just below the little finger there is a `heart line` in the palm. With both the heart lines in one line, check whether the top ends of the little fingers are matching i.ein one line. If not, the navel is most likely displaced.

(vi) Lie down on his back on a hard floor. Apply massaging oil like olive oil or ointment around the navel. With slow circular motions of the thumb in clockwise direction the area around the navel is massaged pushing the area towards the Centre of navel. The misalignment can also be detected, by a string. Lie down on a flat surface - facing upwards. Measure the distance from the large toe of both feet, to the navel centre using a string. If there is a difference in the length of these two measurements, it indicates a shift in the navel position. However, when measuring the position with string, care should be taken to ensure that the body is correctly aligned.

(vii) Nipples Method: The patient should first be made to lie on his back comfortably with the arms at the sides touching the ground. The examiner should place one end of a piece of string on the patient's navel, the other end on one of the two nipples of his/her chest. Then this end of string should be held to the other nipple. The hand holding the string on the navel to remain as it is. If the distance between the navel and the two nipples is the same, the navel is in the right place. If there is even a slight variation in the two distances, the navel is dislodged from its natural position. With the chest bared, measurement is taken with a non-elastic thread or tape from the centre of the navel to each breast nipple. There should be no difference between these two measurements if the navel is in its right place, if there is a difference, and then there is dislocation of navel.

Solar Plexus Shifting and its Problems: Apart from the acute abdomen pain patients experience heartburn and regurgitation, when stomach acid reaches the esophagus. Sometimes the upward movement of the Solar Plexus compresses the diaphragm which the protective layer around the heart and it may be wrongly thought that there is some problem in the heart. Solar Plexus moves upwards or downwards. Upwards causes constipation and downwards causes diarrhoea. While in most cases the navel will move in an upward or downward direction, a sideways movement is also sometimes noticeable. The displacement is directly connected with the navel, nerves, and stomach muscles and will affect each of these in some manner. When navel shifts towards left hip, the person complains of pain and tension on the right upper side of the body and this could affect the liver, gall bladder, abdomen and right kidney. Sometimes the person also complains of pain in lumbar region (waist part) or left leg. When navel shifts towards left side, it affects the right side of the body. It causes stiffness in kidneys, intestines along with pain. When navel shifts towards left side, it causes pain, tension and stiffness in the right lower part of the body. It affects the pancreas, spleen and left kidney. It could also lead to menstrual disorders in women. When navel shifts towards right side, it causes pain and tension on the lower side of the body, and affects liver, gall bladder, and left kidney along with intestinal problems.

Medicines: Medicines don't work for cases of dislocations because it is due to the displacement of a nerve from its usual place in the body. Physical intervention is a must. However medicines do help in maintenance and upkeep.

Homeopathic Medicines Treatment:

Use Alumina 30 three doses daily (if the navel is abnormally pulled back) and causes constipation.

Use Spigelia 30 three doses daily for pulled nerves, strangulated nerves, or pain around navel.

Use Antimonium Crudum 30 three doses daily for stomach disorders, dioscorea or radiating pains.

Use Arnica 30 three doses daily for regular pains.

Herbal Treatment:

- Rapeseed oil: Take a cloth, big enough to cover the navel from all sides. Soak it with rapeseed oil (Torai ke beej or Tilli ke beej or Sarsoon ke beej) and pour a few drops in the navel and place the soaked cloth on all sides of the navel. Do this once a week.

- Saunf: Take powder of 25 grams of Saunf (Fennel seeds) and take it with Jiggery ("Gud" in hindi). Eat this but do not take water for half an hour.
- Ginger: Pour ginger juice on navel and massage the area to control loose motions and cure all stomach diseases.
- Milkweed: Apply the latex of milkweed (Aak ke patte ka doodh) on the navel region to cure dislocation.
- Bush Lucerne (Desmodium gyroides): It is helpful.

Foods Treatment:

Amla (Indian gooseberry) is considered good as a medicine for this disease.

Most yellow skinned or fleshed foods (fruits and vegetables) are good for energizing the Solar Plexus, such as, are yellow corn, grapefruit, lemons, yellow squashes, yellow lentils, Bananas, Mangoes, Pears, Yellow apples, yellow peppers, Star fruit, quince etc. The herbs and spices belonging to the yellow group are ginger, peppermint, spearmint, Melissa, turmeric, cumin, fennel, Dandelion flowers and chamomile. Eating these foods is beneficial.

Yellow colour foods are instant energy boosters and have great nutritional value.

These are foods good for the nervous system and directly involved with the organs that are a part of the digestive system.

Most yellow skinned or fleshed Essential Oils, such as, Rosemary, Peppermint, Carnation, Bergamot, Cedar wood, Vertivert, juniper and lavender. However it is important to use only therapeutic-grade (natural) essential oils. If you are pregnant or suffering from serious health conditions consult a Doctor before using these Oils.

Seed Mantra Meditation Treatment: Practice: RAM (pronounced as rum) is the seed or beej mantra of the Solar Plexus Chakra. Sit away from any support in cross legged or lotus pose and take deep breaths. Visualise the colour yellow in the region of the chakra and chant 'RAM' three times, then chant 'OM' three times and feel the flow of the energy vibrating from head to toe. Now repeat the chant mentally beginning with RAM then chant OM, three times. This is one set. Continue to chant RAM and OM, till you wish to. The seed invocation is a form of a charged mantra. The sound when chanted resonates and reaches directly to the centre of the solar plexus chakra and immediately opens it. The beej meditation will increase the circumference of the chakra and balance it. Benefits: Problems and diseases related to abdomen like digestive disorders, lack of energy, anger, fear, hatred, or excessive need of authority and power can be eased out.

Solar Plexus Balancing/Correction & Setting right:

(1) The Toes Method: Lie on your back, keeping your arms straight on your sides. Let the patient lie down on back on a flat surface. Keep the legs straight and the toes upright and look at the toes. The two big toes must be level. If they are not, it indicates a disturbance in the solar plexus. Put arms straight on side, feet straight. Check the toes then keep your one hand on the knee of the leg whose big toe is on lower level and with other hand keeping the long finger between two big toes try to pull the one which is lower. Check again. If the thumbs are equal in height, thus the solar plexus has been corrected. Do it twice or thrice a day. Repeat this action 2 to 4 times till both the big toes comes in level.

(2) Lie down facing floor Method: Ask the partner to lift up your left hand and the left leg catching from ankles and wrist. Ask him to place one of his legs very firmly in the centre of your back at around L5 position. Carefully and slowly start pulling both leg and hand simultaneously upwards and towards centre perpendicular to your back. Do the same way with the other hand and other leg. Do it one or two times. It should correct.

(3) Lie down on the floor facing the floor Method: Catch both the ankles of the legs with respective hands like the way we do in Dhanurasana. It should be very firmly caught with a good grip. Ask the partner to stand in the middle portion of your body with his both legs on both sides of your body firmly earthed to the floor. He should be a strong person. Ask him to catch your ankle or your leg or wrist of your hand and ask him to lift you upwards whole body from the floor. It should be done very slowly. Do it once only. It will surely bring the navel in place.

Toes Method	Candle Method	Vacuum Method

(4) Raising both legs Method: The patient raises both legs while inhaling in shalabhasana position. In other words, the patient while lying down flat on his back rises up both legs to 90 degrees while

inhaling. Then bends fully both the knees, and tries to bring the knees towards the chest. While both the knees are held in this position the person doing the treatment, standing at his feet puts his palms one on each knee exerting a little pressure on both knees equally. Supposing the measurement of the right nipple is higher, and then holding both the knees exert pressure on the patient's right knee to push it towards the navel, while keeping the left knee undisturbed. Repeat these two or three times. The patient then returns his legs to the original position lying flat. Again the nipple measurements are taken to confirm that there is no difference. If the difference is still there, the treatment is repeated. Supposing the left nipple measurement is more, and then the left knee is pressed, and so on. With the grace of GOD, this is a very sure and effective treatment.

(5) Massaging Method: Another method involves an herbal pack placed on the stomach. These latter methods are local Indian methods, usually practiced in the villages. They provide good treatment, but fail to prevent recurrence. They can be used successfully in conjunction with Yoga Asanas. The person getting massage should lie down on his or her back. The massager should then put his three fingers excluding the little finger-and the thumb into the depth of the navel to feel the pulsation. The pulsation shall be registered by the middle finger. In case of every healthy person, if pulsation is not felt, let the subject relax, and relax your own fingers. Try to feel it again if no pulsation is registered by any of the three fingers the subject will be having problems of stomach-and intestines. Some effort to bring the dislocated nerve back in its original position is to be made sucking the air through a blower-causing vacuum set the nerve in its right position. This method should be properly learnt from an expert before exercising it on any subject in massage. Then the massager should pour the oil into the navel until navel is full. There is a folk belief that a deep navel is a good quality navel. Protruded navel is supposed to be demonic-and persons having bulging navels are eternally dissatisfied. The navel is also the Centre of gravity. Inhuman body there are many lymph nodes in this area, and circular movement clockwise given by the massager helps circulation of digestive fluids in this area. The massager should then press on both sides at the place where the ribcage ends. On the right side of the person getting massage is the location of his or her liver and on the left side his or her stomach is located. Pain experienced by the subject on any side during the gentle pressing by the massager indicates problem in that organ. Pain experienced on the right side indicates problem of liver, and pain experienced on the

left side indicates swelling on the mouth of the stomach. The massage in these areas should be gentler than the normal massage done by the massager. Massage the navel area in increasing circles thoroughly. Then massage under the rib-cage from inside to outside. After working in the area above the rib-cage pay a little attention to the cartilage bone which is joining the last few ribs in the centre of the chest. Circular movement here helps depression. Massage the top of the chest in circular movement going downwards on the inside, and upwards on the outside. Massage of the breasts is slightly different from the massage of the chest. While massaging breasts go around the breasts in circular movement making your circles gradually smaller till you reach the nipples. This gives proper shape to the breasts. Pull the nipple both in men and women with a little pressure given by the thumb and the forefinger. The pulling should be done lightly, but excite all the fine capillaries of blood vascular system, and increase circulation of lymph as there is a network of lymph nodes in this area. End the front massage by asking the subject to sit down comfortably. Massage the shoulders and neck of the subject from the back side. Also do the armpits and put oil there through your fingers.

(6) Candle or Lamp Method: Lie down on bed. Give a light massage of oil (any oil will do) in region around navel. Light an oil/ghee lamp, whose size should not exceed one inch by one inch base, 2 inches height. If oil lamp is not available, use a short piece of candle, stuck to a coin not exceeding 1 inch by 1 inch size. Light the lamp and put it on navel, cantering on navel. Now take a water glass (300 ml) and put on the lamp, such that no air flow to lamp is possible. Apply light pressure to avoid leakage of air inside. The lamp will extinguish due to lack of air and the vacuum resulting from this will make a tight seal between glass edge and skin. Now if you pull glass away from the nozzle in vertical direction, the skin of stomach will also get stuck to inside of glass and will get lifted. Pull with large force, and after few seconds, the air leakage will release the skin back. In this process, the displacement of Solar Plexus (Nabhi-Chakra) gets corrected. This experiment can be done by patient himself, without anybody's help and is safe. Precautions: The oil quantity in lamp should be very little; else hot oil may spill on the sensitive skin of the stomach. Transparent glass is desirable instead of stainless steel glass. However, steel glass produces better seal.

(7) Jump Method: Stand on the edge of a bed, facing the bed on your toes only and jump to the floor, landing on your toes only (not full feet). Do it 2 or 3 times. You can give time gaps in between each jump. This will cure the displacement of Solar Plexus. You have to

jump from a height of 1.5 to 2 feet depending upon how high your bed is. Yes you have to jump backwards on your toes only, not full feet, on the hard floor so that your toes get the feel of an impact by which the nerve slides back into its original place. You can also stand on a sofa and jump to the floor from it. Keep trying as many methods as you want, but there is no better way. You can give time gaps in between each jump. This is a simple and proven method of relief restoration and it works. Repeat it again after one week for a lasting cure. There is another method using the same principle. Stand erect with your back to a wall. Slowly raise your heels alongside the wall to a maximum height. Suddenly let the heels fall with an impact on the floor. Do it several times. The impact of the heels hitting the floor does the reset of the navel (solar plexus).

(8) Vacuum Method: The vacuum method can be tried with empty stomach at any time. This method can be tried together with another technique which is used is creating vacuum for setting the Solar Plexus back and there would be no issues. Make the patient lie on a flat surface with the navel exposed upward. Place a burning lamp on the Navel and carefully cover it with a glass tumbler. Lamp is useful to make vacuum for navel imbalance. Based on vacuum therapy, use on fatty -flabby area to remove fats. Place the cup exactly in the centre of navel and create suction slowly with the help of the pump. When the cup sticks to the body, allow it to remain until it gets removed by itself. This suction created pulls the navel to its original location. Try a couple of times and then test.

(9) Talah (Tibb Arabi) Method: Apply black seed oil and massage the area around the navel by gently pushing it towards the centre with your thumb. Apply the following bandages to strengthen the

(10) Other simple Methods: Whenever the complaint about constipation or loose motions comes, first check the solar plexus and correct it, if necessary. For any problem of any organ below the diaphragm or above the diaphragm like heart, please check up the solar plexus and correct it, e.g. pain in abdomen, stomach etc or pain in chest/heart or even in case the medical adviser informs that the heart is enlarged.

a) When you are empty stomach stand straight then put your thumb on your nose tip and then bend down and try to touch your navel with your smallest finger. b)

b) Lie down and join both feet and try to raise them and see if you feel any kind of stiffness in your navel. Remember to eat something soon after doing exercise and stop stressing about it, because more you are worried about it more stressed you will be and more bloating and burping will happen.

c) While most experienced Vaidya correct nabhi displacement by just inserting thumb or first finger inside and moving it towards head or legs of the patient depending on the requirement, such a technique is difficult for a patient to adopt on himself or for a relative to carry out.

d) Some people cure this by massaging the area near navel, pulling some muscles of armpits, tightening some thread around toes

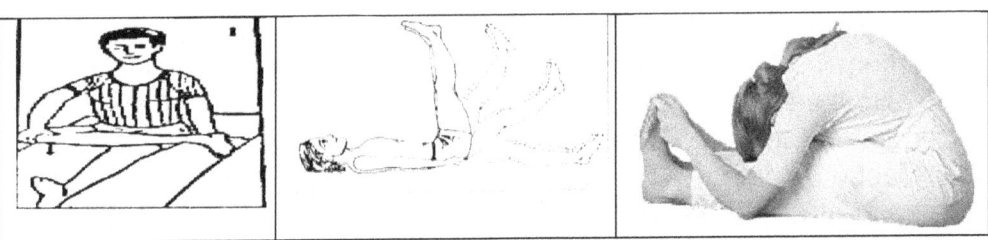

Figures: Solar Plexus Balancing/Correcting Asana:

e) Copper rings are placed at the neck of the toes, so that a little pressure is applied to the neck of the toes, but at the same time no discomfort should be felt.

f) Lie down on back on a flat surface without pillow. Put arms straight on side, feet straight together. Draw your breath in. Now raise both feet together to 90 degree. Don't allow the head to lift. While exhaling, without bending knees bring both feet together slowly on ground. Till you feel the vibrations in the central place of navel, repeat 5-6 times. Feel the throbbing. Some people may not be able to bring it at 90 degree. Let them rise as much as they can.

g) Lie down on back. Put arms straight on side, feet straight together. Exhale and then inflate the stomach to the maximum. Keep in this pose till it is comfortable. Does it daily for say up to 10 times till the navel comes back to normal position. In between puts light pressure on top and bottom side of navel.

h) Sit down on ground or bed. Feet spread straight. First lift right leg and fold and keep it on the left leg. Then with right hand press the right knee towards ground. Repeat it with left leg also.

i) Lie down on back. Put arms straight on side, feet straight together. Exhale. Then expand the stomach like a balloon while inhaling. Remain in the pose till it is comfortable. Repeat at least 5 times.

Solar Plexus Balancing/Correcting Asana:

In normal day-to-day life we do a lot of forward bending but not much backward bending, therefore it is good to practice for a healthy back and to give general balance to the body. Yoga poses, when regularly practiced, are intended to benefit your overall being, from your physical to spiritual well-being and all points in between. Adopted asana, meaning "seated posture," yoga poses for the solar plexus chakra help to clear blockages, and also promote the opening, healing and balancing of the third energy centre.

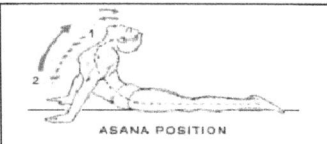
ASANA POSITION
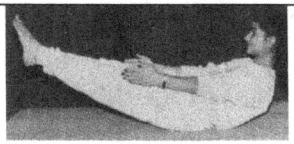
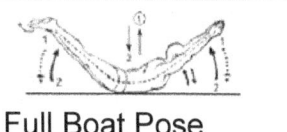
Full Boat Pose

Precautions and Contra-indications: You should not be practiced by those with severe problems of the spine, stomach ulcers, hernias or pregnant women. It should be practiced with care for those with stiff backs and for those who are menstruating. Also it is not recommended for people with heart diseases. It should not be practiced by those who have undergone surgeries of spine, brain, abdomen, heart and lungs.

Duration: To begin with this asana should be held for 5 to ten seconds. It can be repeated 3 to 5 times, depending on the individual's capacity. With practice the number of repetitions can be increased. At this point reduce the number of repetitions but increase the time. Gradually increase the time to 1 minute. After more practice the time can be increased up to 3 to 5 minutes.

Agnisar (Churning of abdomen) Kriya: Agni means fire and Sara means wash so it literally means to wash the fire chakra or Manipura Chakra (Solar Plexus). Practice: Be seated in any comfortable pose like Easy pose, Thunderbolt pose or Lotus pose, place the hands on the knees and breathe in a normal, rhythmic fashion. Focus on breathing for a while, then take a deep breath and exhale slowly. Without inhaling, expand and contract the abdomen 5-10 times or more. Each time you contract, try to suck the belly in deeply, like you are touching the abdomen muscles with back muscles. While coming back, keep a steady stance, gently and slowly inhale deeply. Take a couple of breaths and try again. Ensure that this Pranayama practice is done on an empty stomach, i.e. minimum of 4 hours of fasting. People suffering from high BP, hernia or disease related to intestines should avoid this pose. Why to: Instantly activating the Solar Plexus, it stimulates the digestive system and is a great way to balance the Solar Plexus chakra. Helps with constipation, tones the stomach and even low appetite, this exercise generates and circulates energy in our whole body. The video below will guide you with this breathing practice.

Ardha Matsyendrasana: Ardha Matsyendrasana/ Half lord of the fishes pose Practice: Sit in Staff pose or Dandasana, now gently bend the right knee and place the right foot flat over the left leg. Now, bend the left knee and place the leg on the floor with the heel touching the right hip and toes pointing outward. The leg on the floor will point 45 degrees (refer to the image above). Take a deep breath and twist the torso towards the right side. Place the left hand elbow outside the right knee. The right hand will be pressed to the floor, behind the hips. The spine should be erect at all times, while you hold the pose for 5-7 breaths and looking back. Gently untwist and repeat on the other side. Targeted towards the digestive system and abdominal twisting, it accentuates the feeling of comfort and relaxes the spine and the back. Pressing the abdomen, it strengthens our will power and develops a balance in the right and left sides. Seated twists are generally directed towards harmonising the body and increasing elasticity of the spine.

Bharadvaja's Twist (Bharadvajasana I): This twisted, seated posture stretches and strengthens the spine and shoulders while energizing the abdominal region to open and activate the third chakra.

Dandasana: Practice: Be seated in staff pose or Dandasana, gently bend your knees while you have your hands on the side and pressed to the floor. Following the variations mentioned in the image above, lean back slightly and lifts your feet, bringing your shins parallel to the floor and lifts your arms up with palm facing each other. Take a deep breath if you can and gently straighten the knees, so that the legs form a 45 degree or a V shape. Bring your hands to the front, facing each other. Try to pull the abdomen in to support the spine and create greater balance. Hold for 5 to 7 breaths while you focus your awareness within.

Dhanurasana/Bow pose Practice: Lie on your stomach with arms by your side, palms facing upwards. Inhale, place the chin on the floor, exhale, and bend your knees, so that the feet move towards the buttocks. Grasp your ankles with your hands. Inhale and lift both your chest and thighs up, while still holding your ankles. Ensure your knees do not separate and keep them hip width apart, while you continue breathing deeply at all times. With each breath press the heels back and up, gradually increasing the back bend, keeping the spine long. Hold for 5-7 breaths and slowly release the feet. For beginners, a belt can be used to hold the ankles, if your hands do not reach the legs completely. Why to: Generating a sense of equilibrium in the body, the whole weight along with the blood flow is transferred to the abdomen area. This movement strengthens the abdomen as well as stimulates the digestive system, thereby empowering the Manipura chakra.

Firefly Pose (Tittibhasana): This advanced arm balance asana strengthens your arms while toning your core to activate and balance the solar plexus energy centre.

Full Boat Pose (Paripurna Navasana): Good for stimulating the kidneys and intestines, this seated position helps open and balance the third chakra. Lie down on your back. Take a deep breath. Lift your legs, arms and trunk and balance yourself on your hips. The head, hands and feet should be one foot above the ground and at the same level. The body should assume the shape of a boat. Hold the position for as long as you can hold the breath. This would be ideally to the point where the abdomen starts quivering. Return slowly to the supine position while exhaling. Rest till your breathing becomes normal. Repeat 5 times. The body achieves the shape of a yacht or boat in asana.

Paripurna Navasana: Paripurna Navasana is a great core strengthening the Solar Plexus. Stimulating the digestive system, it balances the whole body and creates self confidence. Enhancing the sense of personal power, it awakens the go-getter attitude.

Paschimothasana: Lie on your back and inhale deeply. Now sit up - with your legs straight in front of you and your toes pointing to the ceiling. Stretch your arms above you. As you exhale, keep your back straight and bend forward from the pelvis. Only bend downward as much as your body permits. Stretch out your arms and reach to your feet or whatever part of the leg you can comfortably reach till. As you bend down, try and keep the heels, calves and thighs touching the floor, the spine straight. Then rest your forehead on the knees (as far as possible) and continue normal breathing. Try to rest the elbows on the floor. Hold the position for a few seconds. As you inhale, start raising the head, and come back to your normal position and relax. Benefits: It is very useful for sufferer from Solar Plexus (navel) disorders, functioning of lungs, intestines and other glands is disorder. This pose also reduces obesity. It stretches the hamstrings on the back of the legs and lengthens the entire spine. It massages the internal organs, especially the digestive organs. It relieves digestive problems such as constipation, relieves problems with sciatica, invigorates the nervous system, stimulates Manipura chakra (Solar plexus centre), balances the prana within the body, calms the mind and improves concentration.

Urdhva Prasarita Padasana or Upward Extended Feet Pose: Practice: Lie on your back with the hands on your sides. Now, inhale and raise the hands, placing them back on the floor above your head. If you need extra support, you can place the hands underneath your hips as well with palms facing downwards. Lift your leg up gently at 30 degrees and hold for 3-5 breaths. Keep your toes flexed. Now repeat the same process at 60 degrees and 90 degrees. Hold the pose at all the three phases for 3-5 breaths or more, if you can and come back in the same pattern. Why to: Builds the strength of the core muscles and improves posture. This pose will challenge your limits and can build massive strength in the abdominal area. By extending and lengthening the abdomen muscles, the pose will involuntarily direct the focus towards the centre as it blurs of all other distractions.

Uthit Padasana (Balancing Pose): Lie on the back with legs outstretched. The hands should be beside the hips. Raise the body above the hips and below the waist, about a foot from the ground while inhaling. Raise the hands from the ground and bring them to the side of the thighs. Hold this posture for a while and then revert back slowly to the lying position while exhaling. Benefits: Uthhit Padasana is essential for maintaining the navel in its normal position. Any displacement of the navel results in a variety of abdominal disorders such as pain, flatulence, indigestion, diabetes etc. For restoring the displaced navel to its original position and to prevent it from further displacement, Uthhit Padmasana is extremely useful. Precautions: Persons suffering from ulcers and lumbar spondylitis should not perform this asana.

Uttanapadasana: Lie on your back, keeping your hands on the sides on the ground, palms facing upwards. Breathe in normally, then keeping legs straight lift them about 8 inches from the ground and hold. Now swing them upwards and downwards, between 6 to 12 inches, above the ground. (e g left leg up 12 inches - right leg down 6 inches - then reverse). Movements should be controlled and slow and without jerks. Do this for a few seconds. Do not exert yourself. Exhale and come back to normal position and relax. Benefits: Thigh muscles and stomach muscles are stretched. The strain reaches inner organs like small intestines, enzyme producing glands and other organs. This asana is also best for _weight reduction, toning loose muscles of the stomach and shaping the belly.

Uttanpadasana: Lie down straight on your back, with the palms flat on the floor, legs straight, and toes together. Inhale, and raise both legs upwards - up to 30 degrees - and hold it for 10 seconds. Then, 60 degrees; again hold it for ten seconds. Then, 90 degrees; and hold it again for 10 seconds. Then, in the same way, come back while exhaling. While returning, place the feet slowly on the floor - avoiding any jerks. After resting for a while, repeat the exercise 3 to 6 times. This Asana helps in keeping the dislocated navel in its proper place.

Virabhadrasana I and Virabhadrasana II: Both standing asanas stretch and strengthen the arms, legs and core while activating and balancing the third chakra. Precautions: Those suffering from acute backache - should practice it using one leg at a time. Benefits: This Asana strengthens the intestines and makes them free of diseases. It removes constipation, gas formation, obesity, and improves the digestive system. It is useful in preventing displacement of the navel, heart disease, stomach pain, and respiratory problems. It is especially useful for backache - when performed using one leg at a time.

Basic Gemstones for balancing the Solar Plexus Chakra:

Gemstones/Minerals affecting Solar Plexus are Citrine, Gold Topaz, Amber, Tiger Eye, Gold Calcite and gold. Citrine and Tiger's eye gemstones resonate with the solar plexus chakra and can help mobilize and balance it. Just having these powerful gems in the room with you, on your desk at work, or holding it while you earth, relax, or read (or even placing it on your solar plexus while you meditate!) are all fabulous ways to increase the flow of energy through your solar plexus chakra. The solar plexus chakra is associated with the colour yellow, and with yellow gemstones. These include:

Citrine
Amber
Sunstone
Yellow jasper
Golden tiger eye
Yellow jade
Golden calcite
Yellow topaz

Acupressure Points for Solar Plexus (Energy Point No.32): Solar Plexus is the "abdominal brain". The solar plexus reflex point is one of the most powerful points in foot reflexology. Within the physical body, the solar plexus is found right in the middle of the upper half of the trunk of the torso, where the rib cage comes together at the stomach level in front of the diaphragm.

On the feet, it can be found if you draw an imaginary line from the sec ond toedown, below the ball of the foot, right within that hollow. It can also be found if you gently squeeze the top of the foot inward. You should find a "little dimple space", that's the solar plexus point.

You will find that if you soak your feet in hot water it will give you a delightful sensation of relaxation at the level of your solar plexus. This is why there is importance for the "foot bath". It's a wonderful way to influence the solar plexus. While seated, bring the foot of your choice up and over the opposite knee and allow it to comfortably rest there. With the opposite side hand, use your thumb to press in and slightly upward on the point (hold for 20 seconds). As you slowly release pressure, don't lose contact with the point; just relax the pressure. Repeat this 3 times and then move to the opposite foot and strengthen the solar plexus.

5.23 Summarized Lifestyle Approaches to Constipation Treatment

1. Drink enough water: If you're suffering from chronic constipation, there are changes you can make to your daily habits which can improve your bowel habits. Your first, and easiest, step is to ensure that you're drinking enough water. As the stool travels through your intestines your body removes water. If you are well hydrated, less water may be removed, leaving the stool softer and easier to pass. Drink enough that your urine is straw colour. If it's dark yellow then you're dehydrated and if it's colourless you are drinking too much.

The fibre in your stool will help to draw more water and keep the stool soft. This is why your doctor recommends increasing the amount of fibre in your diet to help relieve constipation. However, if you're eating a high-fibre diet but not staying hydrated the stool will still get hard and be more difficult to pass. The recommended amount of fibre in your diet is 20 to 30 grams per day; I believe that 32 grams each day is ideal.

Organic psyllium dietary fibre is important to the health of your colon. Psyllium also has other health benefits, including helping to control your blood sugar, reducing your risk of heart attack, stroke, gallstones, kidney stones, and diverticulitis, improving your skin health and helping you to lose or maintain your weight.

Vegetables are the best way to fortify your diet with fibre. If you can't reach the recommended amount of fibre per day then supplementing with organic whole husk psyllium is simple and cost effective.

Regular exercise can also help reduce constipation. The movement helps increase the motility in your digestive tract and can stimulate the urge to have a bowel movement. When you do feel the urge, don't wait. The longer the stool sits in your colon, the more water is removed and the more difficult it is to pass.

2. Reduce the risk of Constipation: There are several ways to reduce your risk of constipation. I strongly recommend eating traditionally fermented and cultured foods on a daily basis to help to "reseed" your body with good bacteria. It's easy to make them. For a demonstration, please see the video above. If you don't eat fermented foods, taking a high quality probiotic supplement is advisable.

The uses of probiotics are so important to your overall health that some researchers are comparing them to a "newly recognized organ." Research links the health and variety of the bacteria in your gut to your behaviour, diabetes, gene expression, autism, and obesity. The bacterium in your gut plays an essential role in the digestion of your food, the motility of your intestines, and ultimately the development of constipation.

Another way to reduce your risk is to speak with your physician about the medications you're currently using. Explore options to reduce the amount of medications you may need or the brands you're currently using if they are linked to triggering constipation. Be particularly wary of using laxatives on a regular basis, as it may exacerbate constipation.

Remember, when you travel your daily regimen is often disrupted. The differences in food, changes to your regular exercise routine, or reduction in water intake can all negatively impact your body's ability to maintain a healthy bowel routine. Try to stay as close to your regular routine as possible. Bring organic whole husk psyllium to supplement your diet on the days you don't get enough fibre. Try to get your regular exercise each day and drink enough water to keep your urine a light straw colour.

3. Squatting can help to prevent Constipation: The last thing most people think about when using the bathroom is position, but this can significantly impact the ease with which you eliminate and even increase your risk of bowel and pelvic problems, including constipation, haemorrhoids, and more. Most of you reading this probably sit to evacuate your bowel, but this requires you to apply additional force (straining), which has some unwanted biological effects, including a temporary disruption in cardiac flow.

Sitting on a modern toilet is designed to place your knees at a 90-degree angle to your abdomen. However, the time-honoured natural squat position (which is still used by the majority of the world's population) places your knees much closer to your torso, and this position actually changes the spatial relationships of your intestinal organs and musculature, optimizing the forces involved in defecation. Squatting straightens your rectum, relaxes your puborectalis muscle, and allows for complete emptying of your cecum and appendix without straining, which prevents faecal stagnation and the accumulation of toxins in your intestinal tract. It is instructive that non-westernized societies, in which people squat, do not have the high prevalence of bowel disease seen in developed nations; in some cultures with traditional lifestyles, these diseases are uncommon or almost unknown.

If you have trouble with bowel movements, especially constipation, I urge you to give the squat position a try. Squatting does involve strength and flexibility that adults tend to lose over time (but children have naturally). Special toilets and stools that get your body into a more "squatty" position can help you get closer to the ideal even if you've been sitting for decades.

4. Medical Treatment Options: In some circumstances these lifestyle choices and preventative measures are not enough to alleviate constipation. Talk with your doctor about being tested for hypothyroidism. In hypothyroidism your body doesn't secrete enough of the thyroid hormone. This hormone has a significant impact on the motility and movement of the intestinal tract, which is why constipation is one of the hallmark symptoms of hypothyroidism.

While it might be tempting to use over-the-counter remedies and laxatives, these remedies are not without risk. When too much is taken, too much water is drawn into the intestines, resulting in dehydration and an abnormal number of electrolytes in your blood. Both dehydration and imbalanced electrolytes can lead to kidney and heart damage, which can lead to death.

Your body can also become dependent on the use of laxatives to have a normal bowel movement. This is especially true of laxatives that use stimulants to increase the motility of the intestines and digestive tract. Stimulant laxatives include medications like Exlax, or laxatives marked as "natural" and include senna or cassia laxatives.

An underlying cause of constipation can also be a magnesium deficiency. Although primarily thought of as the mineral that affects your bones, magnesium plays a role in smooth muscle relaxation and contraction, production of neurotransmitters, building blocks of DNA, and the digestion of carbohydrates, proteins, and fats. The recommended daily amount of magnesium is 310 to 320 mg for women and 400 to 420 mg for men, although this amount may be just enough to prevent outright deficiency.

If your muscles that coordinate defecation are not working together, called dyssynergic defecation, then an anrectal biofeedback mechanism may be the most effective treatment to reteach your muscles to empty the rectum completely. In other cases of rectal prolapsed or a rectocele caused by chronic constipation, surgery may be indicated to repair the area.

5.24 Constipation Remedies for New Born:

Constipation is a problem that most infants face, during the first few months after birth. Some simple home remedies can help alleviate this condition and regulate the bowel movements of the baby. With the arrival of the newest member of the family, you will have to face a lot of new situations that you probably have not prepared for. One of them is the problem of infant constipation. If you are a first-time parent, you might panic at the thought of your baby being constipated. But, it is nothing to worry about, as infant constipation is very common. Almost 50% infants go through constipation and it can be treated easily. You will need to watch out for the signs and symptoms, and once you are sure that your baby is constipated, you should start the treatment immediately.

Causes and Symptoms of Newborn Baby's Constipation

In general, bottle-fed babies are more likely to get constipated, since formula milk is hard for them to digest, as compared to breast milk. Constipation in infants can also be caused by a change in the diet from breast milk to baby formula, or due to dehydration. A change in the components of the baby's diet can cause constipation too. In older babies, introduction of solid foods can sometimes cause mild constipation, which is quite normal.

There are several signs and symptoms, that can tell if your baby is constipated or not. Watch out for the following newborn constipation symptoms, to make sure your baby is actually constipated.

Hard and dry stool pellets in the diaper

Reduction in the baby's bowel movements

Bloating of the stomach

Fissures or cracks on the opening of the anus

Streaks of blood in the stools

Grunting and crying before passing stools

Remedies for Newborn Baby's Constipation

Breastfeeding: Breast milk has the perfect balance of nutrients and makes stool softer. The hormone, motilin, found in breast milk promotes bowel movements in babies.

Stomach Massage: Gentle tummy message can be given to a newborn baby, to relieve constipation and gas. To give a tummy massage, first place your baby on his or her back. Now, gently massage the stomach in a clockwise direction at the navel region and then slowly move outwards in circles.

Leg Bicycling Exercise: This is a gentle exercise that can be employed for relieving infant constipation. For this, place your baby on his or her back, hold the legs and then gently bent them at the knees. Now, move the legs in a forward and cycling motion, by pushing and pulling the legs alternately.

Warm Bath: Consider giving your baby a warm bath, so as to relax him or her. You can also massage the stomach, while giving a bath. This will help your baby pass stool easily.

Water: Babies can get constipated due to dehydration. Ask your paediatrician, if you can give water to your newborn baby, in order to increase his or her fluid intake. If your paediatrician permits, you can give a little amount of cooled, boiled water to your constipated baby.

Examine the Formula: If your baby is on formula, then check whether you are using less than the recommended amount of water, or adding more powder than what is required. In either case, your baby can get constipated. So, always follow the instructions given on the package, while making the formula milk.

Sometimes, changing the formula can cause constipation in babies. If such is the case with your baby, then it might be better to go back to the original formula. In general, it has been observed that, some infants tolerate soy-based formulas better than the cow milk-based formulas. Formulas that contain prebiotics may also help to reduce the incidence of constipation in babies. However, be sure to talk to your paediatrician, before changing formula milk.

Changes in Diet: Babies, who are old enough to eat solid foods, can be given foods that are rich in fibre, after consulting their paediatricians. Cereals like oat and barley, and pureed fruits and vegetables, can be added to a toddler's diet to promote regular bowel movements. Fruit juices, especially, prune, apple, and pear juice, can also provide significant relief in constipation.

385

Medications: As far as medications are concerned, several types of over-the-counter stool softeners and laxatives or enemas, are available for constipation relief. Never use laxatives and mineral oil to treat infant constipation, without the approval of a paediatrician. However, you can ask your baby's paediatrician about using stool softeners for constipation relief. For a severely constipated baby, paediatricians may suggest the use of glycerine suppository. However, continuous and long-term use of suppositories is not encouraged or recommended, as it can lead to dependency.

If the aforementioned remedies do not cure your baby's constipation, then be sure to seek medical assistance. You can consult your paediatrician about giving the baby a glycerine enema. Many people use milk of magnesia and flax oil to treat constipation. Make sure that you do not use them, without asking your baby's health care provider.

5.25 Do & Don't

Constipation is an avoidable condition. Simple intervention that would entail a slight change of lifestyle can be done to help alleviate constipation and prevent it from re-occurring. Maintaining a well-balanced, high fibre diet, drinking plenty of water, regular exercise, and setting a regular bowel habit can help. Don't ever ignore the urge to defecate when your body tells you need to, it is never healthy.

In case that the natural approach doesn't help with your constipation problem, enemas and colonic irrigation help trigger peristaltic movement in the bowel. If these still don't work, laxatives are suggested to stimulate bowel movement.

If laxatives and other measures fail, manual disimpaction is performed on the sufferer. This entails manually removing impacted faeces from the rectum. This may be done with or without sedatives or anaesthetics. In cases that the constipation reaches intestinal perforation, immediate surgery is required to remove spilled faecal matter from the abdominal cavity.

In today's fast-paced lifestyle, it is easy to ignore what your bodies are telling you. People think they have more important things to do and therefore put off for later the need to expel bodily wastes - be it urine, gas or faeces. In the end it will just cause more inconvenience. Too bad people learn their lessons a bit too late.

Do's

Make a habit of bowel evacuation early morning everyday
Drink 8 to 10 glasses of water regularly
Exercise regularly, preferably yoga.

Develop a regular eating habit and chew the food before swallowing

Intake plenty of leafy vegetables and salads

Eat fibre-rich fruits and vegetables like papaya, orange, beans, asparagus etc

Drinking lemon juice mixed with warm water in the morning useful in cleaning the bowel.

Don't

Avoid Hurried Meals and Irregular meals

Avoid smoking and alcoholism and also avoid drinking strong coffee/tea

Curing constipation through exercises is the best option to get relief from this unpleasant disease.

Don't exert pressure to empty your stomach

Don't take excess stress or tension

Foods which constipate are all products made of white flour, rice, bread, pulses, cakes, pastries, biscuits, cheese, fleshy foods, preserves, white sugar, and hard-boiled eggs.

Hurried meals, fast foods and meals at odd times should be avoided.

Intake of fried foods and beans and vegetables like cabbage, cauliflower, potatoes. Nuts and dried foods should be avoided along with non-vegetarian foods

Laxatives medicines are sold over the counter that may offer constipation relief but they don't really address the cause of the problem.

Pregnancy is one such condition in which natural constipation remedies work just best as effectively and is highly preferable particularly when dealing with constipation during pregnancy or constipation after surgery as constipation medicines like laxatives for passing stools. In such situations and individual is incapable of passing any bowel movements without consuming laxatives.

Restrict your intake of low fibre and high fat foods like red meats, cheese, and other processed or refined foods like Maida products.

Say no to processed foods

Sugar and sugary foods should be strictly avoided.

Do not use HCL supplements while using medication such as corticosteroids or anti-inflammatory medicines like Advil, Tylenol or other NSAIDS. These meds can damage the GI lining and increase the chance of a stomach ulcer if HCL is introduced. Do not use HCL if you have stomach ulcers. In that case, heal the stomach lining completely with Gastrazyme, manuka honey the other suggestions here before HCL supplementation.

Only take HCL with a meal containing protein. You will not need HCL if you are eating an apple for a snack.

As you continue to heal your stomach lining, you will be able to gradually reduce and eventually eliminate need for HCL.

Often, when stomach acid is chronically low for a long period of time, even the minimal dose of HCL will cause a burning sensation in the stomach. In this case, focus on healing the stomach lining with the steps above first, then try to re-introduce the HCL after 2-4 weeks of intensive healing.

Grain fibre contains large amounts of phytic acid, a compound which "locks" onto minerals like zinc, copper, iron and calcium. Processed grain products, such as bread and cereals, are not properly prepared and contain high amounts of phytic acid. Soaking and fermenting your grains, as practiced by traditional cultures and explained in Nourishing Traditions, reduces the phytic acid levels.

When stomach acid is optimal, the acid helps to break down the little phytic acid and mineral bundles, rendering some of those previously stolen minerals available to the body. But the body cannot reclaim these nutrients with low stomach acid. Reducing fibre and thereby reducing phytic acid intake, minerals are more efficiently absorbed.

Don't over-hydrate: Mainstream health dogma hounds us to drink 8+ glasses of water per day for "hydration" and to "flush toxins." Actually, over hydrating does neither of things and actually slows metabolism and can cause cellular dehydration (I discuss the topic in more detail. In addition, drinking large amounts of water before or during meals waters down stomach acid and therefore inhibits digestion. If desired, drink a cup of warm, home made bone broth to stimulate digestive juices desired during meals. You may also find it helpful to drink 1/2 cup of water with 1 tsp. raw apple cider vinegar before or after meals. I also suggest drinking a small amount of raw, homemade yogurt with meals to provide probiotics and enzymes to support digestion.

Avoid the Following Refined Sugars and Sweeteners.

Table: Avoid the Following Refined Sugars and Sweeteners

Sugar	Glucose	High Fructose Corn
Aspartame	Galactose	Syrup
Sucralose	Lactitol	Crystalline Powder

Saccharin	Lactose	Monosaccharides
Sorbitol	Levulose	Polysaccharides
Sorghum	Suamiel	Date Sugar
Splenda	Sucanat	Carob Powder
Alitame	Maltitol	Corn Starch
Carmel	Maltodextrin	Tagatose
Corn Syrup	Maltose	Talose
Cyclamate	Ribose	Trehalose
Sucrose	Naturlose	Disaccharides
Dextrin	NutraSweet	Monosaccharides
Dextrose	Polydextrose	Malts of any kind
		Acesulfame-K

Natural Tips/ Remedies for Constipation

If you are doing yoga for constipation, diet control and lifestyle change are a must which will add up to the benefits of yoga for curing constipation. You can benefit by using some or all of the tips/ natural remedies listed below:

Immediately after waking up early in the morning, drink two/ three glasses of water at room temperature. Another better option is to drink fresh lime juice prepared with Luke warm water and by adding one teaspoon of honey. Walk around for 10-15 minutes at a leisurely pace to stimulate bowel action.

If above method does not help, still try to establish a daily routine for bowel movements. Sit on the toilet for 10 minutes at the same time. This may take some time say a month to produce results.

Drink an adequate amount of water each day (six to eight glasses).

Regular physical exercise is also important for maintaining proper bowel movements. Regular yoga practice is the best exercise to avoid constipation.

The diet taken during constipation must be easily digestible so that it does not overload the digestive system. Take light meals including fresh foods, vegetables, sprouts and salads. These will provide natural source of daily requirement of fibre. Psyllium seed husk and wheat bran are good source of natural fibre.

Eat two to three hours before going to sleep, so that the food is digested before you sleep.

Drinking a glass of warm milk before going to bed helps in easy evacuation in the morning. In case of severe constipation, mix two teaspoons of castor oil in the milk.

You should eat food in a relaxed manner. Digestive process depends on how we eat food. If food is eaten in hurry or in a state of stress, anger or fear, it produces a toxic effect in the body and promotes indigestion. Also, chew your food properly and slowly.

A common Ayurvedic medicine for constipation is Triphala Churna. It is a powder made by grinding three kinds of herbs. A teaspoon of this powder taken with warm water or milk at the time going to bed is beneficial.

Try to avoid laxatives.

Sleeping hours should be regulated and efforts should be made to have a sound sleep.

A warm-water or mineral oil enema can relieve constipation.

Do not delay going to the toilet when you sense natural urge for defecation, this can result in constipation.